DATE DUE

LET LIKE
CURE LIKE

LET LIKE CURE LIKE

The Definitive Guide to the Healing Power of Homeopathy

VINTON McCABE

ST. MARTIN'S PRESS

NEW YORK

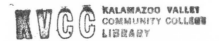

Design by Chris Welch

Library of Congress Cataloging-in-Publication Data
McCabe, Vinton.
    Let like cure like : the definitive guide to the healing power of
homeopathy / Vinton McCabe.
        p.   cm.
    Includes bibliographical references.
    ISBN 0-312-15566-2
    1. Homeopathy.   I. Title
RX71.M33 1997
615.5'32—dc21   97-3018
                                                               CIP

First Edition: September 1997
10 9 8 7 6 5 4 3 2 1

"Let Like cure like," the words of the German physician Samuel Hahnemann, reveal the heart of homeopathy: that we must never seek to deny our disease, and to suppress our pain, but we must always acknowledge the symptoms that we call illness and work with those symptoms; that we might not only heal ourselves but also transform our lives in the process.

—*Vinton McCabe*

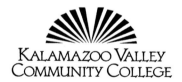

CONTENTS

CONTENTS

PART THREE   EXPERIENCING

ACKNOWLEDGMENTS

In writing any book, and especially a first book, the author has to be able to lean back and trust that there will be someone to catch him. This author is especially thankful for the supporting arms of good friends: David Dumas, Mark Filippi, Marc Grossman, Michael Mendribil, and Lalie Gilmore. I also wish to thank and acknowledge the board and members of the Connecticut Homeopathic Association for their understanding and support.

Further, I must thank my editor, the well-named Joy Chang, for her patience, humor, and insight. I want also to thank my agent, Bob Silverstein, for getting me started on this whole thing; Zinta, who established my work at the Wainwright house; and Roseanne, who opened the doors to the Open Center of Manhattan for me. And to all the McCabes, especially Ann, who would have taken the calls collect, if need be.

PREFACE

All arts lie in man, though not all are apparent. The awakening brings them out. To be taught is nothing; everything is in man, waiting to be awakened.

—*Paracelsus*

I was born sick. As were millions of babies during the baby boom follow-ing World War II, as many millions more have been in the generations since: babies born with already weakened immune systems, with chronic allergies to their home, to their mother's milk, to bottled formulas.

I was born allergic. In those days of the mid-1950s, I was thoroughly tested for my allergies. The list went on for three pages but narrowed to specific major allergens: dust, pollen, milk and all dairy products, animal hair, wheat, corn. I was treated with the treatment of the day, injections of minute amounts of these toxins, the very things that caused an allergic response. The hope was that my body would build up a resistance to these substances to the point that they would no longer trigger an allergic reac-tion. While this treatment was itself parallel to the treatments offered in homeopathy, it failed to treat me as a total person and look at the totality of my symptoms.

Throughout my childhood and early adolescence, I continued these treatments. They began when I was three or four years old. I lived in a small town in western Pennsylvania, and my father and I took the train to Pitts-burgh every few days. I received injections up and down my spine, and each time I cried in a mixture of fear and pain. After a time, the injections were shot into my arms, and the length of time between injections grew to weeks and then to months. Finally a local doctor took over the injections. No more trips on the train. All this time I was also being treated for chronic upper respiratory infections, ear infections that climaxed with a major inner ear infection when I was twelve, youthful skin conditions and sore throats, and a bout of whooping cough that seemed as if it would never end. I was treated for all these things—with antihistamines and cough medicine, with antibiotics of many different types.

By the age of ten, I was told that my allergies were gone, and I could eat anything I wanted. At this time I began to have digestive problems, but no one seemed to think that they could have had anything to do with the allergies, as they had been "cured." By age fourteen, my skin began to break out, and I began a three-year cycle of antibiotics to clear my complexion. And all the while, my seasonal allergies grew worse. What had been simple rhinitis for two or three weeks in May and June now began in early spring and continued until the first frost. For these allergies, a doctor decided I needed cortisone injections, and I received these regularly for another two or three years.

By then I had colitis. No one seemed to find any link between this chronic digestive disorder and the allergies I had had at birth. In fact, no one who treated my colitis ever asked me if I was allergic to anything or even asked me about the foods I ate. I was, however, given tranquilizers and told that my problem was stress. I should learn to calm down.

At age twenty-nine I was told that I could expect to have colon cancer by age forty. I was also told that I should consider an operation to remove the inflamed part of my colon. The surgery need not curtail my lifestyle. Much.

At that time, although I exercised regularly and ate carefully, I could no longer digest the simplest food. I felt hot and sloppy. I had trouble breathing and couldn't concentrate. A friend suggested that I try a system of healing known as homeopathy. I felt that I had nothing more to lose, so I went to see a woman, this homeopath, whom I considered to be perhaps one step above a witch. She made a living by handing out things she called "remedies," things made from herbs and minerals and such.

I was not prepared for her modern office or for the fact that my health insurance paid for the visit. But most of all, I was not prepared for the fact that, within a week of taking my remedy—Sulphur—I was able to digest foods. My movement toward healing had begun.

I am still in the process of healing, of largely undoing what was done to me by allopathic medicine. Homeopathy, when classically used and the remedy wisely selected, is *always* at least as effective as allopathy. And it is effective without side effects, the dangers of chemical dependence, or the suppression of the body's own natural ability to heal.

Today, many children are born with chronic allergies. In many families the members are as linked by illness as they are by blood—linked by arthritis and heart disease, by alcoholism and drug abuse, by chronic fatigue and other forms of immune disfunction, by crippling anxiety and other forms of mental illness. We are a society that becomes more angry, more violent with each generation. In order to understand the causes of this situation, especially the recent explosive growth of immune-depressed disorders such as chronic fatigue syndrome and AIDS, we must take the time to understand the philosophy of homeopathy. And we have to look again at Western medicine, at allopathy, and honestly ask ourselves if allopathic treatments actually improve or weaken our total health. Homeopaths tell us that genetic weaknesses are often caused in children by the allopathic mistreatments of simple illnesses in their parents. Allopathic treatments suppress the body's own natural ability to heal itself and, in doing so, weaken the total system. This weakness is inherited by succeeding generations. Allopathic treatments have become all the more painfully and chronically damaging to the total system by the increased use of chemical superdrugs such as antibiotics.

Since the discovery of the so-called miracle drugs beginning in the 1950s, we have seen an increase in all major chronic conditions. We live longer than people did two hundred years ago, but we live far less well. We are now forced to take a new look at the way we run many aspects of our lives, from the rules of our economy to individual rights. We also must look at the ways we deal with illness and health. Could it be that our very method of attacking disease is in error and could actually weaken us as it supposedly heals us?

This book attempts to explain the basic theory and philosophy of homeopathy in simple terms. Accepting homeopathy requires a willing suspension of disbelief. It demands that we unlearn all that we "know" about medicine and medicine treatment, that we take responsibility for our own health, and that we accept the fact that any collection of symptoms in our body and mind must be connected.

In the pages that follow, I present the core philosophy of homeopathy, a philosophy that I believe is more healing than the remedies themselves. Samuel Hahnemann developed a wonderful method of getting our bodies and minds and spirits well, a unique way of working with the life energy that can give us the great gift of health. But perhaps more important,

Hahnemann rediscovered principles of healing that had been discussed by physicians as far back as Hippocrates, the father of medicine himself. Hahnemann presented these principles to the modern world, naming them homeopathy and using them to cure thousands in his day.

As this is a practical guide, information is included on the remedies themselves and their specific uses. In homeopathy, this is called studying the materia medica. And it is certainly an important part of this study.

Those of us who would be well, who would truly walk on a path of healing, must remember Christ's words that we be "wise as serpents and gentle as doves." We must be open to a change in our thinking and willing to learn a new way of seeing, but we must also be practical. We need to know what to do in acute situations in which our goal is to return to our status quo, and to know how to work transformationally for the sake of our long-term healing. Again, as Christ says, we must be "in this world, but not of it." Our focus may be philosophical, but our lives are rooted in our need for air, for food, for drink.

This book seeks to fulfill both needs, to be a true guide to the use of homeopathics and a philosophical statement of transformational healing. It is written as I continue to walk on my own healing path and struggle with the aches and pains that I myself create while walking through my life. It presents homeopathy as I have learned it and experienced it and seen it practiced. That means it presents, to the best of my ability, a method by which we can all learn to be well.

This book is divided into three sections: Unlearning, Learning, and Experiencing. Even before birth, as we grew within our mothers, we were already hearing philosophy on health and healing. We were born into a nation that is more in agreement about medicine than it is about anything else. We are all going to the same kinds of doctors and swallowing the same kinds of pills.

So, when we begin to tackle homeopathic philosophy, we must first unlearn a good bit of what we have already learned. We must look at our health and our illnesses differently. We must explore the notion that we just might have a good deal more control over the healing of our bodies, the healing of ourselves, than we ever dreamed.

And, having gotten back to our wombs, back to the unlearned state in which all things are possible, then we can look at the philosophy that is the basis of homeopathy. Then we can learn to trust and to experience the remedies, and, more important, we can learn to transform our lives.

INTRODUCTION

Life is short, art is long; occasion is volatile;

experiment is fallacious; judgment is difficult. It is not

enough for us to do what we can do; the patient and

his environment, and external conditions have to

contribute to achieve the cure.

—*Hippocrates*

To begin, we must look at ourselves as whole beings—humans composed of body, mind, and spirit. We are unique in the whole universe, with unique thoughts and needs, unique strengths and weaknesses. Unique illnesses. Because we respect each human as the first and only of his or her kind, we must also respect each person's own needs in terms of healing. For this reason, we must always look to the person— the *whole* person—in seeking healing. We must never look to the disease alone.

As long as our efforts are directed solely at the disease, we work on the level of curing that disease, and we fail to heal the person. Think about it. When we cure a specific condition we seek a direct action: the eradication of a symptom or set of symptoms that cause discomfort. This becomes interesting if we stop for a moment and ask ourselves if it is really and truly possible for us ever to cure anything. That is, is it possible for us to affect four or five "negative" symptoms in our bodies or our minds without also affecting every other aspect of our being? If you slam your finger in a car door, for instance, you directly hurt that finger. But is it only the finger that experiences the trauma? Of course not. Your entire being is affected by the pain in the finger. In the same way, when we try to cure anything, when we pretend that we can isolate a specific part of the body and detach it from

1

the rest of the being, we are playing "pretend." No form of medical science can ever promise that it can affect one area of the body without affecting the whole. The changes that an allopathic drug brings about in the rest of the body are called side effects and have become an accepted part of medical treatment. But the very presence of side effects, of the multiplicity of effects on the human system that any allopathic drug creates, is proof that we really can never cure anything. There is no such thing as a magic bullet that will attack only the source of our pain. Instead, the allopathic drug is more of a scud missile, a device that attacks anything and everything in its path.

We must learn to work systemically. We have to turn our attention to healing our beings instead of curing diseases. When we seek to heal ourselves, we must work with a new philosophy, that we are whole and can never be treated as anything but whole, and with a more diffused goal, that we seek to become not only a healthier being but also one who is more whole.

All of this is homeopathy: seeing that we are unique individuals, that we are whole beings, that we cannot take one pill for a sore throat and another for insomnia. In a whole being, all symptoms are interrelated. All healing is organic to the whole.

The best metaphor I can think of for true healing is breathing, simple breathing, in and out. We all do it all day every day, or at least we think we do. Most people are as starved for air as an anorexic is for food. We hold our shoulders, our necks, and our chests tight, taking in just enough air to survive, never enough to relax or to really live. Yet the air is all around us; it's there to nourish us. We just don't take advantage of it.

In the same way, we don't take advantage of all that surrounds us in terms of healing. We struggle with our aches and pains, trying to bury them, trying to cut them out, but never trying to learn from them. We don't work with a principle of true healing. We sell ourselves short by trying just to get over this cold or that headache without doing anything to change the fact that we will one day get our *next* cold or *another* headache.

To move our central focus from curing to healing demands that we allow the possibility of change to enter into our lives. All healing involves change—*all* healing—a change in our thinking, a change in our living. If some aspect or aspects of our lives didn't need to change, we wouldn't be sick to start with.

And yet, although most of us are chronically ill, many of us with two or three different afflictions that a doctor has told us we "will have to learn to live with," we still don't see the need for change in our lives. We just want that doctor to fix us, to give us something that will take away the

INTRODUCTION

pain. Too many of us are like wild animals who, finding themselves suddenly trapped in steel-jawed traps, gnaw off their own leg out of terror and pain. Too many of us are willing to do anything to get out of pain, enter any drug-induced stupor, have any surgery—anything except take the time to work with the pain, to learn from the pain, anything but actually change our lives in such a way that we can release the pain, and release it permanently.

But if we are to be well, if we are to work toward transformational healing in our lives, the first thing we need to do is to open ourselves to the concept that our illnesses, acute and chronic, are pointing our way on the healing path. They are showing us our own need for change.

The second step toward healing is to begin to know ourselves better, physically as well as mentally and emotionally—what makes us feel better, what makes us feel worse. We have to respect our bodies, minds, and spirits enough to believe that they are doing the best they can to keep us functioning and alive. And that takes us back to our breathing.

Try this simple exercise. Take a moment and feel your body in the chair you are sitting in or the bed you're lying on. Take a deep breath. Feel the air fill your lungs. Feel what that muscular motion of breathing does in your body. Let the air back out. Take a moment to feel what it feels like to exhale.

Now take another breath, breathing as deeply as you can. Hold it. Hold it some more. Hold your breath as long as you can. Make your hands into fists and puff out your cheeks. Keep holding your breath.

This is what it feels like when you suppress a symptom, when you hold onto an ache or a pain by treating it with painkillers instead of working directly with that pain symptom as an avenue of change. This is what we do in traditional Western medicine, which I refer to as allopathy. At first it's fine. At first you wonder what all the fuss is about. You have a headache and you take an aspirin. You have depression and you take a mood elevator. Take the pill and the pain is gone.

When the pain comes back, you take another pill. Repeat as needed. Over time, you can't help thinking that there's a headache under there somewhere, or that somewhere deep inside you are still very depressed, but you can't get to that part of you or feel that part of you. But you know it's there. Every moment of every day, it's there. And the pressure builds like the breath you're still holding.

Let out your breath. You feel free. The pressure is gone. That's homeopathy. It's all about learning to exhale. It's learning about expressing the symptoms that we have suppressed for so long.

We go through life holding our symptoms like we hold our breath, cov-

3

ering our pain with pills that don't remove the source of our illness but only disguise it, trying to trick the body into believing that all is well. Homeopathy teaches us how to let go of the cause of our illnesses, to let go of our pain totally and completely, once and for all. Samuel Hahnemann, the founder of the philosophical school known as homeopathy, promises us that our cure should be "rapid, gentle, and permanent." This promise was revolutionary in eighteenth-century Europe when it was first made. It remains revolutionary today.

Therefore, when we study homeopathy, we are studying deep breathing. A way of living our lives that allows us to exhale our misery, to remove it from our body and spirit. With homeopathy we may do much more than treat a common cold. We may transform our lives and become the people we now have only the potential to be.

When we think about homeopathy, indeed, when we think about healing, we must first think about ourselves. Homeopathy is often called holistic medicine, medicine that works on a theory of wholeness, that each of us is a merger of the visible and the invisible, the tangible and the intangible. That all of us are comprised of body, mind, and spirit.

Hahnemann himself wrote of the wholeness of our being. He believed that when illness manifests itself, we must work with not only the physical body but also with the mind and spirit to attain healing. Hahnemann tells us that illnesses of the physical body, which are by far the easiest to clear, are actually the least important in terms of healing. In fact, Hahnemann tells us that ultimately *all* illness has its beginning in our spiritual selves, and all healing must take place on this level.

Yet many books on homeopathy perpetuate what I consider to be our cultural madness: the desire for an instantaneous result, even if that instantaneous result will be to our long-term detriment. Inevitably, these books focus on the disease and on specific cures while ignoring the more profound healing that is possible—and necessary.

But let's try for a moment to look at things differently, to recognize a more profound possibility: We need to work for long-term transformation. Sometimes this might mean that you have to learn to have that cold. Just brew some ginger tea and rest and let your body expel its toxins and recharge your energy and let you get well.

This thinking is the heart of homeopathy. There is a wisdom in your body and in its illnesses. If you work with an illness instead of wrestling against it, it can guide you through the expression of your symptoms to a life that is truly healthy in body, mind, and spirit.

To the allopathically minded, it is quite the opposite. The symptoms that cause us discomfort are, by their nature, bad. They are also "other." We have somehow got the notion that equates illness with invasion and presumes that, if the invasion is successfully repelled, the illness will stop.

The allopaths have taught us that our world has many enemies in it. Viruses and bacteria are all waiting to attack us like muggers. Certainly some illnesses are more potent than others. But our readings in homeopathic philosophy remind us that we tend to catch, or are susceptible to, the illnesses that are "on our wavelength." Perhaps they are mirrors of our lives. Perhaps they are created not outside of ourselves but are somehow the very product of ourselves; the virus or bacterium is only the fuse and not the bomb. Catastrophic plagues aside, our illnesses tend to have some rhyme or reason to them. They have much to teach us.

It has always been my belief that we should deal with any illness, especially chronic illness, by first asking, "What is the blessing of this disease? What does it have to teach me about myself and about my life? What good things does it bring into my life? Do I get attention and love because I am ill? Do I get to avoid things that I don't like because I am ill?

These are important questions that deserve an answer, or at least an attempt at an answer. Allopaths skip this step altogether and move along with their militaristic model of medicine. Cut it out or suppress it away. The invader must be routed.

In most cases, our belief in this tactic is total and unquestioning. If you asked the average person whether he or she believed in God and then whether he or she believed that a certain headache medicine was good for pain, I am certain that more would believe in Tylenol than in God. We have heard this message again and again from birth. Try to count the number of advertisements recommending a specific medicine in a half-hour television show. In terms of our health and healing, we have placed all of our eggs squarely in one basket, building a powerful cultural dogma and a multibillion-dollar industry in the process.

What if we're wrong?

Think of how much of our thought and our energy, to say nothing of our money, we have spent on health and medicine. In no other area of our lives—relationships, finances, religion, politics, and career—do we narrow our viewpoint to one set of possibilities, one possible outcome, without considering alternatives. We may have several accounts in different banks. We may seek God through different churches and even differing faiths, taking Zen wisdom and applying it to a Christian faith, for example, or blending the Judeo-Christian with the teachings of reincarnation. And most of us explore a number of relationships of various sorts before settling down into a committed lifelong relationship.

But when it comes to our own bodies, and the health of those bodies, we often consider only one point of view. We never for a moment consider the question, What if we're wrong? And no matter how many millions die of cancer, of AIDS, of heart disease, it never seems to enter our minds that we might actually be looking at health in the wrong way, that we might want to consider the way we work with the symptoms that we call disease. Instead, we seek a new doctor who looks at our body and works with us in the same old way.

Many leading "alternative" practitioners are supposedly working to find complementary methods by which their techniques can be combined with standard treatments. But what if we're wrong? What if those treatments cannot be combined? What if we are not even looking in the right places to find the answers we need to achieve our healings? What if we are not even asking the right questions?

Think about it. There are many messages in our lives that seem to have been programmed into us since birth. The topics include morals, religion, relationships, self-worth, politics, bias—and medicine. Throughout our lives, we often find ourselves beginning to question the messages we have received and wondering whether there is another way. Many turn away from their parents' faith or politics. Many more choose to enter relationships with people who will do the challenging for them. But few of us reach the point at which we begin to question not just our doctor but also the philosophical base from which our doctor works and the arena of medicine in which he acts.

We have created a medical arena in which any number of experiments may be tried, any number of guesses may be made, and any number of patients may die from their treatment, and yet those numbers of failures are considered acceptable.

Think of it in terms of a very simple example: eye doctors. You walk into your optometrist's office to have your eyes examined for corrective lenses. He prescribes a set of lenses that are supposed to allow you to see correctly. And yet in a year you go back to get new, stronger glasses. That doctor failed to correct your vision; in fact, he actually weakened your vision by giving you strong lenses to act only as a crutch for your eyes rather than as a corrective measure. He did nothing for your vision except weaken it. If you ask him about this, he will likely tell you that as you get older, your vision just gets worse, and there is nothing to be done about it except to increase your prescription.

What if he is wrong? What if he could do something about your vision, something more than just adjust the lenses in front of your eyes?

Similarly, what if we are wrong about pain? What if it has more to do with what is going on in our lives than we care to admit? And what then can we expect to happen ultimately if we continue to treat our pain by deadening it away, by denying that we have it?

Think of the industry we have built around the notion of pretending that we are not in pain. Look at your television set and watch how many commercials come on in any given hour that promise you that, for a period of four to six hours, you can pretend that you don't have a headache. How many billions of dollars are spent in any given year in the war against pain, a war that is waged always in the same manner: by doping the patient so that he or she cannot feel that pain for a period of time? But what about the cause of that pain, and what about its context? What if we are wrong in the method by which we deal with our pain?

The first step in the process of unlearning is to consider, just for a moment, that we might be wrong. Instead of continuing to work with our health as we always have, maybe we need a more profound change than just a change in practitioner. Maybe we need to consider, just for a moment, that we might be working altogether in the wrong direction. We need a new way of looking at disease, at symptoms, and at our own bodies in illness and in health. We need to work from there on a new path toward healing.

Homeopathy, like acupuncture, represents a wellspring of healing energy. It has roots in Paracelsus's alchemy as well as in modern chemistry. It is a product of Einstein's energy universe. As such, homeopathy is a transformational medicine, a method by which, when the philosophy and the remedy are correct, the patient may transform himself into a new being. I am reminded that modern homeopaths often define the word *health* simply as "freedom." The transformation possible allows us to be truly free, not only of physical ailments but also of their *causes*—anger, fear, guilt, family violence, loneliness, and the like. This is transformation. This is true freedom.

Next, in order to work with our illnesses and to move on to health, we have to revise what we think about medicines, what we think about pills. We have created a culture that largely equates medicine with food. When we take a pill, what is it supposed to do? It is supposed to soothe us, to make our lives easier, to help us sleep, to help us function and prosper in a world filled with terrible enemies. If you think I overstate this point, I suggest that you watch a few television commercials for over-the-counter products. You'll see people smiling through their migraines and mowing the lawn joyfully in spite of their hay fever. In other words, these medicines are nourishment to us, like food. A loving parent gives Nyquil as lovingly as she gives chicken soup.

So our pills are treats that quickly and easily end whatever symptom we are experiencing. On the surface, this seems to follow Hahnemann's admonition that all healing should be "rapid, gentle, and permanent." Well, they appear to be rapid, and as we tend to be at least partially unconscious after taking them, they seem to be gentle as well. But do they ever offer permanent cure? I don't think so.

It is not enough to just rail against allopathy here. If we switch our attention to homeopathics and begin to swallow these sweet sugar pills (homeopathic remedies have a mild sugar taste) but don't work with what pills mean in our lives, we will still spend our lives chasing symptoms around our bodies.

We have to be careful in what we expect from our pills, homeopathic or otherwise. This is not to say that we should lie awake all night with a toothache, but that we should know when we are working for short-term relief and when we are working for long-term good. And we should not go after too many short-term goods when we are seeking a long-term solution.

Many people have become homeopathic junkies. I went through that stage myself. I would take my first cold remedy minutes after the symptoms began, then a second remedy within an hour or two, and a third and fourth in rapid succession. I would then wonder not only why I was unable to get rid of the cold but also why I kept getting cold after cold throughout the winter. It was simply because I had taken my eyes off my mind and was looking only at the illness.

That's the danger of acute treatments and of simply trading the bitter pills of allopathy for the sweet pills of homeopathy without adjusting our thinking along the way. We run after symptom after symptom, illness after illness, and somehow never get around to dealing with ourselves as a whole. In other words, after happily acknowledging that we are body, mind, and spirit, we spend our time only with our body's aches and pains and forget to make the changes in the parts of ourselves that truly matter—our minds and our spirits. This makes little sense to me.

Go back to the colds. If you are getting cold after cold each year, at some point sit down and ask yourself why. Ask yourself what you can learn about this syndrome and what changes you might have to bring about in your being to move past it. Remember, all healing involves change. If we did not need to change in any way, I guarantee that we would not be ill in any way. Yet the person with the illness so often does not see that any change is needed in his life. The angry man with constipation and insomnia does not want to deal with the fact that, in order to get better, he will have to lay down that anger that he perceives as a wellspring of personal power but that is in reality draining off his life energy and slowly killing him. Each of us needs to become aware of the changes that need to be made and to become willing to make them.

This is what homeopathy at its best can help us to do: make actual profound changes in our lives, if we are willing to work on the level of transformation, putting our time and energy into the process of healing and the process of change, instead of spending our time deciding which pill, allopathic *or* homeopathic, to swallow next. Take a remedy called Lycopodium, created from a form of moss, for example. It's a real guy remedy, for men with feelings of insecurity in their manhood, father issues. One man took Lycopodium and, after ten years of having no relationship in his life, suddenly was able to enjoy a happy relationship with a woman. He did not see that as part of the action of Lycopodium in his life, but I absolutely did. He took the remedy primarily to help with his digestion, which it did, but more profoundly, it allowed him to come into a creative and centered sense of himself. It helped him to solve his very deep riddle of self-confidence and manhood and to get on with his life. To him, it was a matter of finding this particular woman. Sheer coincidence. To me, it was a matter of him finding *himself*. There are wonderful mates to be found at all times if we allow ourselves to perceive them and love them.

The true power of homeopathics—and, indeed, of any healing tool—is mysterious and unknowable; true healings are always invisible. They are the ongoing healing of our riddles of self. This is why there can be no remedies for diseases, but instead remedies only for the people who, for whatever reason, have those particular diseases. This is why no doctor, homeopath or allopath, can truly predict the impact of any medicinal substance on the patient but can only give the indicated medicine, like lighting a match to a candle, and trust the healing process to begin.

Part One

UNLEARNING

The action of these remedies is to raise our vibrations
and open up our channels for the reception of the
Spiritual Self. . . . They are able, like beautiful music or
any glorious or uplifting thing which gives us
inspiration, to raise our very natures. . . . They cure, not
by attacking the disease, but by flooding our bodies
with the beautiful vibrations of our Higher Nature, in
the presence of which disease melts away
as snow in the sunshine.

—*Edward Bach*

1

VITAL FORCE

For the vitalist, there is a kind of music, an almost audible hum, that permeates all of creation. Each part of creation, each creature, each plant, even each of the basic elements of creation, is a part of that music. For the vitalist, all creation is one, just as each of us is one whole being, body, mind, and spirit. All creation shares the basic spark of life.

To understand homeopathy, you must first understand vitalism, a philosophy of healing that dates back to the time of Hippocrates in ancient Greece. Vitalism is based on the concept that the world, and everything natural to it, is alive.

The life spark is infinitely creative and ever changing, and it is through this spark of life, called *dynamis* by the Greeks, that we are able to heal ourselves. *Dynamis*, the root word for *dynamite*, encapsulated the ancient Greek concept of life. The word meant "divine breath"; for the Greeks, the concept of life was one of God breathing life into His lifeless creation. Just as modern charismatic Christians have taken the term *dynamus* to name the infilling of humans with the Holy Spirit, the early vitalists believed that, while life still existed within a person, the possibility for healing was present. Further, vitalists past and present believe that as all creation is alive, all creation is self-healing, and that, by making proper use of the life energy of other parts of creation, be they animals, vegetables, or minerals, we can use that spark to empower our own healing energies.

Samuel Hahnemann, the father of modern homeopathy, was, like Hippocrates, a vitalist. On the subject, Hahnemann wrote, "The material organism, without the vital force, is capable of no sensation, no function, no self-preservation; it derives all sensation and performs all the functions of life solely by means of the immaterial being (the vital principle), which animates the material organism in health and in disease."

But this concept of an invisible force that carries and contains the life energy of the living being neither originated with Hahnemann nor is unique to homeopathy. Or to the Greeks, for that matter. In fact, every healing system contains a concept parallel to vital force, or *lebenskraft*, as Hahnemann named it in his native German. This same energy was named *entelecheia* by Aristotle. For Henri Bergson, it was *élan vital*, "the momentum of life." And perhaps it is best known today through traditional Chinese medicine, in which system it is referred to as *chi*.

Whatever it is called, there is a flow of energy that pours through us all, that allows the meat and bones from which we are created to get up and run around. When that force leaves our body, the meat first becomes rigid and then begins to rot. For some that force is the human soul. Others call it the immune system. For the homeopath, this vital force represents the energy that maintains life in the individual. And more, it is considered to be a force that is unique within each individual, with each system manipulating and mutating the force with its own peculiar qualities. The vital force must be considered as an energy flow that is different from any other chemical or physical phenomenon within the individual being. Therefore, it is neither soul nor immune system; it is a unique flow that sustains, heals, develops, and learns. It would be, for Hahnemann, a gift from God and not God Himself alive within each of us.

As homeopath William Boericke, in his *A Compend of the Principles of Homeopathy*, writes: "The connection between the immaterial, spiritual and immortal being, and the body is supposed by him [Hahnemann] to be effected by means of the vital force which he designates Dynamis. We have then, in Hahnemannian physiology, (1) the spirit, the true man, (2) the material body, receiving its life and health through (3) the vivifying force, the dynamis."

Therefore, for the homeopath, this "vivifying force," our vital force, is the connection between our invisible and visible selves. It is the conduit of the energy of all eternity within our mortal bodies. Hahnemann believed that the spirit within each of us was perfect and would always remain so. No illness or evil could destroy the perfection of God's spirit within each of us. But the vital force, as the connection between the eternal and the temporal, not only was vulnerable to ailments and attacks of all sort but also was the seat of creation for all forms of disease.

In all of us there is the visible and the invisible, tangible and intangible. We all have muscles, bones, fat, and blood. We have eyes and ears and noses. But also we have emotions, intellect, and spirit. We have an invisible nature that defies chemical compositions and that allows us understanding of more than just physical creation. This invisible nature is dominant over the physical, and that which disrupts the invisible nature, the mind, and the emotions must ultimately also disrupt the physical body.

Modern science often reduces us to being meat machines, made of many parts that can be manipulated or removed or replaced like parts of a car. But we must never forget that there is an invisible being driving that car, and if that being is in a state of disruption, the meat machine is bound to run off the road and smash into a tree. For Hahnemann and for all homeopaths, all healing must take place on the level of vital force if healing is to take place at all.

If we can accept that illness begins in our invisible nature, then we can quickly move to the next step: By treating symptoms and looking only to the physical body in terms of treatment, we can never bring about a true healing. Take for example the angry man who has colitis. The usual treatment for this disease involves only the pain and not the anger. Even if this "treatment" seems to be successful, that still-angry patient soon needs treatment for migraines or some other disease. While the physician sees these new problems as unconnected to the earlier digestive disorder, the homeopath sees them as the logical progression of illness for this particular patient.

In other words, if we refuse to look to the vital force and to the invisible nature, we spend our lives chasing ailments one after another, as the weakest links in our system break down and more and more serious illnesses set in. But if we clear the block in the vital force with a homeopathic remedy (just as an acupuncture needle clears the flow of *chi*), we work on a more profound energistic level, one that treats the underlying cause of the ailment rather than its symptoms. Homeopathy, like acupuncture, is a form of energy medicine, one that relates to the invisible nature and, through it, to the physical body and its ailments.

Sooner or later, someone always gets the idea of taking a homeopathic remedy and running it to a lab to see what's inside. The results always come back that nothing is inside. The implication is always that, because there is nothing in the remedy, the remedy does nothing and homeopathy is quackery. But put the remedy in its proper context and you will see that it holds great healing potential.

Far from denying the basic principles of science as we all learned them in high school, the basic tenets of homeopathy fit very nicely into the realm of science. In fact, the scientific principles set forth by Newton and Einstein form the foundation for our understanding of homeopathy.

The basis for both homeopathic exploration and practice is the idea that nature is knowable. If we cannot believe that creation is governed by set principles instead of a sort of functioning chaos, then we cannot look to any form of medicine, homeopathic or allopathic, to be of any consistent assistance in the restoration of health. It is only by believing that we can uncover a set of unchanging rules by which creation functions that we can proceed.

Newton's philosophy tells us that to every action there is an equal and opposite reaction. He states that "action and reaction are ceaseless, equivalent, and reciprocal." All action has response. It is by working with this tenet that homeopathic remedies—our *actions*—bring about healing *reactions* from within our vital force. This is the heart of the Law of Similars: "Like cures like." It is this principle by which homeopathy functions. Homeopathy is a reactive medicine, one that places the healing impact on that "equal and opposite reaction," rather than an active medicine, such as allopathy, that places the force of the cure on the first medicinal action and calls that equally potent reaction a "side effect."

As Einstein's discoveries enhance our view of creation, they also enhance our understanding of homeopathy. Einstein gives us this tenet: Matter and energy and essentially interchangeable and their transformations are eternally continuous. All matter, therefore, is energy. It is all made up of swirling bits of energy of different sizes and speeds. The chair you are sitting on is made up of energy, as are your clothes. As are you. You are an energy being.

Further, Einstein tells us that matter/energy is indestructible and persistent and infinitely divisible. Take a handful of dirt and try to destroy it, take it out of existence. You can smash it into smaller and smaller bits, but it's still there. We are forever proving this tenet to be true; as we look into the atom, we are finding that the smallness of matter/energy is as eternal as the vastness of the universe. It follows that there is no lower limit to the quantity of action that is necessary to effect any change. In other words, a minute amount of energy may well be as efficacious in bringing about a change as is a large amount of energy. Therefore, even if you cannot find molecules of a remedy within a remedy, perhaps molecules aren't really necessary to effect a change toward healing. What if there is something smaller, something as yet invisible to our best ability to look within creation, that, while invisible, has an action still potent enough to effect a reaction within our human system? The universe is a wonderfully crafted spiral that is eternal in its vastness and its smallness.

As we are spiritual beings, energy beings, then hasn't science itself taught us that we are eternal in our natures, as our final tenet states it, "indestructible and persistent"? Perhaps it is our perception that is at fault, or the lessons that we have been taught: We should pay attention to our physical symptoms and deal with what we can see and touch and cut in terms of medicine and healing.

If we accept what Einstein has taught us, then we must begin to see our allopathic tradition of medicine as old-fashioned, mired in a universe made up of only what we can see and taste and smell. The universe of acupuncture and homeopathic medicine is an energy universe, one that is alive and harmonious in creation. These philosophies, both thousands of years old, have yet to be proved scientifically because of the limitations of science, not because they are not true.

If we accept the principle of vital force, then we must look elsewhere for our healing. Not to our meat and bones, blood and phlegm, but to our eternal selves—our spirits.

2

SYMPTOMS

Most of us equate symptoms with disease. If you ask a person to give an example of a symptom, he is likely to say "sore throat" or "stomach cramps" or "fever." But symptoms are a more profound phenomenon than this and are the most important tools we have in guiding our healing process.

In considering symptoms, realize that we all are experiencing symptoms at all times. As H. I. Hayakawa tells us in his book *Language in Thought and Action*, we "cannot not communicate," and we communicate our likes and dislikes in many ways other than in sentences. There is also not one single moment in our lives when we do not have some sort of symptom group present.

Symptoms, to the homeopath, are the ways the vital force manifests itself within our beings at all times. Symptoms can certainly be sensations of pain—the sore throat or the stomach cramps. But they can also be benign—the amount of thirst we have, and for what kinds of drinks; our sleep positions; our sex drives; the high- and low-energy times of day. None of these involve pain or disease directly, and yet these symptoms are as profound as any sensation of pain.

In understanding symptoms, we also seek a new understanding of disease.

Most of us think that there is some distinct boundary within us that is either "well" or "sick," as if some switch were thrown or some line were crossed. And, at times, particularly with acute illnesses such as colds and flus, this line seems almost tangible. We have all experienced a moment in which we knew that we were "getting" something. But with the more profound illnesses, with chronic conditions, this line becomes a bit harder to trace. How many cancer cells, for instance, need be present before the patient has cancer? How many headaches does one need to have in a year before the headaches are to be considered chronic?

Most of us feel that we are well unless at the present moment we are beset with pain. This simplistic notion guides most of what we think about health and healing. How many of us go through life day after day with a chronic condition or conditions, having had a pain for so long that it no longer even is considered a sign of illness? How many people judge their days by how much they can accomplish before exhaustion sets in, allowing their lives to be defined by that exhaustion without even questioning it as anything other than normal?

Illness and good health are more intricately involved than we would like them to be. It is our own unwillingness to look at ourselves and to become familiar with the ways we tell ourselves that all is or is not well within that allow us to go into a doctor's office thinking that we are totally well and learn that we harbor a critical condition.

We need to begin to look at ourselves and to listen to the warnings that are coming from within. We also need to come to understand that, as unique beings—and remember, we are unique to such an extent that even our vital force, our connection to spirit, is unique within each of us—there is no rule book of how we can and should function. Instead, we need to write our own rule book, for each of us is the true expert on his own state of being. But too many of us simply do not pay attention to ourselves, do not listen to the wisdom within.

This whole idea of *uniquity* can be difficult for us to grasp. We have all our lives been told that we are, in terms of health care, unique beings to the extent that we take the amount of cold and cough medicine that is appropriate for our body weight or age. So we don't stop to consider that we are truly unique beings, whole universes unto ourselves. And we miss the point that the methods that might be curative for a set of illness symptoms for you might cause me harm or do nothing at all. In short, in the field of medicine in which we were raised, if we have a cold, we would all take the same medicine for it, varying only the amount taken by the individual patient. In homeopathic medicine, if twenty people all had colds, they might well need twenty different medicines to treat those colds, because they are unique beings and as such need medicines that reflect their uniquity.

The only other term that applies to all our symptoms and beings is *wholeness*. Body, mind, and spirit, we are one being. No matter how science tries to divide us into parts, we are, by nature, indivisible. If we have a set of symptoms that include ringing in the ears, insomnia, and rash, then these symptoms must be interrelated; they are being experienced by a unique and whole being. To consider it coincidence that these symptoms are all happening at once, or, worse, to treat these symptoms individually as if your ears do not know what your skin is doing, is to court disaster. Only by respecting the wholeness of each unique being can we treat that being in a truly healing manner, focusing not on the individual symptom or pain, but on bringing harmony to that whole unique being.

In the words of British homeopath Margery Blackie, we must always consider "the patient, not the cure." We must always treat the person who has the symptoms of illness and not the illness itself. Treating the illness alone suggests that we are not whole beings, and paradoxically that it is possible to subdivide ourselves and to promote total health by dealing with a specific system or organ. It denies the context of our illness. Instead, we think some villainous microbe got to us and mowed us down.

To treat the whole is to move a living creature from one state of being to another. In improving the whole, we create circumstances that allow for health, rather than creating the illusion of health through the suppression of pain. To treat each person as a unique individual is to place the healing process within his own unique context instead of demanding that each sick person fit into one general pattern.

We've looked at symptoms in a new way, as important information about ourselves and how we are living our lives. Now let's look at illness with new eyes. Think again about vital force. The spirit within us is perfect and cannot fall ill. It is only in those moments in life in which we are divided from the spirit that we can become ill in our bodies or minds. Hahnemann believed that all illness begins on the level of vital force; when this connection between our selves and the eternal spirit of God becomes blocked, it allows illness to set in.

Homeopath Elizabeth Wright Hubbard gives us an important clue when she writes that homeopathy's "concept of disease is a protective explosion manifesting in an individual as a particular set of symptoms." In other words, illness is a sign that the vital force is intact and is attempting to push whatever is blocking the self from the spirit out of the body. This push to remove the block may become wedged within the system in the body, the mind, or both. And these sets of painful symptoms that we consider illness are therefore actually positive signs, signs that a healing is possible or has already begun.

As we do our symptoms, we must place our illnesses within the context of our lives, respecting that our selves contain all states of being that are at once unique and whole. Physicians call this "the wisdom of the body," the vital force within us, within the context of any illness, removing a deeper block that has manifested on the energy level within our body.

On the subject of health, modern homeopath George Vithoulkas writes that "Health is freedom from pain in the physical body, having attained a state of well-being; freedom from passion on the emotional level, having as a result a dynamic state of serenity and calm; and freedom from selfishness in the mental sphere, having as a result total unification with Truth." We may simply define *health* as "freedom." When we are in a state of total health, we are totally free, not needing to have our lives defined or held in check in any way by symptoms that pain or trouble us. A person in this state of freedom would, therefore, have symptoms of health: a hearty appetite, a generous and loving nature, and so forth. Further, a person in this state of freedom would also be in tune with his spirit within. As Hahnemann puts it in the ninth aphorism of *The Organon*, "In the healthy condition of man, the spiritual vital force, the dynamism that animates the material body, rules with unbounded sway, and retains all the parts of the organism in admirable, harmonious, vital operation as regards both sensations and functions, so that our indwelling, reason-gifted mind can freely employ this living, healthy instrument for the higher purposes of our existence."

What blocks this state of perfect freedom, then, and causes illness to set in? According to Hahnemann, all these blocks must take place on the dynamic level before they can manifest on the physical: "In disease, it is only this immaterial, automatic Vital Force, pervading the entire organism, that is primarily deranged by the dynamic influence upon it of a morbific agent inimical to life. Only the vital principle, thus deranged, can furnish the organism its abnormal sensations and set up the irregular processes we call disease; for, as a power invisible in itself and only known by its effects on the organism, its morbid derangement only makes itself known by the manifestations of disease in the sensations and functions of those parts of the organism exposed to the senses of the observer and physician—that is, by morbid symptoms, and in no other way can it make itself known."

Illness, then, begins in the realm of impulse, of thought. To find the meaning of our illnesses, we often have to do no more than to look at our motivations. The person who is motivated by anger, who is fueled by it and feels empowered by it, incurs the illnesses of anger. The person who chooses the victim role chooses also the illnesses of the victim. The person who insists that he is motivated solely by love and peace and yet is still nearly overwhelmed by illness and pain would do well to look into his own denial.

Finding what motivates us as individuals is difficult, and most often it is a discovery that comes in the process of homeopathic healing rather than at its outset. As we begin a homeopathic healing, we look at the symptoms that are troubling and put them in the context of all the other, more benign symptoms that are also being presented. This complete picture is called *the totality of symptoms*, which represents the patient's true state of being and a road map for the homeopath to follow in the selection of appropriate remedies.

This totality of symptoms helps us accept our symptoms as the expression of the vital force in our lives and bodies. It allows us to rejoice in the belief that our symptoms *are* ourselves, an expression of self, and not some invader within our space. Modern science tries so hard to make us believe that disease is always *other*, some new germ that cruelly attacks our innocent body. This scientific belief gave rise to the 1950s notion that if we could just keep ourselves hermetically sealed within our perfectly cleaned and germ-free homes, we would become stronger beings. We tried it, and it didn't work. The opposite, in fact, is true. While cleanliness is certainly a good thing, those evil germs are as much a part of creation as we are and have a place in our lives.

Look at our children. We have, through the use of vaccines, removed the childhood diseases from childhood, ignoring that simple fact that those childhood diseases belonged in the childhood experience of each of us. They would have built the immune system that supports us for the rest of our lives. And now some forty or fifty years into our policy of vaccinating everything that moves, we have not only a present generation but also a previous generation that was vaccinated and did not get childhood diseases. So we have adults who not only did not get measles when they were younger, but who also did not receive antibodies for measles from their mothers, who also were vaccinated. So when they as adults are faced with measles, they are faced not with an unpleasant week in bed but with a life-threatening disease. This is because we have tried to deny the disease instead of placing it within the context of our lives. And so it works with tuberculosis and with every other disease that we, in our ignorance, believe we can control and destroy.

I am quite aware that to all those who have come to see science as the answer to all our problems, most of what I am writing seems a throwback to the days of the shaman. And in many ways it is.

When science, particularly medical science, began to make a solid effort to eliminate God from the equation, when the rationalists sought to reduce our every emotion to a mix of chemicals within our system, the potential for healing left the field of medicine. It was replaced with the desire for cure. This desire first and foremost insisted that we humans had the power to remove disease, a power that has again and again been shown illusionary. We are no closer to the cure for cancer now than we were fifty years ago. Tuberculosis, which was thought to be gone for good, is back and more powerful and less treatable than before. The occurrence of infectious disease has grown greatly in this generation, and these diseases become more and more potent as time passes. And our powerful drugs, most notably antibiotics, are less and less effective in treating disease.

Perhaps it is time for us to stop worshiping science and begin again to worship our creator. Perhaps we must put God at the center of our healing and, therefore, at the center of our medical science, if healing is ever to take place. And perhaps it is time for us to put aside the paternalistic and flawed notion of curing if we are to be healed. Let's return science to being a tool, a method by which we might test our universe and stop making it an end itself. Often the information that we intuit, that we receive without external validation or provable source, is the most powerful.

Look at it this way. Science says that we use only 10 percent of our brains. This angers me. What it should say is that science can account for only 10 percent of what the brain is doing. It certainly could be doing a good many things that the scientists cannot measure.

We need to stop worrying about the details. Science looks for the exact food that we should all eat, the exact moment at which the embryo becomes the person. Therefore, we are in a constant state of flux. The food that was good for us yesterday is bad for us today. Instead, we need to seek the eternal principles of life and of healing and not the ever-changing details specific to the scientific dogma of the moment. Medical and scientific martyrs such as Galileo, Semelweiss, and Sister Kenny remind us that yesterday's scientific heresy is today's scientific truth.

Perhaps we need to get away from our whole medical model, which replaced the blended notion of mystic and healer with the military leader of the surgeon general. Perhaps if we put our time and attention into what can strengthen our healing response before it is too late, we could find a better result than we have with our war on cancer and our war on AIDS. Certainly it must have seemed sensible at the time to replace the religious notion of healer with the scientific and political notion of medical warrior, but surely time has shown us that the tactics we use to make the world safe for democracy do not make it safe from cancer.

Perhaps it is time for the surgeon general to be replaced in Washington with a shaman.

All of us, at all times, are expressing ourselves in terms of symptoms. Some are symptoms of being, or, simply, the ways we express our unique and whole natures, the amount of sleep we need and the kinds of food we crave, that sort of thing. Others, however, are symptoms of pain, or, when they are clustered together, what we call illness. When we look at it this way, we see that illnesses, far from being removed from ourselves—the "evil invader" belief that germs are like Russians invading Hungary—are part of ourselves. A cold, after all, is not a manifestation of the germ in the body, but is rather the manifestation of what our body is doing to the germ that is present within it. If our total system were strong enough, the cold germ would not be enough of a threat to elicit a response that sends us to bed for a week.

As Vithoulkas gives us information on health, he also defines illness: "What is the parameter that defines, for instance, whether an individual with rheumatoid arthritis is in better health than another one suffering from depression? The parameter which enables such measurement of health is creativity. By creativity, I mean all those acts and functions which promote for the individual himself and for others their main goal in life: continuous and unconditional happiness. To the extent that an individual is limited in the exercise of his creativity, to that degree he is ill. If the rheumatoid arthritis patient is crippled to the extent that his ailment prevents him from being creative more than the patient with depression, then the rheumatoid arthritis patient is more seriously ill than the depressed one."

Therefore, our hierarchy of illness is also an illusion. One man may have a heart condition, another may have cancer. In our society, we put a good deal of effort in judging just who is sickest, who has fallen victim to the worse disease. Indeed, the medical establishment lists the ten biggest causes of death in our society, as if were we actually able to remove the number-one cause of death from that list another disease wouldn't immediately replace it.

Also illusionary is the concept of being a victim of disease. We are, instead, victims of ourselves. No disease, no matter how potent, will ever kill us all. Some of us are immune to everything. In other words, a disease can kill some of the people all of the time, and all of the people some of the time, but can't kill all of the people all of the time.

In fact, many homeopaths, especially those who follow the philosophy of American homeopath James Tyler Kent, are reluctant to name diseases at all. These homeopaths feel that the disease name is a fear word, one that predisposes the patient to "act out" a disease drama. Further, they believe that the name of the disease is actually meaningless. For the physician, the diagnosis leads to a systematized form of treatment that, for those who hold with the principles of uniquity and wholeness, is invalid. If we are treating the person and never the disease, then naming the disease only leads the patient to identify with the specifics of that disease and further graft it onto his self and not work to release it.

If our diseases are integral parts of ourselves, our responses to the stresses and provocations we encounter in our lives, then we are victims of our natures and of ourselves and not of our circumstances or germs. We must change the ways we think of illness and health if we are to be well, and we must look again at the treatments that we use to combat disease.

3

TREATMENTS

Hippocrates, the father of medicine, gave us the philosophical basis for how our disease symptoms may be treated. He wrote that there were two streams of medicine that flowed side by side in opposite directions. Nearly two millennia later, German physician Samuel Hahnemann would name these two streams. The first, which worked against specific symptoms with the idea of suppressing the discomfort until the body could heal itself, he named allopathy. The second, which worked with the symptom, expressing the symptom and expelling it from the body, he named homeopathy.

The term *allopathy* comes from two Greek words, *allos*, which means "other," and *pathos*, which means "suffering." The concept here is that symptoms are to be pushed away through the use of their opposites. Therefore, if you go to an allopathic physician with a cold, with running nose and tearing eyes, you are given a medicine that dries up your eyes and nose.

Homeopathy is also formed from two Greek words: *homios*, meaning "similar," and *pathos*. Thus, *homeopathy* literally means "similar suffering." The concept here is that we deal with our disease symptoms by treating them with more of the same. Some homeopaths say that homeopathy involves treatments in which you are given your own poison. Therefore, if that same person with the cold went to a homeopathic practitioner, he would be given a medicine that would make his nose run and his eyes tear, with the belief that this enhancement of the symptoms already being experienced brings about a rapid and total recovery from illness.

This is the difference between the practice of homeopathy and of allopathy. They are polar opposites, not only in their approach but also in their impact on the body.

The action of allopathic medicine is suppressive. The goal is to remove the symptoms of the disease. If you take allopathic medicine for your cold or your headache—and, indeed, the management of pain from headache to arthritis to PMS has become a multibillion-dollar industry—the action of that medicine is to remove you from the experience of the symptom; it doesn't truly affect the symptom itself. Think about it. If you take a cold medicine, does that medicine do anything at all to cure your cold? Or does it merely allow you to pretend for a period of time that you have no cold?

This is a core problem with our stubborn reliance on allopathic medicine: We have created a society of denial. Our medicine is the medicine of denial. This denial of illness runs all through our society. We also use our credit cards to pretend that we have enough money to buy that new stereo when in fact we do not. We want it all now: health, wealth, and happiness. Anything that cannot deliver the goods immediately is suspect at best and a total failure at worst.

The problem with this engine of denial that is driving us is that it will not run forever. It will break down. While we can certainly take an aspirin for a headache or fever once in a while without any harm to our systems, the reliance on suppressive measures in the long term is much more harmful than it is helpful.

Think about denial in terms of emotional and mental health. Have our health care experts told us that if we hate our parents and refuse to deal with the issue, sweep it under our emotional rugs, we become stronger and better people? Quite the opposite. Any psychologist, from Dr. Joyce Brothers onward, insists that you can become stronger, you can become truly well, only by facing the issue, talking it out, and removing the block from your mind and heart. Until you do this, they insist, this block colors your life's work, relationships, and behavior patterns.

In the same way, this use of suppressive treatments for the purposes of denial of illness weakens the overall system if used repeatedly. And the stronger the suppression, the greater the overall impact. Therefore, the use of an occasional aspirin is far less toxic to the system than is the use of an occasional antibiotic or steroid. As our society's medical practitioners become more and more liberal in their use of potent allopathic drugs, drugs that mask symptoms but do not heal them, the cost is tremendous. With each generation we become weaker and weaker, both as individuals and as a society, more dependent on these drugs and less resistant to illnesses as a whole.

A century ago, children were not born allergic to everything in their environment. They were not hyperactive. A diagnosis of attention deficit disorder would have been meaningless. It is representative of our weakened condition as a whole that these disorders not only exist but grow in number and potency with each new generation. The same is true for chronic fatigue syndrome and its related disorder, Epstein-Barr virus. These ailments and other autoimmune disorders signal a weakening of our ability to live healthy lives.

The flaw in the thinking that lies behind an allopathic treatment is within the concept of disease itself. For the allopath, the symptom is just a symptom; it has no meaning and no particular reason to exist. Further, since the time of Greek physician Galen, when the human body began to be subdivided into its many parts, the treatment given by an allopathic practitioner focused on one symptom or one part of the body. Therefore, if you have more than one symptom, you must be treated with more than one drug, likely by more than one practitioner. This leads to the polypharmaceutical approach to medicine in which many substances, which may or may not combine in a healthy or wholesome fashion, are used in the treatment of a single person's multiple ailments. Your single or multiple symptoms may improve, but your overall health will surely decline.

Suppressive treatments are palliative; they merely remove the pain while leaving the cause intact. This means that although the pain remover may seem to stop an individual headache, it does nothing to strengthen the overall system and make it more headache-resistant. Indeed, in time, the need for painkillers will be greater as the headaches become more frequent or more potent. Therefore, the use of suppressive treatment on any part of the body acts only to hook the patient into an endless spiral of symptom and treatment. From antacids to skin care products to antihistamines, we are bombarded with the promise that the product is "stronger than ever."

I say that if the product worked in the first place, its strength would not need enhancement.

The deepest legacy of allopathic treatment lies in the use of polypharmacy. Here the interactions of multiple medicines, each with its one level of suppression, actually create new diseases from the drugs that supposedly cured the old diseases. The whole system is left weaker than it was before treatments were begun.

Modern medical science even has its own term, *iatrogenic,* to describe these diseases that are created by allopathic treatment, as if by giving them their own category it was making these ailments less shocking and unacceptable. The legacy of allopathic medicine, finally, is the weakening of our individual systems and, through the passing on of these newly created flaws to generations to come, the ultimate weakening of humanity.

I always think about it in terms of gym class. If you hated gym as much as I did, then you know that even if you can get a note to get you out of gym for a day or a week, you must ultimately go to class. You must ultimately climb the rope, no matter how spindly your arms are. You must ultimately run the required twelve-minute mile.

It is the same with our lives. Each time you suppress a symptom, each time you deny an illness rather than respect it, you are getting a note for gym. But each time you do that, you are allowing your arms to become more spindly and your overall system to become less and less capable of running the good race.

How much better if we could learn to become conversant with our bodies, our minds, and our emotions. How much better if we could learn just to have a cold, go to bed and sweat out the toxins in our system, instead of putting our jobs and our need for attention ahead of our need for healing. This is to say nothing of the fact that, by denying that cold and suppressing it, we take it with us into the workplace. Just because we have suppressed the symptoms does not mean we are not contagious when we sneeze or shake our mucus-covered hands with someone else's. In this way, we spread the need for denial along with that cold, as the next person rushes out to the drugstore to buy something that allows him to deny his ailment and continue to spread it through the community.

A true understanding of homeopathy demands that we become conversant with ourselves, that we respect the fact that we are whole beings—body, mind, and spirit—and that we are also unique beings, with thoughts, feelings, and symptoms unique to ourselves.

Hahnemann stated the central tenet of his homeopathic philosophy as "like cures like" (*similia similibus curenteur*), which he called the Law of Similars, one of the Three Laws of Cure that I discuss later in this book. By this he meant that there is a reason underlying each of our symptoms, that something, some issue or block in the vital force, is being expressed within the being. Only by working with the symptom, by listening to the message that it brings, can the symptom be released from the body.

Perhaps British homeopath Edward Bach, developer of the healing system of flower essences, expressed the Law of Similars best when he referred to it as "like repels like." If as a child you were ever taken on the Pennsylvania Turnpike, as I was, and stopped at any of the rest stops, you likely were given either one of those giant multicolored lollipops or the salt and pepper Scottie dog magnets. If you got the lollipop, you got only a brief sugar high, but if you got the Scotties, you got a gift that represents the Law of Cure. If you placed these little plastic dogs, one black and one white, both with dual polar magnets glued to their feet, with the north pole of one facing the south pole of the other, the dogs rushed toward each other and stuck together. If, however, you put the north pole of one to the north pole of the other, the dogs repelled each other, and you could make them do a little dance driven along on invisible forces.

That little dance is the dance of similars. As Bach states the Law of Similars, if you have a set pattern of symptoms of disease and you take a homeopathic remedy whose energy pattern is the same as the one that you are experiencing, that internalized remedy will repel the symptoms out of your body.

If you don't want to think about homeopathic remedies as little magnets, Hahnemann tells us that we can also think of them as vaccinations. And, as Edward Jenner, the discoveror of the smallpox vaccine, was familiar with Hahnemann's work, it is widely believed in homeopathic circles that the whole idea of vaccinations is a bastardization of homeopathic principles.

Hahnemann tells us that all medicines, homeopathic or not, create "artificial diseases" in the human system. Think about this for a moment. As we have already defined diseases as just a set of unpleasant symptoms, don't our traditional medications simply create within us artificial symptoms that are in opposition to the symptoms that we are already experiencing? Just take Nyquil when you *don't* have a cold, and you'll see what I mean. The difference in the types of medicines, homeopathic or allopathic, is not whether or not they create artificial diseases but rather what kind of artificial diseases they create.

Allopathic remedies create artificial diseases that work in opposition to the natural disease. They dry up running noses, stop you from sneezing, and so on. Homeopathic remedies, on the other hand, create artificial diseases that are similar to the disease that is already on hand. And the more similar the artificial disease to the natural, the better the remedy will work.

Why is the artificial disease of homeopathy more effective than the one set in place by allopathic methods? The allopathic artificial disease fades as the antihistamine fades. In a few hours, your cold comes back, and since your whole system has been knocked down by the power of the remedy, your cold comes back stronger than ever. When, however, you set up an artificial disease that is working in concert with the natural disorder, you work with the system as a vaccination works. As the system as a whole rises up against the artificial disease, whether it is a homeopathic remedy or a vaccine (often these are much the same thing), it overcomes the "artificial disease" caused by the remedy or the vaccine. In doing so, the system overcomes the natural disease. In addition, as with a vaccine, as the system overcomes the "bit of poison" placed within by the homeopathic remedy, it becomes stronger as a whole and more resistant to the disease in the future.

This brings us to the concept of the *microdose*. When Hahnemann was developing the philosophy by which homeopaths would come to practice, it was central to his work that allopaths were incorrect in their use of more and more natural or chemical substances in treating disease.

Hahnemann saw the toxic side effects of allopathic drugs and sought a better way. He did the logical thing: Instead of using more arsenic to treat a disease (he was working in the late 1700s, after all), he began to use less. In doing so he discovered two very interesting things. As you diluted more and more, the toxic effects faded away, and as they faded away, the healing power of the remedy increased just as dramatically.

In fact, modern homeopaths now know that at a certain level all the substance contained in a given remedy disappears and only the energy signature, or vital force, of that original substance remains. In this way, in homeopathic remedies, the vital force of any of a million other parts of creation—animal, vegetable, or mineral—may be used to harmonize your own vital force in a time of weakness, and it may do so without the toxic side effects of the original substance. Thus the toxic arsenic becomes the benign remedy Arsenicum, and strychnine becomes Nux Vomica. Both of these remedies, and many others like them, which are poisonous in their substance state, become healing when the substance is removed by dilution and only the vital force remains.

So in terms of treatment, homeopathy works in direct opposition to allopathic medicine, the so-called scientific medicine of the Western world. It uses less and less of a healing substance, whereas allopathy, when faced with an unsuccessful cure, uses more and more. Think: "New and Improved!" And where allopathic drugs cause a new set of symptoms that are in opposition to the natural disorder, homeopathic remedies create an artificial disease that is as close to the natural disorder as possible.

It is important here to clear up a possible confusion I have created. I just compared homeopathy to vaccines, yet earlier I deplored the widespread vaccination of children against measles. Why? The answer is fairly simple: There is a great deal of difference between the concept of vaccination and the way it is practiced.

First, the *concept* of vaccination is a good one. Instead of using more of the disease substance, we use very little, just enough for the body to notice. Very homeopathic in concept.

The problem is that this homeopathic concept is being used allopathically. The scientists creating vaccines ignore the fact that you and I are unique and whole beings, that person one is not person two is not person three. One vaccine does not fit all. If we all took a flu shot today, some of us would have no response at all to the shot, some of us would be saved from getting the flu, and some of us would get the flu because of it. It all has to do with our unique natures and our unique responses.

Therefore, when we are dealing with truly evil, life-threatening diseases and we vaccinate against them, we are opening a can of worms. Unless we create vaccines with the individual in mind, and I don't know how we go about accomplishing this, then we have to accept a certain number of failures. And in some cases these failures can be fatal.

To vaccinate or not to vaccinate. This is a decision that can be reached only individually. There are, unfortunately, as many cons as pros to the notion. Homeopathic remedies, of course, offer an alternative method by which we can become disease-resistant. But laws and cultural dictates are powerful reasons to make decisions slowly and clearly.

It is time to mention herbs. Many of the people who enroll in classes in homeopathy think that they will be studying herbal remedies. They always are crushed when they find out that they won't.

Many homeopathic remedies are, of course, taken from herbs, and the homeopathic pharmacy is largely based on the herbal remedies that were in use in Hahnemann's time. But remember—homeopathic remedies are energy remedies, not substances. They have gone through a two-step process, which Hahnemann called *potentizing*, in order to unleash their healing power and remove their toxic nature. (More on this process is discussed in the section that follows.) Herbs, no matter how lovely they look and smell when they are growing, are largely allopathic in their behavior.

This is to say that our herbal tradition is largely suppressive in its action. Taking valerian for a nervous disorder is no "healthier" than taking Valium for the same disorder. Both suppress your symptoms, dull your senses into a denial of illness, and weaken your overall system at the same time. One has to wonder, then, about modern "alternative" practitioners who give their patients both herbs and homeopathics, subjecting them to an internal tug-of-war.

It can be valuable to study herbs and their actions on the body, in order to compare the actions of those herbs with that of the remedy taken from them. But the use of herbal remedies alone ultimately brings about the same systemic response as a lifetime of over-the-counter medicine: depletion, suppression, and chronic illness.

I am reminded of Woody Allen's film *Sleeper*. Woody Allen is frozen in a medical procedure and is awakened many years later, only to find that the doctors in his hospital are feeding him a diet of fried foods and chocolate cake. When he asks about this, he is told that everything he knew about nutrition in his time has been superseded by new scientific discoveries that have proven that chocolate cake is good for you.

The truths of allopathic medicine are forever shifting. Leeching promotes health, leeching causes death. Eggs are good, eggs are bad. And on and on. Modern science has replaced the permanent principles of creation with constantly changing scientific studies. The principles of homeopathic treatment are unchanged from the time of Hippocrates. They follow from an understanding of nature's healing process and work with and promote that process in the human system. Because they deal with immutable principles, the practices of homeopathy do not and will not change. The methods and treatments are the same today as they were two thousand years ago and as they will be two thousand years from now. Homeopathy, in truth, has less to do with taking little pills that have been infused with the energy of other living things than with coming to understand the regenerating, healing nature of all life, all creation.

So to understand and to practice homeopathic medicine we make an adjustment in our thinking and understanding of ourselves and our very natures. We must unlearn the ways we consider ourselves to be ill and to be well, reconsider our overwhelming desire just to be rid of any pain that we feel.

We have mortgaged our ability to live lives that are free from illness, denial, and suppression because we look only at the present moment when we are unhappy. Homeopathy demands that we also consider the long-term goal of balance and transformation. This does not mean that homeopathic remedies cannot be powerful tools in acute situations. But it does mean that, even in these emergencies that can crop up and overwhelm us, we remember who and what we are and what our true nature is. We remember that our spirits represent our true beings, and that any illness that cannot touch this true being really represents only a momentary problem to be dealt with and released.

What, then, have we unlearned?

- Sick or well, we are more than meat. There is more to us than can be seen or measured, and within our nature there are both visible and invisible aspects, tangible and intangible. The invisible nature is dominant over the visible flesh. We have been told again and again that we are physical beings and that we have physical ailments. The truth is that we are energy beings, and wherever our energy nature is blocked, illness begins. Einstein has already shown us that all matter is energy.
- We are filled with symptoms every moment of our lives, and these symptoms are just expressions of our unique nature. We all have symptoms of the body as well as of the mind and emotions. We have symptoms of disease as well as symptoms of our state of being, which are often benign in nature. In fact, the totality of our symptoms, in body and mind and spirit, reveals the state of our being. When a group of those symptoms are unpleasant enough, we seek to trade them in for a more pleasant set of symptoms. That is why we got to the hospital. We can either work with or work against those symptoms in seeking to alter them. To work against them is to suppress them deeper into our system. To work with them is to help the body to continue to express them until they are removed from our system.
- Whatever has been suppressed in our being must, by the nature of our being, be expressed once again. And as you increase suppression by stronger and stronger treatments, the expression comes from a deeper and more painful place. Thus, the diaper rash that is suppressed by antibiotic cream comes back as earache, which, treated by antibiotics, moves into the more painful situation of allergies, and so on.
- As energy beings, we must be treated energistically in order to be well. The use of physical substances as treatments only induces the state of suppression. Energy treatments such as homeopathy and acupuncture offer methods by which disease symptoms can be removed from the body in a manner that is rapid, gentle, and permanent.

If we can unlearn all that has been programmed into our hearts and minds in a lifetime of living allopathically, if we can learn to not be limited in our healing by the fears of the well-meaning world, then transformation is in our grasp. Homeopathy is only a tool for that transformation, because all healing, like all creation, is an act of God. And within all aspects of creation is the ability to heal in body, mind, and spirit, and an ability truly to change, to transform as a caterpillar transforms.

34

We have so many solid reasons for not attempting transformation in our lives. We have our fears. We have our righteous indignation that tells us that we are better off if we are correct than if we are simply happy. We also have our society, which so often leads us down any number of garden paths with its new treatments and rules. And we have our denial, the denial that we clutch to our hearts at the slightest hint of pain. Parents, doctors, teachers, friends—all add their voice to the notion that we should leave well enough alone and let the addition of new technologies be enough. Just try not to notice that we have left God out of our plan for healing.

With all this, there is only one reason to move toward healing, toward transformation: because you are finally ready. Usually this means that you have already tried everything else—diet and exercise and pills and machines and spas and biofeedback—and still you are bound by your ills. Still your life is limited, even defined, by ailments and symptoms that you have not only named in the form of the disease name but also have taken into your mind and heart, to the point that you know more about your illness than you do about your country, your religion, and your spouse's favorite movies.

So many of us are professionally ill. We have taken our illness on as our careers. This is especially true of senior citizens, many of whom define their lives by their multiple ailments, as they once defined their lives by the office they entered every day. How the professionally ill's eyes glow at the notion of a doctor's appointment. Finally, a chance to show one's true profession: suffering. And, sadly, it is often a chance for the professionally ill to have someone pay them a little attention.

Few people who enter this pit ever climb out the other side. Those who do have reached the point in life where they know that it is just not working, not only that something is lacking in their treatment but that something is lacking in their lives. They are ready for a fundamental change. They are ready for transformation.

For some, the path to change comes easily to their body and mind. For others, and I was one of them, the path is long and hard, involving education and requiring an act of dedication and an act of will.

The philosophy of homeopathy intertwines with this process of change. The core philosophy is actually amazingly simple. It can be contained on very few pages. The practice, however, can be amazingly complex. Let us turn our attention to the history and the hands-on practice of homeopathy.

Part Two

LEARNING

The cure of the part should not be attempted without

treatment of the whole. No attempt should be made to

cure the body without the soul, and, if the head

and the body are to be healthy, you must begin by

curing the mind. . . . For this is the great error of our

day in the treatment of the human body, that

physicians first separate the soul from the body.

—Plato

4

A HISTORY OF HOMEOPATHY

History is a hard thing to get right. We have only paper trails of journals, letters, and notebooks to follow. We often can find any number of source materials that give us a third party's opinion of our subject. This makes it easy to bend, fold, and spindle our history to match our own opinions and biases.

But it is vital that we consider homeopathy within the context of the cultures in which it was developed. Like the miniskirt and the laptop computer, homeopathy was very much a product of its day.

THE MESSENGER AND THE MESSAGE

The ancients had a way of confusing the messenger with the message that he brought. If a field commander who was locked in battle saw that the war was likely lost, he sent a messenger running to the commanding officer with the news. The commanding officer, if he was displeased with his living memo, had the messenger killed, as easily as a corporate boss might today delete E-mail. It was not an effective method of warfare, but it cut down on the negative news from the front.

In two thousand years, we haven't learned to separate the messenger from the message. However, today we tend to kill the message rather than the messenger.

Perhaps we think a political leader has a good plan that will make our lives better. Then we read in a magazine that someone claims to have had sex with that politician, or to have smoked pot with him twenty years ago. This tends not only to change our opinion of the politician but of his plan as well. We not only won't vote for him, but we will vote against his agenda as well.

The same holds true for our religious leaders. The message may be helpful for us, but we can't seem to forgive them their humanity. When they seem to fail us by being frail humans, we turn our backs on their churches as well.

This seems to me to be a terrible waste. The media glare of our day has made more and more messengers reluctant to deliver their messages or has caused them to be willing only to post them anonymously on some Internet bulletin board. We can't afford to kill either the messages or the messengers. Just as that ancient runner had not chosen to dash toward death, it is often true that our messengers of change for society have little choice in the matter.

As evangelist Oral Roberts writes in his autobiography, "The message is greater than the messenger." This message may be considered by some messengers to be a miracle and a blessing, an inspiration no more or less mysterious than the inspiration required to paint a painting or compose an opera. By others it may be considered a curse, as any other form of inspiration may be considered a curse, as with Sylvia Plath or Vincent van Gogh.

Not liking the messenger is just one way of avoiding listening to an important message. Too often we want to shrink our messages to fit our attention spans, our concepts of the universe, and our personal preferences. If the message isn't immediately interesting, we just change that channel. In this way, we overlook and refuse to hear the messages that might change our lives. Or we get caught up in a maze of details, worrying about exactly what potency of a homeopathic remedy we should take, for example, rather than learning about why we should consider taking any homeopathic remedy in the first place.

Or, perhaps worst of all, we judge the message by the messenger. If the physician cannot heal himself, then it must be true that his healing philosophy cannot heal anyone. We do not consider it possible that a less-than-brilliant physician could have a brilliant philosophy, or that the reasons why a person is not healed have nothing to do with the physician.

This attitude is certainly nothing new. Because God chose to send Moses, a stutterer, to tell Pharaoh to let the tribes of Israel go, it was easy to ignore his message. It took a few miracles before Pharaoh would pay attention.

We have to learn to test the messages we receive, not by how they are presented or by how the presenter looks or sounds, but by how they live in our own hearts. It is not enough to judge the message by the life of the messenger. Although it certainly sounds hypocritical to say, "Do as I say, not as I do," that doesn't mean that the do-as-I-say message isn't valid. Certainly if I prove as an individual messenger to be unable to lift two hundred pounds above my head, it does not mean that it is not humanly possible to lift that weight.

Remember, if the ancient messenger stumbled on his long run, it did not make his message any less important to the commanding officer.

HOMEOPATHY IN CONTEXT

Homeopathy as a science was developed by Samuel Hahnemann in the years following his 1789 breakthrough on the subject of healing. But its principles have been explored throughout the very history of medicine and healing. This is an important concept: The principles of the method of healing that became known as homeopathy are as ancient as any other concept of healing. They are a part of a philosophy of wholeness and of working with symptoms instead of suppressing them.

Therefore, if the first caveman who put a leaf on an itch "discovered" allopathy by suppressing a symptom, then the first caveman who said "leave that alone" when someone tried to put that same leaf on his rash "discovered" homeopathy. In coining the word, Samuel Hahnemann lays claim to the formalized concepts of homeopathy, but he no more invented them than Columbus invented America. He merely was the first to recognize that the principles that he would name homeopathy represented a coherent practice of medicine.

When we study the history of homeopathy, especially in the days before Hahnemann, we are studying a thread, an idea, as it winds its way through the lives of individuals. The practice of homeopathy was to these men and women the same spark of inspiration that it was for Hahnemann. It was for some the logical outgrowth of the study of nature. For others it was the irrational and illogical product of intuition. Either way, for centuries homeopathy was like footprints on a beach. The paths laid down by the early practitioners of homeopathy were washed out of human history, often because their work predated written history.

In this section, I consider the lives of some of those who shaped homeopathic philosophy over the centuries. Like any true healing philosophy, homeopathy is a message that is bigger than its messengers, and it is a message that has been brought to humanity again and again over thousands of years. The people who brought this message were no less flawed or, in some cases, bizarre than other people; they were just willing to speak their message.

For some, the bringing of the message meant fame and fortune. For others it led to a lifetime of poverty and discord. Because, like politics and religion, healing philosophies have the power to separate lovers, destroy families, and influence cultures. No other core philosophy so reveals the truth of a culture than what that culture does with its sick and dying.

HIPPOCRATES: HEALER AS DEMIGOD

The Greek physician Hippocrates (460–370 B.C.) was the first to voice the possibility that similars may cure, although he also explored the possibility that contraries cured. He wrote, "That which produces strangury cures strangury" and "by similars the sickness develops and by the employment of the similar, the sickness is cured."

While it is possible for us to grasp the meaning of Hippocrates' words, it is nearly impossible for us to understand the importance of his work to early culture. For thousands of years, our ancestors believed that illness was just another of life's experiences. A person became ill and either got better or died. It was a great leap of belief and understanding that first allowed our ancestors to try and intervene, to try putting that leaf on a rash to see if they could change the circumstances of the illness. This placed people in a role that had formerly been filled by God.

In this role, Hippocrates had an advantage. He was the son of Heraclides, himself a noted physician. And the bloodline of Heraclides and Hippocrates was believed to be traced back to Asclepius, the god of medicine. Therefore, the man who would become the father of medicine was almost a demigod in the eyes of his patients, a patriarchal figure in whose veins flowed the diluted ichor of the gods.

In his early years, Hippocrates, having mastered the healing arts taught him by his father, traveled throughout the region of his birth, teaching, speaking, and practicing medicine. He is said to have brought about nearly miraculous cures, becoming one of the most powerful and influential physicians of his day. In fact, Hippocrates would become one of the most wealthy and powerful men in the world, establishing early on that a skilled physician can and should be able to earn any and all money that his skills allow. Given the belief of his family history and the cures that were attributed to him, it would be hard to find a comparison to Hippocrates in terms of wealth and influence in today's culture without venturing into the realms of rock music or pro basketball.

Hippocrates was also very much a man of his times. It is important to note that his contemporaries included Sophocles, Aristotle, Euripides, and Plato, whose writings give us much of the information we have on the life of Hippocrates. As these others were, each in his own craft, exploring the nature of life and the rules by which creation evolves, so too was Hippocrates making his own inquiries into nature and forming his own conclusions.

The island of Cos, Hippocrates' birthplace off the western coast of Asia Minor, became the center of the Hippocratic school of medicine, one that was much copied in its day and one whose traditions live on today in the words of the Hippocratic oath, if not in the hearts and minds of modern medical practitioners. It might be said that Hippocrates invented the modern health spa on Cos. The sick, who were used to having their doctors make house calls, much as we Americans were in the 1950s, were invited to come to the island to recover their health. In what would become known as the Asclepian School of Medicine, the sick were removed from their daily lives in order that they might receive some insight into their lives. It was central to the philosophy of the medical academy that the sick must receive some insight, some revelation in order to become well.

Treatments certainly included diet and exercise, but one was also as likely to be given the prescription of seeing "two tragedies and a comedy" as to receive a bitter herb. The Greeks were great believers in epiphany, releasing the emotions by witnessing the lives of others. Another way to look at this is that for Hippocrates and his followers, a great part of healing was in helping the patient to overcome self, to allow and encourage that patient to consider others ahead of considering self. By coming to care for the other more than the self, even for an instant, and even in as artificial a setting as a theater, the patient could experience an emotional release. This release, joined with some new understanding of self from the vantage point of the other person's mind and heart and experiences, might then result in a healing moment for the self.

Dreams were also highly important at that health spa on Cos. They were much considered and discussed, as it was believed that the gods often gave us their most important messages while we were deep asleep. And it was not until the patients had had their insights, their dreams from the gods, that they left Cos. Not until they felt ready to leave the care of the priests, doctors, and artists, all of whom worked hand in hand on that sunny Aegean island to restore health and restore spirit, did the patients take up their lives as they had left them and transform them into platforms for health and change.

Hippocrates saw disease as an event not only in the life of the individual but also in the life of the society and the planet. Often he felt that the healing of the individual also involved the healing of the environment in which he lived. Hippocrates' healing process often involved a great deal of doing on the part of the patient working to reestablish a healthy connection to society and to the planet, and working to carve out a healthy life in that society and on that planet. This made the patient a partner in his own care, empowering him to make the changes necessary for the health of himself, his society, and his planet. Nobody got off without responsibility in this healing process. Nobody got to be the victim in the disease.

Hippocrates refused to look at a specific disease or name it by its chief symptom or symptoms. Instead, he looked at the person, his life, his surroundings, and harmonized all. This was a medicine of balance and of wholeness. And it was this emphasis on wholeness, and the allowance of uniquity, in that each and every patient sought his own unique insight from the gods and his own unique cure, that brought Hippocrates such success as a physician. Therefore, Hippocrates, while he may or may not truly be the father of medicine, surely is the father of holistic health.

Hippocrates believed that nature holds first and foremost with a principle he called *stability*: All things in nature seek in every moment of creation to be in balance with all other things in nature. This is true on a universal level, on a global level, and on a personal level. If all things are in balance, Hippocrates would say, then all things are in a state of health. It is only when the stability is disturbed, when a state of excess or deficiency develops, that illness begins. And it is the physician's goal and task to restore stability to the system and balance to all things.

For the ancient Greeks this balance was essential to health. Their physicians held the belief that the human system, if healthy, was a balance of four humors: blood, yellow bile, black bile, and phlegm. A predisposition toward an excess of any one of these humors led a person to be susceptible to the illnesses associated with that humor. Further, this excess, in a chronic state, would color the patient's own personality with the humor's own disposition. Thus, even today we use the words *sanguine* and *phlegmatic* to describe people's personalities.

The tool that Hippocrates and his followers used in the restoration of balance was something they called "innate heat" (what homeopaths know as vital force). It was the innate heat that kept balance and order among

44

the humors, that kept the body in a state of health. It was by working with this invisible energy system of innate heat that the physician could restore and promote continued health.

Further, Hippocrates was the first to sit down and consider what practitioners and patients could do in treating the symptoms of disease. He reasoned that you could do only three things with a pain: drive it in to the system by suppressing it, drive it out of the body by expressing it, or leave it alone and see what happens. Since humanity had already given the third method a few thousand years of trial, and it hadn't worked sufficiently well, he looked into the other two methods.

These were, he believed, two streams of healing that flowed side by side in opposite directions. At no point in their flow did they touch or relate to each other. The one, homeopathy, worked with the symptoms, seeking to understand their message and, in doing so, bring them out of the body, expressing them out of the human system. The other, allopathy, worked against the symptoms, palliating the pain and driving its cause deeper into the human system.

In his life and his work, Hippocrates seems to have selected expression as the method by which healing can and will take place. For him, as for us, this expression also involved the "aha!" insight into self that allows us to let go not only of our illness but also of our ego. It was because of Hippocrates' work, and because he and his followers kept logical and concise records, teaching their methods to succeeding generations through case studies and clinical lectures, that Hahnemann would one day be able to take this philosophy to the next level.

CELSUS: HEALER AS REBEL

Aulus Cornelius Celsus (25 B.C.–A.D. 50) was a Roman patrician who defied the cultural codes of his day by becoming a physician. At that time, physicians were considered servants on the level of barbers, and no patrician considered such work. But Celsus held firm that he would work in the healing arts and would elevate them to a higher level within the Roman culture.

He is the father of plastic surgery and became respected for repairing lips and ears, and for creating the world-famous Roman noses. His contribution to the concepts of homeopathy had to do with his own belief concerning the symptoms of illness. It was Celsus who first believed that these symptoms could actually be a sign that the immune system was functioning and that the body was trying to cure itself. He worked specifically with fevers, believing them to be the body's method of burning toxins from the system. He said, "Give me a drug that will produce a fever and I'll cure every illness." He further noted that a drug that could cause a fever in a well person could cure one in a sick patient.

Celsus's literary output was encyclopedic and greatly advanced for his time. He was among the first, with the Roman physician Galen, to favor the dissection of cadavers for the sake of increased medical knowledge, and he presented clear, thorough anatomical descriptions in his writings. He is best known for his descriptions of illness, and his description of malarial fevers is yet to be surpassed.

But he is most important to us for his view of symptoms as a sign of a functioning immune system seeking to balance the overall system, and for his excellent writing on that view, particularly in his work with fevers of all sorts. His writings, like Hippocrates' before him, would enlighten the work of Hahnemann and others in the centuries to come.

DIOSCORIDES: HEALER AS NATURALIST

Pedanius Dioscorides (first century A.D.), both a naturalist and a physician, traveled extensively with the Roman army. In fact, it is said that he joined the Roman legion in order to be able to travel throughout the known world, so great was his desire to learn about healing plants.

In his travels, Dioscorides gathered information on six hundred different plants that were used medicinally by the many different types of healers he met along his way. When his travels ended, he gathered the information together and published his De Materia Medica, which was used throughout the Arab, Greek, and Latin worlds for 1,600 years. This was the first gathering of information on the "materials of medicine," and it laid the basis for the practice of herbal medicine.

He is considered the father of botanical science. Many of the names he gave to plants are still used today. His concise descriptions of the plants, often including habitat and distribution, were very accurate. The herbal remedies he wrote about formed the basis of herbal medicine as it is still practiced today. These herbal remedies would also become the basis of homeopathy; Hahnemann created his remedies from the existing herbal pharmacy that was available to him in his day-to-day practice.

Dioscorides believed that as God allowed the creation of illness, so too did God create healing power within all living things. He wrote, "Where disease is, there is the remedy also."

GALEN: HEALER AS WARRIOR

By all accounts, Galen (A.D. 129–199) was a difficult man. Although he was among the most brilliant men of his day, he was no one you wanted to have angry with you, and it was all too easy to get him angry.

Galen, a Greek physician, developed his own system of medicine based on the theory *"contraria contrariis curentur,"* or contrary cures contrary. In doing so, he established the methods of practice that would become known as allopathic, the form of practice most popular in the Western world today.

His system of healing, like that of the Greeks before it, divided the human body into four humors: blood, phlegm, yellow bile, and black bile. When the humors were balanced, health resulted. When they were thrown off balance, illness resulted. These four humors also represented the human traits of wet, dry, hot, and cold and their constitutional natures as sanguine, phlegmatic, choleric, and melancholic. At the heart of Galen's treatment was the premise that if you had been thrown into a wet state, you could be cured only by the use of a dry substance. This system is practiced today; when we have seasonal allergies and our nose is running and our eyes tearing, we take a substance that will dry up our eyes and nose.

Galen held powerful influence over his fellow physicians, and soon they began to see symptoms as something to work against, always giving substances that caused an opposite reaction within the system to the circumstances that already existed. Therefore, while Galen adapted the concept of the humors from the Greeks, he stressed the concepts of deficiency and excess in his medicine, to the point that they overwhelmed the core concept of balance.

To his credit, Galen worked from the basic premise that only by understanding how the body works, and how disease itself behaves as a mechanism, can a practitioner work to restore that body to health. Unfortunately, by being so very true to this core philosophy, Galen created a system of medicine that can do much harm.

Galen turned the world away from Hippocrates' holistic methods. He insisted that the physician must treat only the disease, never the whole being, and treat the disease as a hostile invader. In his quest for knowledge, he was among the first physicians to insist on dissection as the only method by which the practitioner could come to understand how the body was made, how it worked, how it got sick, and how it could be restored to health. It is important to note that all early dissections were performed on animals, with the hope that their structure was close to that of humans.

In moving medicine in this direction, Galen developed the philosophy of the body as a "meat machine" whose parts could be taken out and fixed, replaced at a later time, or exchanged for a better part in the future. In this way, the idea of piecework came into medicine, and conditions were treated, never persons.

Gone is the notion of balance and of the healing process of the individual and his environment. In its place is a militaristic notion of physician as warrior, standing as sort of a thin red line between humanity and death by disease.

Certainly Galenic medicine is to be congratulated in its desire to understand the structure of the body, its anatomy and physiology—the function of its parts. But this process of discovery transformed medicine from a science of *experience*, which stressed the universal principles of healing above and beyond the transitory principles of process and treatments, into a science of *experimentation*, which sees nothing in the way of unchanging principles, which focuses on the notion that illness can be stamped out like communism, and which stresses momentary cure over permanent healing.

PARACELSUS: HEALER AS MADMAN

Perhaps no figure in the history of healing is as controversial as Paracelsus. He alone stands as a figure of such genius that he could have saved an entire village from the ravages of the plague, yet he was so obnoxious that he could have been driven from that town within days of his miracle.

Paracelsus was born in 1493 in Einsieden, Switzerland. He died in 1541. This used to trouble me. It was part of my teaching that the ancients, contrary to our ignorant assumptions, lived a good long time. Hippocrates lived for more than seventy years, as did many others. The combination of sunshine, temperate climate, and clean water allowed for a good long life. It was not until people moved into the cities, with their poverty and filth, that diseases became rampant and life spans were shortened.

So, with all the happy and holistic ancients living into old age, how is it that Paracelsus failed to make it to fifty? Well, here the stories differ slightly: Some say that he was the victim of a murder plot and was thrown to his death from a window; others say that he died in a barroom brawl. Either story could be true, given the life he led and the enemies he made.

He was christened Philippus Theophrastus Bombastus von Hohenheim. The name he assumed, Paracelsus, refers to the great Roman physician Celsus and translates as "above Celsus" or "superior to Celsus."

A friend of his, Dr. Conrad Gesner, wrote that Paracelsus "certainly was an impious man, and a sorcerer. He had intercourse with demons. . . . His disciples practice wicked astrology, divination, and other forbidden arts. I suspect that they are survivors of the Celtic Druids who received instructions from their demons. . . . This school is responsible for the so-called vagrant scholars, one of whom, Dr. Faustus, died only recently."

Indeed, as a man whose nature contained both ancient mysticism and modern science, Paracelsus's life became legend, and legend intertwined with that of the aforementioned Dr. Faustus. Paracelsus seemed so much the embodiment of the man who surrenders his very soul to the devil in exchange for knowledge of the nature of all things that Goethe's *Faust* seems a retelling of Paracelsus's life.

Early Works and Training

Paracelsus was also compared to another legendary individual, Martin Luther. He was called "the Luther of Medicine." This was both an insult and a compliment. As Luther had hammered his theses to a church door, Paracelsus had publicly burned a textbook, *The Cannon of Avicenna*, declaring war against his fellow doctors. He announced, "The patients are your textbook, the sickbed is your study."

In fact, Paracelsus's own study of medicine was unique. He received his first education from his father, who, like Hippocrates' father, had been a physician of some note, and then he went on to earn his medical diploma from the University of Vienna. At that time, the medical program at the University of Vienna included the Four Higher Arts: arithmetic, geometry, music, and astrology. Astrology was particularly stressed, because it was believed that by casting the chart of a patient, the physician could best create potential treatments. It was understood that the human body and its many parts were ruled by the planets. Paracelsus rebelled against this notion, writing that "human wisdom is so great that it has made the stars, the firmament, and the zodiac subject to man. . . . The sky must obey him like a little dog."

Still, he somehow managed to receive his diploma. But on graduation in 1510, Paracelsus felt that the university had ill prepared him for work as a healer. So he traveled the known world, throughout Europe and the Middle East, to Egypt, Arabia, the Holy Land, to Transylvania, Croatia, and Hungary, learning from the barbers, midwives, and herbalists who were the healers of the common men and women. Paracelsus later wrote, "Everywhere I sought certain and experienced knowledge of the art. I did not seek it from the learned doctors alone; I also asked the shearers, barbers, wise men and women, exorcizers, alchemists, monks, the noble and the humble, the smart and the dumb."

He added this folk knowledge to all that he had already learned and came to a conclusion: The ancient healers had been correct in their assumption that "like cured like," and, above all else, Galenic medicine must be overturned. Paracelsus noted that folk doctors had for centuries worked by the creed, "The iron that made the wound also will heal it." The heart of this creed noted that any poison, given in small doses, acts as an antidote. Paracelsus wrote, "Poison is everything and no thing is without poison. The dosage makes it either a poison or a remedy." This concept both mirrors and predates Hahnemann's Law of Similars, that like cures like.

Alchemy and Chemistry

While the concept of similars may be the great link between Paracelsus and Hahnemann, surely it was the fact that Paracelsus was both chemist and alchemist that caused the great rift between their philosophies. Hahnemann felt that Paracelsus's arcane experiments and general behavior were a source of embarrassment for all healers. Paracelsus was the bridge between the ancient art of alchemy and the modern science of chemistry. At first, like other alchemists, he sought to transform lead into gold. But as he became more interested in the nature of creation, he became more a chemist. Paracelsus came to believe that perfection could be expressed in two ways: by transforming crude substances into their essences (alchemy) and by transforming essences into complex substances (chemistry). Paracelsus used cooking and baking as examples of complexities yielding greater results. As he continued his work, he became even more the chemist, specifically interested in the creation of chemical medicines. He wrote, "Medicines were created by God. But he did not prepare them completely. They are hidden in the slag. It is a matter of removing the slag from the medicine."

To the alchemists of his day, he instructed, "Don't make gold, make medicines." And the seven healing arcana of the ancient world—iron, salt-peter, ammonia of sulphur, sodium bicarbonate, sulfuric acid, red and black antimony—became the basis of many medicines he used. To these he added—sulphur, calomel, blue vitriol, and compounds of zinc, arsenic, and lead. All of these would, in due time, become the basis for potent homeopathic remedies.

The Five Diseases

As Paracelsus practiced and developed his art as both a chemist and an alchemist, he codified his findings in a number of books. In all of these writings, he sought to overturn the Galenic model of medicine. In order to do so, Paracelsus turned his attention to nature. In the course of his study, he finally had to admit that, while he still might privately wish the stars to follow our orders like little sparkling dogs in the sky, in reality humankind is powerless to resist the immutable laws of nature.

With a desire to work with nature, Paracelsus developed the theory of the Five Diseases, which illustrates how he believed a person becomes ill.

1. *Ens Astri:* Diseases caused by the influences of the stars and weather. The stars here were meteorological components only. Diseases of this type include such conditions as rheumatic pains that were exacerbated by changes in weather.

2. *Ens Veneni:* Diseases caused by poisonings of all sorts; disturbances of the metabolism.

3. *Ens Naturale:* Inherited conditions that arose from the patient's basic constitution.

4. *Ens Spirituale:* Diseases of the mind, of any or all of the invisible, intangible parts of our nature.

5. *Ens Dei:* Diseases sent by God. Paracelsus felt that, like Job, any of us could be tested by God in the form of disease. This category of disease could be treated only by prayer and could be healed only by God. It was otherwise incurable.

Paracelsus felt that there were also five types of doctors, five types of treatment available, and five viewpoints in the treatment of disease.

1. *Naturales:* Physicians who treated contraries with contraries. Paracelsus acknowledged that this was indeed a form of treatment, but just barely. The *naturales* were the lowest level of physician.

2. *Specifici:* Herbal practitioners who approached disease empirically, who used their own experience and experimentation in treatment. Often self-taught, these were the practitioners of folk medicine.

3. *Characterales:* The wise men and magicians who followed the principle of like cures like, using the seeming magic of similarity in their treatments. In this category Paracelsus also placed all who used the occult in their treatments.

4. *Spirituales:* Those who had passed through the level of alchemist to become chemists, who used chemical drugs in the treatment of mental diseases.

5. The final group had no name, or at least no name that Paracelsus would speak aloud. They were those who called upon the power of "Christ and Apostles for their treatments of disease." Paracelsus thought these faith healers were the highest level of healer.

Oporinus

During 1527 and 1528, Paracelsus was at the height of his career. His fame had spread throughout the known world. He taught, treated patients, wrote, created pharmacies of medicines, and went through one secretary after another.

At this time a young man named Oporinus came to work for Paracelsus. He did not last long in Paraclesus's employment, but he gathered together enough stories to last him a lifetime of dinner parties.

Oporinus wrote to a friend: "As to Paracelsus, he has been dead for a long time and I should hate to speak against the spirit of his death. . . . While he was living, I knew him so well that I should not desire again to live with such a man. Apart from his miraculous and fortunate cures in all kind of sickness, I have noticed in him neither scholarship nor piety of any kind. It makes me wonder to see all the publications, they say were written by him or left by him but which I would not have dreamt ascribing to him. The two years I passed in his company he spent in drinking and gluttony, day and night. . . . All night, as long as I stayed with him, he never undressed, which I attributed to his drunkenness. Often he would come home tipsy, after midnight, throw himself on his bed in his clothes wearing his sword which he said he had obtained from a hangman. He had hardly time to fall asleep when he rose, drew his sword like a madman, and threw it on the ground or against the wall, so that sometimes I was afraid he would kill me."

Surprisingly, however, the fact that Paracelsus was never without his six-foot-long sword, in whose hollow handle he kept his "elixir of life," the laudanum to which he was addicted, was not the reason that Oporinus left Paracelsus's employ. As part of his job description Oporinus had to allow Paracelsus to test his new alchemical potions on him, and he found this particularly trying: "Once, he nearly killed me. He told me to look at the spirit in his alembic and pushed my nose close to it so that the smoke came into my mouth and nose. I fainted from the virulent vapor."

Soon after, Oporinus found a better job.

It is through the letters of Oporinus that we get our best glimpse into the life of Paracelsus. Certainly only here do we get a picture of his sex life: "He did not care for women and I believe that he never had doings with any. In the beginning he was very modest, so that up to his twenty-fifth year, I believe he never touched wine. Later on he learned how to drink and even challenged an inn full of peasants to drink with him and drank them under the table, now and then putting his finger in his mouth like swine."

Like many of the other details of his life, there has always been some question as to Paracelsus's lack of interest in women. Allegedly, Paracelsus was a eunuch. Here again the tales surrounding the condition differ. One tale blames a drunken band of Greek sailors, another credits an angry bull.

Whatever the truth, it does seem to be a fact that Paracelsus lived and died a virgin. Even those who called him any number of names never added lecher to their lists. In fact, he advocated chastity and, perhaps speaking from direct experience, announced often that it was better to be a castrate than an adulterer.

Nuremberg

In the early sixteenth century, syphilis was a deadly disease. While astrologers believed that it was a peculiar conjunction of three planets in 1494 that had created this new disease, it was also thought that perhaps the Spanish sailors who had traveled to the New World had brought the disease back to the Old.

Syphilis was merciless. It caused painful and disfiguring ulcers, in some cases so great that it seemed that the flesh was being eaten away. For this reason, some felt that this new disease was not new at all but was the reemergence of the biblical plague of leprosy. Because the disease seemed linked to sexual behavior, although that had not yet been proved, it took on even more power and was seen by many as the wrath of God. The pope called syphilis "The French Disease."

At this time, Paracelsus rode into Nuremberg. The doctors of the town sought a way to shut the man up and close down his practice. So they challenged him to a debate. But he refused the debate in favor of a greater challenge. He suggested that they bring someone incurable to him, someone with syphilis.

The doctors upped the ante and brought not one but fifteen persons who suffered from syphilis. They gave Paracelsus a prison hospital in which to work, with a full staff at his disposal. Then they sat back and waited.

Just what Paracelsus did in the way of treatment remains unknown. What is known is that he cured nine of the fifteen patients.

Instead of aiding Paracelsus in his cause of overturning the Galenic school of medicine, his work in Nuremberg turned the traditional practitioners against him, branding him a pariah, a warlock, and a madman. The year of this miraculous effort, 1529, marked the height of Paracelsus's influence and the beginning of his decline.

Sterzing

Paracelsus had had a brilliant career, but he had also alienated many powerful politicians and physicians throughout Europe. And suddenly, in 1532, it seemed as if a curse had landed upon him. After a lifetime of miraculous cures, the cures all suddenly seemed to fail and his patients died. With these sudden failures, his opponents at last had the clout to drive him from their lands. Unable to practice, Paracelsus wandered throughout Switzerland and Germany. Poverty-stricken, he said, "I do not know where to wander now. I do not care, either, as long as I help the sick."

He was asked to help the sick in Sterzing. His friend Kerner begged him to help this town that was literally dying of the plague. The plague was, of course, a deadly disease. It traveled quickly throughout Europe, killing off whole communities. Paracelsus saw this outbreak as an opportunity to do good, to heal the sick. Working with the principle of like cures like, Paracelsus created a remedy for plague from the excrement of those who were already sick and dying. Using the principle of dilution, he removed the toxic nature of the substance and enhanced the curative powers. With this remedy, he saved the village of Sterzing.

Once the citizens were saved, however, Paracelsus is said to have celebrated his victory with three days of drinking and a good deal of property damage, after which he was driven out of town.

Conclusion

Paracelsus died at age forty-eight. He had created for himself an image unlike that of any other healer in history. He left behind several books on the philosophy of healing, most notably his 1535 work, *The Great Surgery Book*, in which he quotes the words of Hippocrates: "A physician who thinks that he heals does not understand the art. You may understand for what purpose there is a physician. He provides the shield for nature and protects the injured part against its enemies, so that the force without may not retard, poison, or injure the forces of nature, but may preserve its vital power. He who takes good care of wounds is a good surgeon."

Paracelsus was the first to recognize the vital force within all living things as the source of all healing. As a visionary, he foresaw such inventions as the steamboat, the telegraph, radar, and the atomic bomb. In his lifetime, Paracelsus also worked with healing as an esoteric art and as a science. The color of food substances and healing herbs was of great import to him; he believed in the healing potential of colors. It was this work, along with his general image as a mystic as opposed to a scientist, that infuriated Hahnemann as much as Paracelsus's work in similars interested him. Hahnemann would insist that the work of Paracelsus in no way influenced him. However, Hahnemann did translate the works of Paracelsus and could not have helped but notice the ramifications of his theory of similars.

SAMUEL HAHNEMANN: HEALER AS REVOLUTIONARY

Christian Samuel Hahnemann was born on April 10, 1755, in Meissen, Germany. He was the son of an artist and was raised in the strict Lutheran church. It was the dream of his mother that her son become a doctor. While he showed some interest in pleasing his beloved parent, his earliest notable talent was for learning foreign languages, particularly Latin and Greek.

Like Paracelsus before him, Hahnemann attended the University of Vienna. There he found a mentor, Dr. Quarin, who in turn introduced Hahnemann to Baron Samuel von Brukenthal, governor of Transylvania. The baron, who was wealthy beyond anything Hahnemann had ever dreamed of, offered the young man a job in his family home in Hermannstadt. There

Hahnemann would be family physician and librarian. He would organize the baron's countless books and his prize coin collection. Hahnemann took the job and for two years organized the books and coins, did simple doctoring, and, most important, learned languages. Through the baron's books, Hahnemann became fluent in German, Latin, Greek, English, French, and Spanish. His job done, and everything shipshape, he returned to college to complete his degree.

Hahnemann was awarded a Doctor of Medicine degree in 1779, and became a practicing physician in Hettstedt, a copper-mining town at the foot of the Hartz Mountains. He stayed there only nine months, having noted to a friend that "It was impossible to develop either mentally or physically." He left for the larger town of Dessau in 1781.

By all accounts, Samuel Hahnemann was a passionate man, serious-minded, sensitive, and brave, with an unusually erect posture. But, he was slight of build, pasty pale, and already balding. However, Johanna Leopoldine Henriette Kuchler, the daughter of a pharmacist, saw only his good points when he courted her, and she agreed to marry him as soon as he asked. They married in 1782.

Both families were thrilled with this marriage, which seemed as good a business deal as it was a love match. With Hahnemann treating his patients, and his father-in-law making the medicines, it seemed a medical dynasty in the making. But it was not to be.

It was the traditional medicine of the day, bloodletting and leeching in particular, that first began to repulse Hahnemann. Hahnemann believed, quite correctly, that patients died more often from their treatments than from their diseases. He continued to practice medicine in order to support his large family, but he became more and more concerned with medicine as it was then practiced.

The Wilderness Years

Hahnemann published texts and spoke openly in defiance of the medical model of his day. His stand made it increasingly difficult for him to practice medicine and for his family to live in a given village. Hahnemann was beginning to develop a reputation not only as a troublemaker but also as a dangerous quack. The family was often forced to flee in the dead of night.

Hahnemann turned to translating medical texts as an alternative source of income, his gift for languages enabling him to translate both classical and modern works into all the major European languages. It was through these translations that Hahnemann came to study the earlier texts that presented the principle of similars. By 1789, Hahnemann had been away from the practice of medicine for one full year, making a good living from translations and writing. He decided to seek a spot in which he could spend the rest of his life in quiet study and translation.

At this moment, Hahnemann laid his hand upon the future. It came to him in the form of yet another book that he had been hired to translate into German. The book was *A Treatise on Materia Medica* by Scottish physician William Cullen. In its pages, Hahnemann found an account of the drug Chinchona, which was taken from the bark of a tree and was being used to treat the disease then called intermittent fever and now called malaria. It had been discovered that natives of Peru, who chewed the bark like gum, were immune to the disease. Taken with the account, Hahnemann acquired some Chinchona and tried an experiment on himself. Each day for several days he took a high dose of the drug, although he was in perfect health. In a matter of time, he began to experience heart palpitations, quickened pulse, coldness of the extremities, and redness of cheeks—all symptoms of intermittent fever. The symptoms lasted only a few hours but reappeared with each new dose. Hahnemann kept notes on his experiment: "Chinchona bark, which is used as a remedy for intermittent fever, acts because it can produce symptoms similar to those of intermittent fever in healthy people."

Bingo. With this sentence, homeopathy was born. Hahnemann had uncovered the Law of Similars.

In the Hollywood version of the Hahnemann story, we would see pages flying off calendars superimposed over Hahnemann's stern face. And almost instantaneously, he would be seen practicing his new form of medicine, under a wooden sign bearing the painted word *homeopathy*.

In fact, Hahnemann did not realize the full implications of his discovery. Although he continued to ponder what he had seen, he returned to translating and wrangling with traditional medicine for six years before coining the phrase *"simila similibus curentur."* Like cures like.

Throughout these years, Hahnemann wrestled with two other principles that would be central to his homeopathic art.

The first came to him simply enough. Because he greatly feared the toxicity of the drugs available in the medical pharmacy of his day, one based in the ancient herbal materia medica, Hahnemann began to dilute his medicines. And, as he made them more and more dilute, he noticed something mysterious: As a substance became more and more dilute, it seemed at the same time to become less and less toxic and more and more powerful as a healing agent.

Hahnemann worked with two different scales of dilution. The first was the X scale, taken from the Roman numeral for 10. This method involved taking one part substance and diluting it with nine parts water to achieve the level of 1X. One portion of this mixed with nine parts water created 2X. The other scale was the C scale, for the Roman numeral for 100. Here the dilution was one part substance to ninety-nine parts water.

As Hahnemann practiced his craft, he had a second insight. Day after day, as he traveled in his rickety cart loaded with his diluted medicines, he noticed that the person who received treatment at the end of the day seemed to get much more powerful results than the person who was treated earliest. He began to work with the idea that the shaking that each remedy received in that cart somehow increased the power of the remedy.

Hahnemann came to call the process by which a remedy was created *potentization*. This two-step process involved both *dilution* and *succussion*, which was his new term for the shaking that the remedies now received as a matter of form. Hahnemann took the vial of liquid remedy, shook it with two strong twists of the wrist, and then slammed his wrist down on a leatherbound Bible. No other method that he tried yielded results as satisfying.

With his process of potentization and his Law of Similars, Hahnemann was developing, step by step, trial by trial, a new way not only of treating disease but of looking at the very nature of illness.

Because of his temperament and his new discovery, Hahnemann's popularity decreased. Hahnemann and his family were continually uprooted and thrown out of each town in which they settled. Over the next thirteen years, they moved seventeen times. On one of these moves, tragedy struck. As the family fled in their rickety cart, Joanna held her younger son, Ernst, in her arms. The cart struck a rock in the road, overturned, and Joanna fell onto Ernst as she tried to protect him. Ernst's neck was broken, and he died.

During these years in the wilderness, Hahnemann's faith in himself, in his new discoveries, and in God was tested again and again. He was a stern and distant man, particularly with his remaining son, Friedrich. I believe that it was his own feeling of failure, his inability to provide for his family as he wanted to, that colored his ability to reach out to his children and to embrace them lovingly. Surely Hahnemann's dedication to medicine and to his discoveries cost him dearly in his own marriage, as Joanna was forced to divide her loyalties between a husband who followed his own vision, no matter the cost, and her children, who needed, wanted, and deserved a loving and secure environment, no matter their father's peculiar muse.

Duke Leopold

As it would time and time again, fate intervened to keep Hahnemann in his practice of medicine. His brilliance as a physician could not be denied, even when he began to work actively toward the creation of a new medical model. In 1792, the ailing Duke Leopold II of Austria sent for Hahnemann for treatment. After working with Hahnemann and his new, diluted medicines, Leopold improved so greatly that Hahnemann returned home. However, after Hahnemann left his side, Leopold, following the advice of his other physicians, began to mix the homeopathics with allopathic medicines. He soon died.

In a fury, Hahnemann returned for the funeral of the man he considered not only a supporter but also a friend. He followed the casket as it was pulled through the streets. As his anger and grief increased, Hahnemann began to shout out curses, denouncing those who he believed had killed the duke as surely as if they had cut his throat. After the funeral, he began actively to write pamphlets denouncing allopathic medicine.

This outburst only further alienated Hahnemann from his fellow doctors, creating more friction in the medical community and making the mainstream physicians (whom Hahnemann would himself one day name "allopaths") even less willing to consider Hahnemann's new point of view.

Herr Klockenbring

It was in the summer of 1792, when Hahnemann was thirty-seven years old, that he received the case that would finally bring him positive attention. He was given charge of a nursing home for mental patients established by Duke Ernst, a German nobleman. The asylum had only one patient, Friedrich Klockenbring, minister of police and secretary to the chancellor of Hanover. Klockenbring was in a state of violent insanity and was chained in one wing of the duke's palace. Hahnemann was offered the rest of the palace for himself and his family, as well as a full staff, if he would, in essence, baby-sit the duke's crazed brother-in-law, Herr Klockenbring.

Hahnemann took his role as healer seriously. He accepted the position and moved his family to the duke's estate with the idea of actually helping Herr Klockenbring. His first action was to remove the chains from Klockenbring and give him the freedom of the estate.

The staff must have wondered who was crazier, Klockenbring or Hah-

59

nemann. Hahnemann is said to have followed his patient for a period of weeks, without speaking, only watching. If Klockenbring climbed a tree, Hahnemann climbed with him, watching, trying to form a diagnosis from which he could treat the man. Then he began talking to Klockenbring and listening to his answers.

At last Hahnemann reached his decision as to which of his remedies would help Klockenbring. He gave a single dose of the remedy Antimonium Tartarticum, made from the metal antimony. Within six months, Klockenbring had recovered sufficiently to reenter the world. But although Duke Ernst was impressed with Hahnemann's skill, he felt that perhaps Klockenbring should not return to his high-stress job of head of the German police, and instead gave him the position of head of the German lottery.

By curing his only patient, Hahnemann was now out of a job. The family was forced to leave the only comfortable home they'd ever known. But Hahnemann had brought about a cure (deemed impossible in his day) and had begun to build a reputation. After all, every noble family of the day was bound to have at least one member chained up somewhere, giving Hahnemann an almost endless supply of patients.

As he built his practice, Hahnemann continued to explore the Law of Similars. And 1796 may be said to be the year in which homeopathy truly began, for it was in this year that he coined the word *homeopathy* to describe the techniques he was already using.

Jenner and Vaccinations

This was also the year in which a British doctor, Edward Jenner, made another medical breakthrough by injecting a young girl with cowpox and demonstrating the principle of vaccination.

Hahnemann realized that although the idea of vaccination seemed to follow logically the principle of similars, it was a dangerous course because it involved introducing matter derived from disease into the human body. Hahnemann developed methods by which toxic substances, with the toxicity removed, could be used to combat disease. In his writings, Hahnemann states that the use of vaccines had also occurred to him, but he was suspicious of using living organisms in the human body and worried that, like so many other medicines, vaccines might prove to be worse that the diseases they were said to prevent.

Organon *and Materia Medica*

By 1805, having gained a reputation as a brilliant translator and a controversial practitioner, Hahnemann turned his attention to writing and began the first of the six editions of the volume that would be his magnum opus, *The Organon*. Each edition contained the theories of the one before it, along with new discoveries, as Hahnemann developed the techniques of the practice of homeopathy. Each was constructed as a series of aphorisms, short paragraphs enlightening one aspect of homeopathic theory.

In 1805, Hahnemann also began his own materia medica by writing about his first remedies: Aconite, Arnica, Belladonna, Chamomilla, Drosera, Ignatia, Ipecacuanha, Nux Vomica, and Pulsatilla. His *Materia Medica Pura*, containing sixty-six remedies and filling six volumes, would not be published in total until 1821.

Hahnemann clearly enjoyed the fact that, after so many years of struggle, he was finally respected as a practitioner and, for the first time in his adult life, prosperous enough to live without fear. He felt that he had come at last to a stopping point, that finally he could buy the house he would live in until his death, and that, surrounded by his children and grandchildren, he would live out the rest of his years in quiet solitude.

In our Hollywood version, we Fade Out on these happy moments.

Melanie

Fade Up on a stormy sunset, October 7, 1834. Years had passed and Hahnemann had grown to be an old lion of seventy-nine. His wife had died years ago. Before her death, they had found their peace together, and she died in his arms. His children were grown and scattered, except for his two daughters, who acted as his caretakers.

On the night of October 7, lightning crashed around the horizon. Rain poured from the sky. A carriage drew up to the front door of Hahnemann's cottage in Köthen, Germany.

A stranger ran from the carriage and pounded on the door of the cottage, begging to see Dr. Hahnemann. The daughters told the stranger that the doctor no longer saw patients, but the stranger pushed past them. Hahnemann came from his parlor to see the cause of the noise. The figure fell down kneeling before Hahnemann.

Having witnessed such a dramatic entrance, Hahnemann agreed to see the stranger, who removed hat and cape to reveal a beautiful young French woman. The Marquise Marie Melanie d'Hervilly had made the dangerous journey from Paris to Köthen alone to seek treatment for a chronic respiratory condition, tuberculosis. Hahnemann agreed to treat her and insisted that Melanie stay with the family during treatments.

As he treated her, the two fell in love. Although she was only thirty-one, the two were soon talking marriage. Melanie, a woman of noble title and independent means, suggested that Samuel Hahnemann give his daughters their inheritance and the cottage and return with her to Paris. There she would take him into her own home and support his continued work in homeopathy. He agreed.

His reputation preceded him, and soon there were lines of Parisians around the block waiting to see the master homeopath. But Hahnemann could not treat everyone who sought his care and still proceed with the work that interested him most: the formation of a homeopathic philosophy. While he wanted to help all those who sought it, he also wanted to work with the continuing evolution of *The Organon*.

The solution to the problem was Melanie herself. Since her own healing, Melanie had proved an adept practitioner. Her knowledge of materia medica came to rival Hahnemann's own. Soon they practiced together, with Melanie actually selecting remedies and their follow-ups.

Satisfied that all was well with his patients, Hahnemann turned his attention to his writing. He did something unusual. Although it is said that Hahnemann had a success rate of about 80 percent, he looked back at the 20 percent, asking himself what he might have done to bring about cure in those cases as well.

The answer to the question was to work deeper, to look at not only the disease but also at the whole system under the disease, including the family and the genetic pool from which the patient had come. Hahnemann wanted to find the predisposition for specific diseases that the patient had had from birth. These he would call *miasms*, and his work in this area would distinguish his last seven years of life. In these years Hahnemann also would consider the potential actions of remedies far more diluted than it was possible for him to create in his own laboratory. And he would establish a protocol for the use of these remedies.

Had Hahnemann lived another decade he would have no doubt added much to his philosophical foundation. In these Paris years, he moved from the mind-set of pragmatic scientist closer to that of mystic. His vision shifted from the visible to the invisible, almost as if he had begun to see ultraviolet.

But his life ended suddenly, in midsentence, as most do. Samuel Hahnemann died in the early morning of July 2, 1843 at the age of eighty-nine. His heart had given out, as hearts do.

The day of Hahnemann's funeral was again a stormy one: slate gray and breathlessly hot. The funeral procession was small, mourners were few. Behind the horse-drawn carriage walked Hahnemann's daughter, Amalie. She walked with her head down, singing softly to herself. With her was her son, Leopold. Behind them walked Melanie, her head held high, her jaw clenched. Behind her were servants and business associates.

The morning had started poorly. When the bearers came to remove the body, they brought a coffin up the narrow stairs to the bedroom. As they carried the body down the stairs in that coffin, one of the bearers lost his grip for a moment and the coffin nearly flew down the stairs. Melanie, certainly overwrought with the circumstances at hand, became very angry and lectured the bearers on their work responsibilities. She was worried that they would, in their carelessness, damage her banister.

Melanie's fortune had been spent supporting her husband's work, and so Hahnemann was buried like a pauper. His body was laid to rest in the Montmartre Cemetery in Paris at Public Grave #8, where the coffin was placed in an ancient trilevel vault, resting above two strangers. Not until Hahnemann's followers in the United States raised money themselves would Hahnemann receive a proper resting place.

Historians are divided as to Hahnemann's relationship with his second wife and her influence on him. It was in these last few years of life that Hahnemann began to experiment with high-potency preparations and antimiasmic cures. For some homeopaths of his day, this work was the culmination of a career of genius; for others it was the sad loss of a once-great intellect into senility. For many, Melanie was, quite simply, the Yoko Ono of homeopathy.

Hahnemann had decided, because of his poor relationship with his son Friedrich, that Melanie would be his heir. He trained her in homeopathy, and, in these final years, it was Melanie who treated the vast majority of people who daily lined up outside their door. Upon Hahnemann's death, however, when Melanie applied for a license to practice homeopathic medicine in order to support herself, the male homeopathic practitioners of the day barred her from doing so.

This created a problem not only for Melanie, who would never stop her study and sometimes secret practice of homeopathy, but also for homeopathy itself. The sexism of the day denied the world an heir to Hahenmann's work, leaving a worldwide homeopathic movement fractured and weakened.

Melanie would adopt a daughter and raise her herself. Her daughter would marry the son of a respected homeopath, and Melanie would become an adviser in her son-in-law's practice. But she would never fill the void in her life created by the death of Samuel Hahnemann.

HAHNEMANN: HEALER AS HEIR ·

Friedrich Hahnemann was born in 1786 in Dresden. As the elder son, Friedrich should have been heir to Hahnemann's work and fortune. This became particularly true after the death of Ernst, when Friedrich was the only son. However, a strained relationship haunted father and son, almost from Friedrich's birth.

Many of the problems in their relationship began when Friedrich as a child fell from a horse. Friedrich's shoulder never healed correctly, and he developed something like a hunchback from the accident. His father was unable to cure him. For Samuel, Friedrich became a visible and tangible example of the limits of homeopathy—and of his own limits as a healer.

This seems to have made Friedrich almost obsessive in his desire to earn his father's love. But the more he tried, the more his father seemed to disapprove of his son. Friedrich dutifully entered the family business, graduating from medical school in 1812 and opening a pharmacy. He followed homeopathy faithfully, perhaps hoping that this would earn his father's approval, and this practice opened him up to ridicule by the local doctors. But, unlike his father, Friedrich refused to give up practice or move away.

Friedrich married a widow with a young daughter, named Adelheid. Once more he attempted to secure a relationship with his father, believing that if he showed himself to be an adult, supporting his family and making a good living in homeopathy, surely his father would at long last give him the love he had withheld. Samuel, however, refused to bless his son's marriage, asking him why he would take on some other man's wife and child rather than find a woman of his own.

The years wore down on Friedrich. Finally, he seems to have had some sort of emotional breakdown. One day he literally disappeared without a trace. He deserted his wife and child and never returned to his home.

Like his father, Friedrich had a multitude of gifts apart from medicine, chief among them a gift for languages. Friedrich spoke Greek, Latin, French, English, Italian, and Arabic. He also played both guitar and piano.

Unlike his father, Friedrich put his talents to use in order to travel around the world. In 1818, he was seen in the Netherlands. In 1819, in

England. In 1823, in Dublin. In 1828, he was in the United States, where he was seen again in 1832 in St. Louis and 1833 in Galena, Illinois. Wherever there was a plague, whether the flu or cholera, Friedrich seemed to appear. He traveled the world fighting disease with great success. Most times he refused payment. He supported himself by playing piano in bars or on ships in exchange for passage.

After traveling throughout the East, he affected the dress of the Chinese, wearing silk pajamas and a straw hat, perhaps in the mistaken notion that the outfit helped hide his hump. It is safe to say that Friedrich was noticed wherever he went, if only as a humpbacked piano-playing coolie instead of one of the world's most talented homeopaths. Back in Germany, stories of Friedrich's travels reached Samuel, each story more alarming and amazing than the last: fighting influenza in St. Louis, mysterious fevers in the South Seas.

We don't know when or where Friedrich died, or if he and his father ever reconciled, even by post. It has been written that he died in Scotland and in Dubuque, Iowa. His two trademarks remained his hunchback and the fact that, as his father put it, "He dressed rather freakishly in Oriental clothes."

I like to think of him as a sort of Lone Ranger, appearing mysteriously when needed, refusing payment for his deeds, rejecting all thanks. And disappearing just as quickly and mysteriously as he'd appeared, his work done, leaving those whose lives he'd saved to wonder, "Who was the hump-back with the pills?"

HERING: HEALER AS DISCIPLE

Homeopathy, at least in the United States, owes more to Constantine Hering than perhaps to any other person. Born on the first day of 1800, Hering became not only Hahnemann's friend and most constant follower but also the major force behind the development of homeopathy in North America.

Hering attended the University of Leipzig with the goal of becoming a physician in the Galenic mold. While in his final year, Hering was assigned a paper disproving the ideas of healing as set forth by Samuel Hahnemann. Hering did comprehensive research before drawing his conclusions. Unfortunately for his grade point average, Hering's conclusions were that Hahnemann was on to something, and instead of being censured, he should be consulted concerning healing practices.

Hering was in a panic. He couldn't turn in the paper he wanted to write and still graduate from Leipzig, and he couldn't turn in the paper his professor expected and still live with himself.

Finally, he turned for help to the only man he felt could truly help him: Samuel Hahnemann. He wrote Hahnemann, telling him of his dilemma. Hahnemann wrote back that he certainly knew through firsthand experience exactly what Hering was going through. He counseled the young man to write the paper that was expected of him, turn it in, get his degree, and then practice medicine as he believed it ought to be practiced.

This was probably the only time in what would become a lifelong friendship that Hering did not do as Hahnemann advised. He turned in no paper at all and transferred to the University of Würzburg, where no one asked him his opinion of homeopathy. He received his Doctorate of Medicine in 1826.

As Paracelsus traveled throughout Europe, learning all that he could from the healers of his day, Hering traveled for five years throughout South America, where he learned the folk and herbal traditions. From these he made many new homeopathic medicines, most notably Lachesis, which was created in Hahnemann's method, from the venom of the bushmaster snake.

With the recklessness of youth, and the valor common to the early homeopaths, Hering tested Lachesis as Hahnemann had tested Chinchona. After placing his wife by his bedside with pad and pencil in hand, he drank the venom and had his wife keep copious notes of his delirium. The symptoms he experienced closely mirrored those of the actual snakebite and gave a clear picture of the actions that the homeopathic remedy Lachesis could create in the human system.

The idea for this remedy was inspired by Jenner's work on vaccines in England. Hering was horrified by what he called "very heavy-handed homeopathy" and sought a way diseased tissue could be made into nontoxic medicine. After his initial experience with snake venom, Hering turned his attention to such potential toxins as the saliva of a rabid dog, experimenting with the notion that diseased tissue and other toxic substances might be used in the creation of new and powerful homeopathic remedies. As Hering stated his theory, "The stronger the poison, the stronger the cure."

In 1833, Hering immigrated to the United States. He set forth with great zeal not only to spread his homeopathic message but also to import along with himself a number of skilled European homeopaths. Within one short year, he had turned the little town of Allentown, Pennsylvania, into a veritable hotbed of homeopathy by establishing the North American Academy of the Homeopathic Healing Art.

Hering then founded the Homeopathic Medical College of Pennsylvania, which in 1880 merged with Hahnemann Medical College in Philadelphia. Most important was Hering's founding, in 1844, of the American Institute of Homeopathy, which predated the American Medical Association by three years and offered homeopaths the same organizational basis that the AMA would offer allopaths. Hering was the first president of the organization, and through his work both as an educator and organizer, homeopathy began to flourish in the United States and would continue to do so for about seventy years.

Hering was not the first homeopath to settle in America. The first was Dr. Hans Burch Gram, the son of a Danish sea captain, who came to New York City in 1828. But it is safe to say that there would likely be no homeopathic movement in America today without Hering.

It is impossible to overstate Hering's skill as an organizer or his talent for working with a group of persons as difficult as homeopaths. While not lacking in passion for homeopathic medicine, Hering was as calm and kind as Hahnemann was manic and stubborn. Hering's motto, by which he lived and through which he spread his philosophy across America, was: "The force of gentleness is magnificent."

Hering was also an extraordinary practitioner of homeopathy and is noted as the discoverer of both the allopathic and homeopathic applications of nitroglycerin as a heart attack remedy. It is ironic that Hering died of a heart attack in 1880.

Perhaps Hering's most important gift to homeopaths is Hering's Law, which traces a general pattern for how healing takes place. Although certainly every practitioner can give specific examples that do not follow this general law, it gives insight into how symptoms usually shift as part of a homeopathic healing.

According to Hering, we can expect healing to take place:

- From the inside of the body to the outside: that is, from the more important organs (the heart, lungs, etc.) to the least important organ, the skin. An occurrence of a rash during a homeopathic treatment is a sure sign of cure taking place.
- From the top of the head to the bottom of the feet: The movement of the symptoms will follow this general pattern. Therefore, the appearance of diaper rash, jock itch, or athlete's foot during a homeopathic treatment is the perfect flow of symptoms, as it involves both movement out to the skin and down from the head toward the feet.
- In opposite occurrence from appearance: In other words, the symptoms that are the first to occur will be the last to disappear. The symptoms that have appeared most recently will disappear most quickly. The chronic con-

dition that you have had for twenty years will be slower in clearing than will the skin condition that you developed last month.

HUGHES: HEALER AS DEMAGOGUE

Every movement has its bully. Dr. Richard Hughes, born in 1836, soon after Hahnemann's death, was a complete student of homeopathy and follower of Hahnemann's method until he learned of Hahnemann's shift of philosophy in his final years. Hughes completely rejected the work of Hahnemann's final years, especially his metaphysical theories and use of high potencies, which Hughes referred to as "airy nothings." As Hughes was the leader of the British School of Homeopathy, his rejection of Hahnemann sent shockwaves throughout homeopathic circles worldwide. It had been unthinkable to this point that any homeopath actively disagree with Hahnemann.

Because of Hughes's denial of the wisdom of Hahnemann's last years, and his strict adherence to Hahnemann's early work, the British practice became restricted to the use of low potencies in repeated doses. Further, Hughes largely practiced homeopathy with Galenic methods. He insisted on the study of pathology and the use of homeopathic remedies in the treatment of specific diseases. Above all else, he insisted that his practice always be scientific in its methodology. Remedies would be given based on their action on specific organs or systems in the human body, not on their general actions on the whole being.

Hughes practiced in the London Homeopathic Hospital. There he continued his reversal of Hahnemann's work and principles, in particular with his fervent desire to have homeopaths become respected coworkers of their allopathic brethren. Homeopathy and allopathy were not philosophically so far apart, he reasoned, especially if you diagnosed and treated your patients with homeopathic remedies but selected and used them by allopathic principles, based on the clearing of specific symptoms and not on the treatment of the whole being.

Because of Hughes's reputation, his large output of writings, and his personal hauteur, his influence on the practice of homeopathy spread throughout the world. Even today, many homeopaths practice a bastardized version, one that places the homeopathic pharmacy within the allopathic arena. The problem with this approach is that it does not work. Homeopathic remedies are homeopathic in two ways: how they are made *and* how they are used. If you take a perfectly potentized remedy and use it allopathically, in the treatment of specific disease and not in treatment of the whole person, then that homeopathic remedy becomes an allopathic drug. Perhaps, as energy medicine, it never is as toxic as a true allopathic drug, but it is just as suppressive.

Today Hughes's followers tell their patients to take low-potency remedies (usually no higher than 12C) two or three times a day, regardless of their individual reactions or their particular system and its unique needs. The patients, while they may receive some palliation of pain, never achieve true healing or transformation. Instead, they enter our medical system through a new door but end up in the same endless spiral of treatments.

Hughes referred to practitioners who blended homeopathy and allopathy as "enlightened." He transformed his homeopathic practice into an ongoing soapbox for medical politics, and he welcomed all who would join in what he called his process of demystifying homeopathy. He even changed the jargon of homeopathy from the latinized terminology that had been handed down from ancient days to one that mirrored the allopathic.

The sheer force of Hughes's personality created a rift in homeopathy between those who adhered to Hahnemann's philosophy and those who practiced only by Hughes's methods. In digging the chasm between those who use high potencies and those who only use low, Hughes weakened the cause of homeopathy globally. As homeopaths channeled their energy into fighting among themselves, they not only looked like fools to those who were more interested in homeopathy itself and not the specifics of individual practices but also drove each other out of business through their ongoing feuds, leading homeopathy itself into a period of decline.

It is ironic that the man who said that he would popularize homeopathy by blending it with allopathic medicine instead made the practice of homeopathy far more obscure through his efforts.

Hughes died suddenly, in Dublin, in 1902.

KENT: HEALER AS MYSTIC

James Tyler Kent (1849–1916) is considered to be America's foremost homeopath. He wrote what is considered the definitive repertory and developed his own school of homeopathic theory along lines similar to those of Hahnemann's last years. Kent stressed constitutional prescribing and the fact that certain types of people have affinities for certain illnesses and remedies. Kent employed high potencies, believing that they work on the highest—the spiritual—level for healing.

Kent was himself a deeply spiritual man. He was known to state, "All my teaching is based on Hahnemann's and Swedenborg's." Kent gave homeopathy a clinical structure that it so greatly needed. And more, he gave it a philosophical structure and looked to the spirits of his patients as well as to their bodies in order to bring about healing. Kent died in 1916, five years before the publication of the sixth edition of *The Organon*. We can only guess what impact the final few additional paragraphs might have had on his work.

Kent began his career in medicine by working in the area then known as eclecticism, as created by French physician Henri Leclerc. Eclecticism was also called phytotherapy, and would today be called naturopathy, as it blended herbalism with dietary concerns.

Kent was born into a large Baptist family in Woodhull, New York, and was said to have been a devout Christian from a young age. He married young, but his wife died soon afterward when she was only nineteen years old. Kent graduated at nineteen from Madison University (now called Colgate), and two years later he received his degree from the Bellevue Medical College. Then he graduated from the Eclectic Medical Institute of Cincinnatti, Ohio. When he was twenty-six years old, he set up in practice as an eclectic physician in St. Louis, Missouri.

Kent quickly built a reputation as an excellent teacher and writer and as a distinguished member of the Eclectic National Medical Association. At this point, his life seemed set in place. Kent married again and, established both in his work and in his home, put his energy into his writing, his teaching, and his private practice.

Kent's life was soon turned upside down when his wife, Lucy, became ill. Just a decade after he lost his first wife, Kent was faced with losing his second. With years of experience in eclectic medicine, Kent vowed to restore Lucy to health, but nothing he tried was effective. In his panic he turned to allopathic medicine, taking Lucy to doctor after doctor, without result. Finally Kent heard of Dr. Richard Phelan, a homeopath. Kent took Lucy to Dr. Phelan. Almost miraculously, she was cured.

Soon after, in the fall of 1878, James Tyler Kent again knocked on Dr. Phelan's office door. He had come to ask the doctor to teach him homeopathy.

Perhaps it was his own medical background and the fact that the herbal remedies he already used were the basis of many homeopathic medicines that caused Kent to take to homeopathy, both the philosophy and practice, as if it were a part of his basic nature. He would become the most influential homeopathic educator and practitioner in the United States. Some argue that he also became our country's best.

Kent and his followers felt that they were the philosophical heirs to Hahnemann, who treated in the classic method with just one dose of a remedy selected to cure all the ills of the patient. Kent always stressed the invisible nature in his prescriptions, emphasizing the symptoms he called "mental" over the ailments of the physical body. Finally, Kent insisted that the practitioner and patient together must learn to wait for the totality of healing, not just for the ceasing of a specific symptom, before repeating or changing the remedy.

Further, Kent gave high potencies of remedies, in direct opposition of Hughes and his followers. Kent believed that for any chronic problem a potency of 200C or higher should be used to bring about cure. But most important, Kent almost single-handedly brought homeopathy back from the state of philosophical bastardization it had reached by the time of Hughes's death, with homeopathic prescriptions based on pathology alone. To ensure the continued practice of classic homeopathy, Kent founded the Society of Homeopathians, a functioning support system for the like-minded and a training ground for those who wanted to learn Hahnemann's homeopathic philosophy.

Over the course of the next few years, Kent traveled the nation, teaching his method to homeopathic medical students. He trained an entire generation of practitioners. He then became professor of materia medica at the Homeopathic Medical College in St. Louis, a position he held from 1881 to 1888. From 1890 to 1899 he was professor of materia medica and dean of the Post-Graduate School of Homeopathy in Philadelphia. He then moved on to the Hering Medical College and Hospital in Chicago from 1903 to 1910.

By all accounts, Kent was a superb teacher, blending his personal knowledge of homeopathic remedies with Hahnemann's written materia medica. Kent's *Lectures of Materia Medica* and *Lectures on Homeopathic Philosophy* are still valuable tools for serious students of homeopathy.

While enjoying an extraordinary professional reputation, Kent's personal life was marred by tragedy. Some twenty years after her life-threatening illness, Lucy Kent passed away. Widowed a second time, Kent threw himself into his society work, claiming to be content in his quiet life. Ultimately, however, he married once more. His third wife, Clara Louis Toby Kent, was a physician. She had a major impact on Kent's thinking, and through her

Kent came to be a Swedenborgian. Through his study of Swedenborg's writings, Kent brought a new mystical viewpoint to homeopathy.

Emanuel Swedenborg was born in 1688, so his work predated even that of Hahnemann. A Swedish scientist, Swedenborg excelled as both a scientific researcher and an inventor. It was his work in mathematics and physics, however, that led Swedenborg down a new path. In 1734 Swedenborg undertook a new profession, as a "seer of divine wisdom." In 1745 he claimed to have had a religious vision, and thereafter he dedicated his life to religion instead of science. He is the author of several books, most notably the twelve-volume *Heavenly Aracana*, a synthesis of religion and science in its viewpoint on creation. Swedenborgian societies sprung up across the globe in response to his writings, and the writings of Swedenborg would become one of the major foundations of Theosophy a century later.

Kent's deep interest in Swedenborgianism is considered a major problem for many of today's practitioners. Like Hughes, most would like to be considered thoroughly modern scientists. Most are given to uttering phrases like, "We should use both homeopathic and allopathic approaches to medicine, each when considered best in a given situation," thus mirroring Hughes's wish for a marriage between the opposing therapies. Because of this, Kent's impact on homeopathic practice has diminished in the last decade, but the philosophical foundation that he laid, and the rules by which he used homeopathics, are still very much in use. In fact, when the phrase "classical homeopathy" is used, the speaker, whether he knows it or not, is most often referring to Kentian, not Hahnemannian, homeopathy. Kent gave equal credit to Hahnemann and Swedenborg for his success as a homeopath, and his work shows the impact of both.

As a pragmatic man, Kent also left the homeopathic world with a powerful tool: his repertory. A repertory is a book that lists symptoms of the mind and body in a dictionary format. With each symptom is listed the remedies that work well for that symptom. By gathering together symptoms and suggested remedies, a practitioner is better able to ascertain the needed remedy.

Before the creation of the repertory, practitioners either knew their remedies or they did not. If they did not know the remedy suggested in a given case, that patient was pretty much out of luck. The repertory gave that practitioner a place to go in order to research a case and better understand it. The first repertories, created in the early 1800s, were simply the notes gathered over a lifetime of cases. But Kent's repertory transcended the others, with its impeccable organization and more than 1,500 pages of information. Even today, with dozens of repertories available, Kent's stands as the basic repertory that every serious student of homeopathy buys first and refers to most often.

Kent's mystic doctrine cost homeopathy the respect of many scientifically minded allopaths and of some homeopaths as well. But Kent left behind a legacy of cases treated and cases cured. He left behind a generation of practitioners whose practices had a philosophical foundation in Hahnemann's own words. And he left behind his writings, which are as much an education today as when they were put down on the page.

After his death, Clara continued his work, editing his repertory through six editions, the last of which is still in print.

BACH: HEALER AS EVOLUTIONARY

In many ways, Edward Bach was the exact opposite of Samuel Hahnemann. Born in 1886 near Birmingham, England, Bach was as calm as Hahnemann was excitable, as gentle as Hahnemann was bold.

Like Hahnemann, Bach studied to become a doctor in order to help those who suffered. Also like Hahnemann, Bach soon saw that medical science offered harsh medicines, cures that often were harder on the human system than the disease they were said to combat. He noticed that even the most successful allopathic "cures" were truly palliative rather than curative. Like Hahnemann, and Paracelsus before him, Bach came to believe that the answer to curing the sick lay in long-forgotten healing arts. And finally, like Hahnemann and Paracelsus, Bach believed that the efforts of the physician, if he is to be considered a true healer, should center on the causes of disease rather than their cures.

Bach attended University College Hospital in London, and he stayed on there as an assistant bacteriologist throughout World War I. Bach worked in the fields of pathology, immunology, and bacteriology. He was especially interested in finding the cures for chronic diseases, because he felt that allopathic drugs were often sufficient in the treatment of acute situations but failed to combat chronic disorders. His research into the impact that intestinal bacteria have on the whole system made his name in the area of scientific research. But it was not until he joined the London Homeopathic Hospital in 1919 that he began to develop this work in a way that would make him famous.

Bach Vaccines and Nosodes

In 1915 Bach began to study strains of intestinal bacteria and their relation to chronic illness. Influenced by the work of Jenner and his small-pox vaccine, Bach prepared vaccines from bacteria found in the bowels of persons beset with chronic illness. These vaccines seemed at first to be of great help in working against chronic bowel disease, arthritis, and chronic headaches.

But Bach, like Hahnemann, became wary of these very vaccines that had brought him wealth and fame as a physician. He came to believe that side effects were inevitable with the use of any vaccine. And he sought a simpler, gentler way of bringing about a cure.

In 1919 Bach took a job with the London Homeopathic Hospital. He immersed himself in the writings of Samuel Hahnemann and was surprised and pleased to find a philosophy so similar to his own. Hahnemann's insistence on treating the patient and not the disease changed the way Bach practiced medicine and became the center of his own philosophy of treatment.

Bach returned to those vaccines that he had already created and from them made homeopathic remedies. Since the remedies were taken from diseased tissue, they belonged to a new class of homeopathic remedies, called nosodes. These seven bowel nosodes still had the healing power of the original vaccines but without the toxicity of those vaccines. They were administered orally and cured chronic conditions for many hundreds of patients. These nosodes were welcomed into the homeopathic pharmacy and are still in use today.

Although Bach had enjoyed a great success with his discovery, he was not satisfied with his work as a healer. He felt that the cures that had taken place had done so only on a physical level without healing occurring also. Once more, Bach sought a deeper and simpler way of working. As Paracelsus three hundred years earlier had sought the nature of the creation, Bach now sought the nature of disease.

The Bach Flower Remedies

Bach returned to the British countryside in order to ponder the issue at hand. Since his boyhood, Bach had always meditated outdoors. In the summer of 1928, Bach took a vacation from his busy London medical practice and traveled to Wales. There, while sitting by a mountain stream, Bach began the next level of his life's work.

Bach gathered impatiens and mimuluses as they grew wild. He decided to work with these plants, to find the healing virtue within them. Bach insisted that as he held these plants and meditated with them, he could feel their life energy and perceive their healing power. These would be the first two of his remedies. Clematis was the third.

Bach explains his choice of plants as remedies:

> Metals are sub-human. The use of animals would necessitate cruelty, and no trace of such must occur in the divine art of healing. Thus we are left with the vegetable kingdom. Plants are of three types. The first group is relatively below that of man in their evolution; of such are the primitive varieties, the seaweed, the cactus, the dodder, etc. Also those which have been used for wrong purposes, some of which are poisonous: Henbane, Belladonna, and the orchids are examples.
>
> A second class, on the same relative scale as man, which are harmless, and may be used as food.
>
> But there is a third group, relatively as high or higher than average mankind. Of these we must choose our remedies, for they have been given more power to heal and to bless.
>
> Moreover, there is no cruelty entailed in this: for as these plants desire to be used for the benefit of human nature, a blessing is conferred upon them during their service to man.
>
> The first group, by lowering the vibrations of the body, renders it unfit for habitation by the Spiritual Self, and hence may cause death. But the last class have the power to elevate our vibrations, and thus draw down spiritual power, which cleanses mind and body, and heals.

The Twelve Healers

By 1930, Bach had identified a dozen remedies, the Twelve Healers, as he called them, and the flower remedies had become the highest priority in his life. He left his lucrative practice on Harley Street in London and, at age forty-three, spent the last years of his life in the same manner that both Hahnemann and Paracelsus had spent so many of their years—wandering. Bach walked hundreds of miles throughout England and Wales, gathering curative plants and developing his system of medicine. As he perfected his system, he found that by placing a flower on his tongue he could feel the healing effects of that plant in his mind and body. He coupled this experiential system with an ongoing study of plants and medicinal herbs, in order to find those flowers that were best suited to healing.

At the same time, Bach was developing the philosophy behind this healing system, one that was based both in the homeopathy of Hahnemann and Paracelsus and in the Theosophy of the time in which he lived. Certainly Edward Bach was aware of the occult revival taking place all around him, especially as the most powerful of the Theosophical circles was based in London. It has been said that Bach was at one point a student of Rudolf Steiner, himself a Theosophist and founder of the Anthroposophical movement. It has been suggested that it was Steiner who first suggested the flower remedies to Bach.

Bach wholly accepted Hahnemann's findings concerning both healing in general and homeopathy in particular. But unlike Kent, Bach did not feel bound to begin and end his study where Hahnemann began and ended his own. Bach said that the tragedy was that Hahnemann had had only one lifetime in which to complete his work. Bach believed that it was up to Hahnemann's philosophical heirs to complete the task of creating a philosophical foundation for healing. Bach restated Hahnemann's Law of Similars as "like repels like." Further, he continued along the pathway that Hahnemann had begun to walk in his last years, working more and more with the symptoms of the spirit and ignoring more and more the symptoms of the body. But the greatest step that Bach took in the evolution of homeopathy was the selection, creation, and use of the flower remedies themselves.

In developing his system of the Twelve Healers, Bach returned to his homeopathic training in order to create remedies based in Hahnemann's system of healing. Bach's plants, once selected, were made into mother tinctures, or zero-potency homeopathic remedies. They are, strictly speaking, homeopathic, although they have been neither diluted nor succussed, as traditional remedies are. Therefore, some schools of homeopathy accept the Bach remedies as homeopathic, others do not. But even if the remedies lack the traditional structure of classical homeopathic remedies, they retain the philosophy of homeopathic cure.

We will not find Hahnemann's Laws of Cure at work here. In fact, cure does not even enter into the equation. Bach was concerned only with healing. He believed that if we put our effort into healing, cure surely follows.

Flower Remedy Treatments

In developing his remedies, Bach felt that he was fulfilling his destiny. All his life he had sought a deeper, simpler cure, a true method of healing. In the ultimate development of thirty-eight flower remedies, Bach created a homeopathic system far simpler than Hahnemann's. Hahnemann's remedies are selected on the basis of a case taking on the levels of body, mind, and spirit. Bach's remedies are based solely on the emotions, the moods of the individual. Hahnemann's system calls for the selection of the single remedy from a pharmacy of more than 2,500. Bach's system calls for the selection to be made from only thirty-eight remedies, with up to seven remedies being mixed together at any given time. Hahnemann's system demands that the correct potency be selected. But all of Bach's remedies are the same potency. For all the beauty of its philosophy, Hahnemann's system is another medical plan by which scientific, professional practitioners prescribe medicines. Bach's system, however, allows for self-healing and intuitive prescribing. And, in that Bach felt that each of us needed all of his remedies, prescribing became a matter more of when than of what.

Illness and "Primary Error"

Edward Bach developed far more than just another system of remedies; he developed a philosophy of healing. His philosophy contains the reasons for the creation of illness and a plan for the creation of health. In his pamphlet "Heal Thyself," Bach writes of his new philosophy that "all disease is created by a 'primary error,' and this error drives the being away from and works against Unity. As we work against Unity, we, like flowers lacking sunshine, begin to weaken and wilt—we become ill." Bach identified seven primary diseases of humankind: pride, cruelty, hate, self-love (selfishness), ignorance, instability, and greed.

Bach goes on to explain his concept of "primary error":

> Disease is in essence the result of conflict between Soul and Mind, and will never be eradicated except by spiritual and mental effort. Such efforts, if properly made with understanding, as we shall see later, can cure and prevent disease by removing those basic factors which are its primary cause. No effort directed to the body alone can do more than superficially repair damage, and in this there is no cure, since the cause

is still operative and may at any moment again demonstrate its presence in another form. In fact, in many cases apparent recovery is harmful, since it hides from the patient the true cause of his trouble, and in the satisfaction of apparently renewed health the real factor, being unnoticed, may gain in strength. Contrast these cases with that of the patient who knows, or who is by some wise physician instructed in, the nature of the adverse spiritual or mental forces at work, the result of which is precipitated by what we call disease in the physical body. If that patient directly attempts to neutralize those forces, health improves as soon as this is successfully begun, and when it is completed the disease will disappear. This is true healing by attacking the stronghold, the very base cause of suffering.

One of the exceptions to materialistic methods in modern medical science is that of the great Hahnemann, the founder of Homeopathy, who with his realization of the beneficent love of the Creator and of the Divinity which resides within man, by studying the mental attitude of his patients towards life, environment and their respective diseases, sought to find in the herbs of the field and in the realms of nature the remedy which would not only heal their bodies but would at the same time uplift their mental outlook. May his science be extended and developed by those true physicians who have the love for humanity at heart.

Many homeopathic practitioners make use of both Hahnemann's remedies and Bach's floral essences. Although the two methods should never be used concurrently, because they interfere with each other due to their similarity, both methods can bring about remarkable healings. In general, the Bach remedies work more slowly and subtly than do Hahnemann's. But their ease of use and their ability to bring about a complete cure of the individual give much to recommend them.

More important than the remedies themselves, however, is that Bach taught his fellow homeopaths that the evolution of both the science and art of homeopathy has not ended. It truly has just begun, with each homeopath being responsible for the information he can share and the healing energy he can bring to homeopathy.

5

CASE TAKING

There are as many methods of homeopathic case taking as there are persons who work with homeopathic remedies. Some boot up their computers to get at their homeopathic software, others get out their pendulum and ask their Native American Spirit Guide Running Fox for advice.

But no matter the method used, the purpose of the case taking is always the same: matching the totality of the patient's symptoms to the homeopathic remedy most similar to those symptoms. The selection is not and must not be based in the concept of *need*. If we give the remedy that we feel the patient needs, we are acting allopathically. We are basing a decision on the concept of deficiency. Instead, in order to best select a helpful remedy, we must become familiar with the patient's complete state of being, with the issues—mental, emotional, physical, and spiritual—the patient is already wrestling with. And we must respect the fact that, by virtue of the appearance of symptoms, the vital force is already at work trying to bring about healing, trying to solve the issues at hand.

Then we can choose a remedy that reflects the totality of those symptoms and that best matches the patient's state of being. In taking the selected remedy, the patient is allowing his own system to heal itself. The remedy only helps present the possibility of healing, of letting go of those symptoms.

It does not and will not fill some hole in that person's being. Were this the case, were homeopathic remedies selected based on some lack in the person's physical being or character, then it would be unlikely that arsenic or snake venom would act in a helpful manner. Instead, the remedy selected is the one that acts as a mirror for the patient to get a good long look at himself and that presents the patient with the possibility of change for the better.

In this way, both in taking the case and taking the remedy, we start with today and work from there. We work with the patient as he sits before us. We do not assume that we know his past or future, but we uncover both in the act of healing.

There are three aspects to the taking of the case. The first is taking the actual medical history. Often, on the surface, this is the easiest part. Many practitioners make use of a long medical history form in order to get the full story. Such a form, filled out by the patient before he meets with the practitioner for the first time, can certainly be helpful.

But there are more complex aspects of information gathering that require the practitioner to set aside his ego and to listen, without judgment or insight, to the words of the patient. It is the job of case taking to uncover the patient's state of being today, his basic motivation or motivations in life, and to see how that state of being has shifted throughout the patient's lifetime and what has caused those shifts.

The second aspect of case taking is research. The well-taken information is worthless unless the practitioner knows how to make use of that information in the selection of the correct remedy and then knows how to give that remedy.

The third aspect of case taking concerns diagnosis itself. Most modern homeopaths make use of the same clinical diagnoses that modern allopaths use, giving a specific name to the disease that the patient's symptoms clump together to reveal. But homeopathic diagnosis also involves other parts specific to homeopathy. Just as we look at disease and treatment differently from allopaths, we also consider the diagnosis in a different light.

All told, case taking is something of a mystery. Like a good sleuth, a good homeopath knows when to keep his mouth shut and just listen. He knows how to look for clues and how to put those clues together to get to the truth.

And, perhaps most important, the homeopath knows timing. Just as the sleuth knows just when to call the suspects together into the drawing room and announce the killer, the homeopath knows how to create an environment of healing and when to give the patient information about his healing process and when to give the remedy.

It is also important that the homeopath and the patient work together as a team, one that has enough energy to get the job done. There is a power created by the healing intent of both the patient and the practitioner. Because of this power, it is vital that the patient work only with a practitioner with whom he can form a solid team. Intellect and learning are not enough. Remember, the practitioner, like the patient, is a unique and whole being and must make use of his own unique gifts. The left-brained, scientifically based homeopath who may be just right for you would be the worst choice I could make for a practitioner. The patient must match the practitioner. The practitioner must match the patient. Then you get the job done.

This means that not only does the practitioner have to be uniquely talented and trained but that the patient must be as well.

THE PATIENT

Those of us who turn to a homeopath for help often do so only after everything else has failed to bring about a healing. We have already tried every specialist that allopathy has to offer. We have also probably already tried the route of diet and exercise without adequate response. And, more and more likely, we have already tried Chinese medicine and perhaps even acupuncture without total success.

Therefore, the patient of homeopathy is likely to be dispirited if not desperate on entering the practitioner's office. His condition is now not only chronic in nature but also deeply suppressed by the treatments he has already received.

The first thing the patient should sense on entering the practitioner's office is that this is a safe place. This is no small thing. For any of us, simply walking into a place in which we feel safe, in which we feel that we can express any aspect of our nature without being judged or condemned, is enough to begin a healing process.

This safe space is just as important for the practitioner as for the patient. Therefore, the space becomes one in which both parties are free to relax and to speak, with full knowledge that nothing spoken will be repeated outside. With this understood, it is the sole responsibility of the patient at this point to tell his story as he understands it.

As the camera adds fifteen pounds to our image, so too do we often get bloated in telling our symptoms. This is allowable, even expected. In the beginning of the process of homeopathic healing, the patient has only to be willing to give it a try.

THE PRACTITIONER

The practitioner's role, especially in these first moments, begins also with a willingness to give it a try. A homeopath who is bogged down with worries and fears or aches and pains of his own is likely to miss something important in the patient's tale. The skilled homeopath yields his ego to that of the patient, yields the center stage of his own life, for the moment, to the patient. Watching that patient in the spotlight, standing as his witness, the skilled homeopath uses every talent at his disposal to gather information. Hahnemann himself considers the practitioner's own psychology in *The Organon*. He describes the five attributers the practitioner needs:

Patience. How many of us have waited in a practitioner's office for a half hour or an hour, only to have that practitioner be unwilling to give us the fifteen or twenty minutes we require to tell him fully about our needs? And after treatment has been given, how many of us have been told, when treatment fails, that it is all in our heads?

How many times have we been made to feel that it is somehow our responsibility to get well not the doctor's responsibility to treat us? There is some sort of unwritten timetable for our healing, and if we don't arrive at health on schedule, we are somehow failing not just ourselves but our doctors as well.

Homeopaths, more than any other practitioners, must be willing to listen to their patients. Listening, in fact, is the basic requirement of case taking. The homeopath must also be willing to enter into a meaningful conversation with the patient. The homeopath who seems hurried or not paying attention to the patient is ineffective. Hahnemann was quite willing to spend as much time with a healing process as that healing process took. He proved this with Herr Klockenbring, with whom he climbed trees. Modern homeopaths should do no less. They should take the time that it takes to gather the needed information, all the while bearing witness to the patient's telling of his life story.

Remember, a homeopathic practitioner is the patient's partner and peer. Both are cooperating around the goal of health and healing. The practitioner who does not display due patience both with the patient and the disease is deeply flawed.

The same is true of timetables and remedies. Some patients move toward health far more quickly than anyone expected. Others move slowly. It is not the job of the homeopathic practitioner to judge the healing process, only to encourage it, however long it takes and with whatever remedies are needed along the way.

Knowledge of human nature. Homeopathic Practitioners deal daily with patients who are depressed, hypersensitive, overly impressionable, timid, angry, fearful, and have a tendency to deny or to exaggerate their symptoms. Wise practitioners know that any or all of these attributes are symptoms of the very nature of the patient. They may be signs of disease as well. But they will, if correctly observed, lead toward a curative remedy.

A practitioner must be able to understand the nature of his patient's illness. To do this, he must be able to discern the patient's being, motivation, and the issues surrounding his illness.

Psychological insight. This requirement is in keeping with the knowledge of human nature. If we assume that there are a limited number of issues motivating humans in general, then it is the job of the homeopath to be able to identify what motivates his patient in particular. Often a practitioner must have the insight to know *not* to trust the case as presented by the patient. Some patients are in deep denial or are in great fear of their illnesses. The practitioner must have the wisdom to take in whatever information he can from another sense—from vision instead of hearing—or he must turn to the patient's family for more information. But he must be on the ball in the case taking, removing all attention from himself and his needs and dealing only with this patient in front of him and his issues and his needs.

Caution. This is a vital component of wise homeopathic care. As Hahnemann notes, many situations that are called chronic diseases are not diseases at all, but are rather the price we pay for unhealthful living—not exercising, or smoking, for example. The wise practitioner knows when to treat homeopathically and when *not* to. He knows the patient's issues and which to challenge the patient with and which the patient may not be ready to deal with.

Above all, the wise practitioner knows and respects the power of homeopathic remedies. If he errs at all, it is on the side of caution, giving a remedy less often or at a lower potency than might be needed. Further, the wise practitioner uses his patience to move the patient toward health at the patient's, not the practitioner's, rate of speed.

Education and skill. Finally, but perhaps most importantly, the practitioner must have the necessary skills to take the mantle of healer upon himself. This may demand a knowledge of pathology, of disease itself, and of physiology. On top of this, the practitioner may make use of whatever tests modern science has made possible to better diagnose illness. In addition, the practitioner needs experience in the use of homeopathic remedies as well as a knowledge of the remedies themselves.

Several states restrict the practice of homeopathy to allopathic doctors, many of them with a partial knowledge of homeopathics at best. Often the layperson visiting that doctor actually knows more about the remedies than does the doctor. Therefore, it is very important to find out about a practitioner's training in homeopathy and his experience in the remedies. Don't be afraid to ask. If he is offended by the question, he is not a good practitioner. Also ask if he has read *The Organon*. Maybe ask his favorite paragraph in it, just to see if he has an answer.

The patient should never be afraid to question the practitioner's methods or practices. Nor should he hesitate to ask for some suggestions of reading materials, for some tools he can use to educate himself about homeopathy. A skilled practitioner is never offended by a patient who is concerned with his own healing process. Indeed, an educated patient is easier to treat homeopathically.

The educated patient is willing to give the practitioner all the information he needs for the selection of a remedy. Cooperation between the practitioner and the educated patient is a must in the correct taking of the remedy and in helping to determine when it is appropriate to stop taking a remedy. All of this creates a healing energy between patient and practitioner, one that stands to evolve the practice of medicine that has the patient entering the practitioner's office with the attitude of a toy: "I'm broken. Can you fix me?"

TAKING THE CASE

The skills involved in case taking are vital to the selection of the right homeopathic remedy, the one that will move the patient toward health. Case taking involves the ability to connect with the patient, to completely listen to what the patient is saying, and through the use of vision, smell, hearing, and, often, touch, to take in all that comprises the "being" of the patient. Remember, in homeopathy we are always concerned with the treatment of the person, not of the disease. Therefore, it is important to know as much as possible about what makes this person unique in all the universe, and what of that unique and whole balanced state that may be called health has been disrupted by the present illness. And specifically how that illness has taken place.

Whether the case is a simple acute situation like a cold, or a long-term chronic condition, it is most important that the homeopath connect totally with the patient, that active communication occurs at all times, and that at no time does the homeopath separate himself from the patient by attitude or even by the intense desire to cure. Healing begins with communication. And communication between homeopath and patient creates a safe place in which healing can begin immediately. At no time should a patient feel hurried or belittled by a practitioner. Such treatment is the sign of a flawed practitioner or, more likely, an allopathic wolf in holistic sheep's clothing.

Case taking begins as the patient walks in the door and the practitioner begins to register important information. The first thing the practitioner is likely to notice is the overall behavior pattern of the patient. Is this a timid person who almost slips into the room, or is this a dominant person who strides into the room and takes possession of it? Either way, the patient is telling some important information about himself.

The way the patient moves in his own body is important. Does the person seem at home in his body? Is there any sign of pain in movement? The speed and strength of movement give the practitioner an important clue to the patient's vital force.

The practitioner also watches the patient's gestures, looking for tics and nervous mannerisms, for particular feelings that are not revealed verbally.

Then, even before the practitioner considers the patient's actual words, he must consider the way the patient speaks them. Does this person speak quickly and easily, or is communication difficult, with pausing, scratching, and looking around the room? These are all symptoms of the patient's being that are every bit as important as are the aches and pains.

The patient's physical being, age, weight, and sex are all important pieces of information that are revealed to the practitioner just as soon as the door is opened. And all of these pieces of information are important guides in the selection of an appropriate homeopathic remedy.

Now the case taking begins, at least as far as the patient is concerned. The wise practitioner speaks as little as possible, asks as few questions as possible. The practitioner tries to keep the case taking in the patient's own words and from his own viewpoint.

It is the practitioner's role to listen, truly listen. Whether the patient sums up his case in two sentences and then stares into space, or jumps into a litany of aches, pains, and injustices that threatens to run longer than an Oliver Stone film, the practitioner should simply listen, taking what notes he finds it important to take and asking few clarifying questions.

When the tale has been told, the practitioner sits quietly for another minute. He knows that often the most vital piece of information is withheld, and that when faced with dead silence at the end of their tale, many patients blurt out this information rather than face the ongoing silence.

Now the questions begin. Having kept notes, the practitioner goes back to the beginning of the tale, asking the patient to fill in information where needed. Again, it is important that after a question has been asked, the practitioner sit and listen to the answer without interrupting.

Patients who have already educated themselves in the allopathic method, who concern themselves with pathologies and chemical treatments—that is, most patients—should be encouraged to express themselves concerning their ailments in their own words and to restore to those words the emotions that have likely been drained from them.

The homeopath works down the list of symptoms reported by the patient, having the patient assist in grading the symptoms in order of importance. The homeopath needs the same information concerning each symptom: sensation, location, duration, and modalities. *Sensation* relates to how the pain feels specifically—is it throbbing, burning, tearing in nature? Or does it have some other sensation attached? The practitioner should never lead the patient by listing the possibilities but should simply inquire about the sensation of discomfort. *Location* also demands specificity. Exactly where does the pain occur? If the patient has a headache, the pain is obviously in the head, but where in the head? The forehead? The occiput? Does the pain move from place to place? Does it, for instance, begin on the right side of the forehead and move to the left? The exact location and the motion of the pain are vital to the selection of the correct remedy. Next there is *duration*. How long has the patient had this symptom? Can he remember when it first came on and the circumstances of his life at that time? And what treatments has the patient already tried for the symptom? This last is vital; some treatments, chiefly steroids and antibiotics, are so suppressive in nature that they may render a symptom incurable by homeopathic standards. And then there are *modalities*, which are very important to the selection of a remedy. Modalities are the factors that make the symptom feel better or worse. An important modality of indigestion may be that it is worse when the patient is lying down.

After all this information has been taken concerning every symptom, the homeopath should ask about how the symptoms combine. For instance, a patient's headaches may get better as his digestive symptoms get worse. These are called concomitant symptoms, and they can help a practitioner select the right remedy.

Finally, it is important that both practitioner and patient agree on the goals of treatment and that those goals be specific. A patient who goes out the door with a notion that he will one day soon "feel better" is likely to be dissatisfied in a few weeks' time.

When all the needed information has been taken, the practitioner begins the process of educating the patient about homeopathy. In general, the practitioner tells the patient how homeopathy works and how homeopathic healing is likely to take place in his life. The practitioner makes sure that the patient is knowledgeable and comfortable with the homeopathic process before the first remedy is given.

As the practitioner has been patient with his client, so now the client must exhibit patience. Most practitioners, unless a particular remedy is clearly and quickly called for, ask the patient to return at a scheduled time to receive the first remedy. During the intervening period, the practitioner revisits the case taking, synthesizes the information, and selects a remedy.

RESEARCHING THE CASE

Repertorization is the name given to the process by which the homeopath assembles the information that has been gathered from the patient and reassembles it in a manner that he hopes will lead him toward the appropriate remedy.

There are many ways to repertorize a case. But most often the patient's symptoms are first divided into symptoms of the mind and symptoms of the body. Each of these groups then is divided into general symptoms and specific symptoms.

On both mental and physical planes, the general symptoms are considered to be more important and are considered first. General symptoms flow throughout the being. They are usually referred to as "I am" symptoms. The patient will say, "I am afraid of the dark" or "I am unable to eat wheat." In vocalizing a symptom as "I am," the patient reveals that he identifies with it and may well define himself by that symptom. The general symptoms often lead the homeopath to the basic motivation of the patient: The person who is motivated by fear reveals himself through "I am."

Specific symptoms are "I have" symptoms: "I have dizzy spells" or "I have a peculiar fear of dogs." They often relate to a specific organ or portion of the body. The patient here does not define himself with these symptoms but rather seems to be carrying them around with him. They have not yet become part of the being and are therefore of less importance.

Just as the specific symptoms are less important than the general symptoms, so too are the physical symptoms less important than the mental symptoms. Mental symptoms relate to any "invisible" part of our being. Therefore, they may be said to be mental, emotional, and/or spiritual in nature. Mental symptoms can be divided into general and specific. A symptom that is mental and general is, "I am afraid of the dark." This symptom appears on the deepest part of our being, the mental, and speaks to the whole being from that plane. A symptom that is mental and specific is, "I have a peculiar fear of dogs." Although this is a fear issue and a deep symptom, it is one that the patient does not identify with but rather merely observes and reports. It is of secondary import compared to the mental general symptom.

Physical symptoms are arranged very simply in the repertorization process. The generals, speaking as they do to the whole physical being, are listed first. The specifics are then listed in order from the top of the head to the soles of the feet.

The final organ of the body considered among the specific symptoms is the skin, which in terms of homeopathic healing is considered the least important organ. When symptoms appear first on the skin, they are most easily expressed and removed from the body. When chronic conditions are brought forth through homeopathic treatment and move, layer by layer, toward healing, they at last appear on the skin as some sort of rash before they are finally released and removed.

The irony of this system of organizing symptoms is that most patients rush in for treatment of a physical specific symptom, the least important or involved form of symptom. Often, a patient has lived for years with physical chronic conditions and has been plagued all her life with emotional ailments, enduring all these long term, and rushes for help when acne appears on her forehead. And, although the homeopath may wish to all but ignore physical specific symptoms in the selection of treatments, he may not do so, because that very little symptom may be of utmost importance to the patient.

While organizing all this information, the practitioner must remember to include the modalities. All of us have modalities that are both general and specific in nature. General modalities speak to the being as a whole and to what factors make the person feel better and worse. Some people always feel better in warm weather; others thrive in the winter cold. Some people feel better in the early morning, others in the late afternoon. These general modalities are the way most people best reveal who they are to their homeopath. They are perhaps the most powerful indications of homeopathic constitution, and many practitioners feel that if they can just pull together a good sense of the patient's mental symptoms and general modalities, they can find appropriate treatment.

Specific modalities speak to the individual symptoms and tell the homeopath what makes that particular symptom feel better or worse. While not as strong diagnostic tools as the general modalities, these too can be very helpful in the selection of a remedy and should not be ignored.

With the pages and pages of information that the average patient gives, the literally dozens of symptoms big and small, the practitioner must be capable of grading symptoms in importance, both to himself and to the patient. Further, he must have some method of winnowing down the sheer number of symptoms. Hahnemann suggests that we put together a case using the image of a common household object. Hahnemann said that just as a three-legged stool is the most solid means of support when reaching to the top kitchen shelf, so too is the three-legged case the most sure.

Many practitioners select the three symptoms that seem most important and base the diagnosis and treatment on these three. Usually they include one general mental symptom that best suggests the patient's basic motivation, one general physical symptom that best defines the physical constitution, and the one specific physical symptom with which the patient is most uncomfortable. The other symptoms are of course not ignored, but these three, along with the general modalities, are stressed in researching the case.

With the case-taking information reorganized, the homeopath must now work to use this information to select a remedy. For this he turns to a repertory, a dictionary of symptoms organized in a manner similar to that which the practitioner uses: first the mentals, and then the physicals from the top of the head to the bottom of the feet.

Each symptom is broken down within the repertory to more and more specific terms through listings called rubrics. Each rubric lists the remedies that have been used appropriately in the treatment of that symptom. For a patient suffering from headaches, the practitioner might first turn to Head: Pain. Under that heading are dozens of pages of rubrics, each speaking to specific aspects of head pain: pain by time of day or season of year, pain in the forehead or in the occiput. The fully repertorized symptom of headache may involve dozens and dozens of rubrics, each listing possible remedies.

The practitioner now gathers the rubrics in order from the mentals to the physicals, and from the top of the head to the bottom of the feet. He works through the rubrics, noting which remedies come up most often and, most important, looking to find a pattern or flow. By this process, the homeopath narrows the list of possible remedies from several thousand to the three or four that have come up most often and seem most able to speak to the case.

The practitioner now reaches for the homeopathic materia medica. This lists the remedies in alphabetical order, giving an overview of the remedy, its actions, and the issues it speaks to, and then listing the individual symptoms that the remedy has action on, again in the top-to-bottom format. He considers each of the handful of likely remedies, looking for the one that is most similar in action and motivation to the patient himself. This remedy and the others similar to it form the basis for the homeopathic drug diagnosis.

DIAGNOSING THE CASE

The first diagnosis, and the most important, is the drug diagnosis. The practitioner takes the name of the remedy that seems most similar to the patient and gives the patient the remedy name. The patient will be referred to as a Lachesis, an Arsenicum, or a Sepia. As the selection of a remedy is based on the remedy's similarity to the patient's state of being, the remedy name is often more likely to express that patient's personality than is his given name.

Next is the differential diagnosis. This is a listing of the two or three other remedies that seem likely to be helpful in the case, which extends the practitioner's concept of the patient's constitution into a family of remedies. Most often, these remedies themselves are similar to each other, as well as to the patient. In other words, the remedy types speak to the same sort of emotions and work out of the same sort of wounds. This allows the practitioner to look beyond this moment and to conjecture, however briefly, on other remedies that might extend the healing process. While not locking the practitioner into a specific course of treatment, the differential diagnosis provides the practitioner with some overview of the case and a possible path to follow.

Finally, the practitioner considers the clinical diagnosis. In homeopathy we tend to look not at illness but at a person with this or that clump of symptoms. We treat the person truly as if no one has ever had this particular grouping before—and unless this is a recurrence of a particular illness in a patient's life, for all intents and purposes no one *has* had this particular collection of symptoms before.

The practitioner's real diagnostic job is to determine the patient's present state of being, his totality of symptoms, and to treat that state with a remedy that best expresses that state of being. From there the practitioner's job is to wait, to watch, and, perhaps, to pray.

In homeopathic treatment, particularly in the treatment of chronic disorders, we always begin with the patient's state of being today and work backward through the patient's life, uncovering and expressing all that has been suppressed.

This is a tall order, and it takes time, patience, energy, and no small amount of skill. Further, it takes a commitment on the part of both the patient and the practitioner, a commitment to change and a willingness to let change take place whatever manner and time span the change itself dictates. The practitioner cannot project what tomorrow will bring. Nor can he try to guess what traumas the patient might have suppressed on the mental or physical planes. The practitioner must wait to see what the patient expresses, wait for the time of treatment, and then treat today and only today.

The practitioner must be committed not only to the patient's case but also to the patient's being. Allopaths are trained to remain objective, to have no emotional involvement in the case. Homeopaths certainly understand the appropriate boundaries of professionalism, but they also know the power of empathy. And they understand that our beings require more than rational medicine if we are to be well.

THE RATIONALE OF THE IRRATIONAL

We humans need a balance of rational and irrational thinking in our lives. Whether we call it faith or instinct or something else, irrational thinking often gives us our deepest insight. The truths that we uncover through our "belief in things unseen" are the most potent. Evangelist Oral Roberts speaks of things that "you know that you know that you know." These are the things that need no proving to you, the realities of life, as you see them. Irrational thinkers stress the invisible nature of life over the visible and tangible, stress knowing over thinking, both as a process and as a result. By this definition, homeopathy is at least as irrational an art as it is rational.

All this flies in the face of modern science, which, instead of knowing what it knows of the universe, tends to attack the realities of life the way a four-year-old approaches the rules and boundaries handed down to him by his parents. He tugs on his mother's skirt, looks up, and demands, "Why?" Science seeks the "why" of the universe and fools itself into believing that that which can be named can be controlled. And of course, thinking that we control something and truly controlling it are two very different things.

Modern medicine follows suit. Instead of working with nature, with the immutable but intangible laws of nature, modern medicine continues stubbornly to demand that if it can name it, it can control it. So it is with the common cold, and so it is with AIDS. Medical science has named a virus that it insists "causes" AIDS, and the search stops there. Now the process is one of taking control of that virus. The fact that medical science has never been able to convince any virus to do anything it doesn't want to do is ignored. The medical science that has failed to cure the common cold insists that a vaccine for AIDS is only time and money away.

Homeopathy, largely thanks to Hahnemann's final years in Paris, blends the physical with the spiritual, the rational with the irrational. The finest homeopathic practitioners are those whose minds can operate on both the rational and irrational circuits of thought. What treatment often comes down to is the practitioner, having done his research and homework, and experiencing the patient as an Arsenicum, simply knows that he knows that he knows that this person, so wracked with fear and yet so demanding and fussy, needs Arsenicum to balance out his energy.

In the sixties, we all read Robert A. Heinlein's science fiction novel, *Stranger in a Strange Land.* In it, Michael Valentine Smith, a Martian who has come to live on Earth, introduces the word *grok* to our vocabulary. By this foul-looking and -sounding word, Heinlein suggests a knowing that is indeed different from our human one, a knowing that is deeper than human understanding, that uses the senses as a secondary source of information rather than as the primary basis of all knowledge. As Smith says, "I am not long out of the nest. For knowing I must see. But an Old One does not need eyes to know. He knows. He groks. He acts." This is the melding of the rational and the irrational, of thinking and knowing.

It could be said, then, that the skilled homeopath must come to grok his patient if that patient is to be made totally well. A case may be made that the patient must grok the practitioner as well. Groking is total understanding, and that's the only thing that really gets you anywhere as a patient or a practitioner.

HEALING AS AN IRRATIONAL ACT

While medicine at its best melds the irrational mind of the practitioner with the rational, the processes that now dominate the field find themselves heavily weighed in one or the other.

Allopathic medicine focuses on the goal of curing—the process of removing disease from the human system. By its very nature, this process is both goal specific and rational. Curing takes place from the outside in. An outside force, most often a physician and his medicines and operations, moves into the body, changing the disease process. He hopes that this force will remove the disease and leave a healthy patient behind.

Most important, curing is a finite act. We wrestle with the demon that is disease and, if we win the war, the patient lives. If we lose, the patient likely dies. No effort is spent trying to put the disease into the context of the patient's life or to look at how the disease differs in its symptoms from one patient to another. Instead, our vision stays focused on the moment of "impact," the moment in which the battle is joined. We look only at how the disease in the individual is like the disease in all others so that we can get a diagnosis, and by that diagnosis have a plan of action to follow. We give our full strength to the resistance against the disease. Sometimes we win, but often we lose.

In truth, the diseases that have been "conquered" have been conquered not by our superior power, but by the disease itself becoming part of the context of our lives and, in doing so, becoming more or less benign. Take for example the influenza epidemic of the early twentieth century that killed millions of persons worldwide. The fact that flu has now become more or less an annual inconvenience has nothing to do with anything that medical science threw against the virus. No, it has to do solely with the fact that the virus itself mutated and became less fatal. All "new" disease, as it comes into contact with our society of humans, comes first in its most deadly form. As it was with flu, so it is now with AIDS. As the virus filters in the human gene pool, it adapts to us far more than we adapt to it. Because it is in the virus's own self-interest that it not kill its host, it "chooses," as it gets to know that host, to weaken rather than to kill. This allows the virus itself to, as a Vulcan would say, "Live long and prosper."

Medical science still harbors the rational hope that it can cure the human patient of any sort of illness. Yet truly, it can only palliate the pain and hope for the best. Look at medical history and see how many other illnesses, including tuberculosis, were thought to be controlled, if not eliminated, only to return again and again, more resistant than before to the rational attempts to combat it.

We read that science has all but eliminated smallpox and that all that remains is some frozen tissue that the scientists themselves debate whether to destroy. The arrogance of the belief that a disease can be held at bay in a test tube at once amuses and frightens me. I believe that something that was made naturally can recur at any moment. Each time we use the rational mind against the problem of health and healing, we live to regret it. The rational mind needs not only to understand our world concretely but also to control all its aspects rather than just live in harmony with them. The rational mind needs to disrupt the laws of nature when it comes to human health; it congratulates a patient who has been scarred, bled, and weakened almost to death's door for having just survived. Giving the concept of healing a chance seems to be not only a wiser but also a more humane method of treatment.

Healing is by its very nature an irrational act. To believe in healing requires me to believe that, whatever is wrong with me and however frightening the prognosis, I can be made whole. To believe in healing is to believe that Christ could call Lazarus forth from the tomb. To believe in healing is to believe that change can come about in your life like spontaneous combustion, that you can "catch" health just as you can disease.

In fact, the more you look to the power of healing, the less interested you are in even knowing what is wrong with you in the first place. When the pain begins, the healing process is the healing process is the healing process. Unlike the rational procedures that guide the act of curing, the irrational process that is healing follows the laws of nature and is unchanging no matter what disease challenge faces the patient. It is indeed irrational to believe that anyone with AIDS will survive the disease. Yet, someone will, and that someone will be the first of many. No disease, no matter how deadly it appeared when it first arrived in our lives, has stayed deadly forever. So telling any and all who are diagnosed with full-blown AIDS that they should prepare for death, while completely rational, is truly incorrect, or certainly will be one day soon.

The rejection of the rational procedures of curing disease makes the progression to the healing path not only irrational but revolutionary as well. It has much to do with the refusal to fear. It involves turning down the volume on all those who tell you that they know what the future brings for you and your disease. As we live in a society that is fear based, to reject the fear and to demand that change can always happen, that we can truly and fundamentally change for the better, not only as individuals but also as a group, is to reject society's most basic teachings. It is to stamp your foot and to remind yourself that that which society calls supernatural is just that which society cannot legislate or control. It is no more out of the ordinary than is childbirth or your heartbeat; it is merely unpredictable and uncontrollable. Yet, as a tool for healing, the supernatural—the power of prayer, remissions, and the like—is the most powerful we possess.

Healing is the yin to curing's yang. Healing involves a willingness to trust. To trust not your doctor, but God.

Healing is less an action than a process. Unlike curing, it is not particularly goal oriented. It involves a movement toward health and toward wholeness, but it does not seek to spell out just what that movement should entail. Healing involves an internal process and is always internally motivated, no matter how many others come along as helpers to the process. While the average person on an average day may call himself well and say that he needs no cure of anything, he is in fact always in the process of healing. Healing does not require some ache or pain or other.

This thought of healing as an infinite process ties into our own purpose in this life. If we cannot become aware of any work that we are called upon to do, any lesson that we need to learn, we can always certainly call upon the healing process to guide us in our life.

Healing demands that we acknowledge that disease is us and that we are our disease and not its victim. Healing demands that we learn from our disease and understand that we can be made well only by letting go of that disease. While it can be difficult, even seemingly heartless, to leave a patient to wrestle with the reality of a migraine or arthritis, how much better is this process than one that says, "Don't even think about it, just take this pill."

Healing also demands that we be willing to change. So many chronically sick people think that no aspects of their lives need to be changed. They see illness as akin to a scud missile attack. The missile either hits your house or it doesn't. Thus they are innocent victims of illness. But even if we believe that the illness was like the train that struck us down as we picked wildflowers on the tracks, don't we have to take some responsibility for being on the tracks in the first place?

All illness involves susceptibility. You have to have some chink in your armor to let the illness in. Some illnesses, especially when the strain of the illness is fresh and new, find that the vast majority of persons in a given population are susceptible. Good for the germ, bad for the people. But most illness, especially chronic illness, is geared to a person and that person's particular lifestyle and thought process. There is good reason, after all, why the red-faced abusive man ends up dying young of a heart attack. What is surprising is that, if we can all agree that this particular man basically killed himself by the way he lived his life, we cannot extend the metaphor to include more people. To me a good use of taxpayers' dollars would be a medical study to look at what all persons with rheumatoid arthritis had in common in terms of personality traits. The same for prostate cancer, and so on.

The very fact that a person has an illness, from a basic cold to a chronic disease, says that there is something in his life that needs to change. With a cold, it may just be a small adjustment; that person needs a rest or a more healthful diet. With a more complex situation, the need for change is more complex. This is why, in homeopathy, the patient is a full partner in the process. The patient needs to come to identify the changes that must be made. The changes cannot be assigned by the practitioner, the priest, or the judge. They are part of the internal mechanism of healing.

Healing as an irrational process demands that we be less rational, less guided by our perception of events and of the nature of our lives, and more willing to learn the truth of events and of our lives. The physician who is also a healer has returned, in his own mind, all the healing power to God and uses God alone as the source of all healing. To do this is to work not as the revered Father but as the servant to the patient, the one who listens and assists in the healing process.

The most damaging trait that a physician can have is cynicism. True, physicians are well educated, and after years of practice, many have seen it all. When I walk in for my appointment, the doctor may have seen the very condition that I experience time and time again in many other patients. But he has not seen *me* before and does not know, no matter how good he is at guessing, what that disease is like in my own unique and whole system. He does not know the outcome; he can only play the odds.

In the end, it all comes down to the individual and how he perceives his life. And how that individual fits into his community, how he helps to shape his society. The majority of us still tend to stay with the rational and believe that where there is smoke there is fire. Society in general consists of rational people doing rational things. We have adapted to our lives and to the seemingly random events that fill them. We have come to see our illnesses as just more random events, events without meaning. More important, we have formed a culture that demands that others share this opinion, this same lack of meaning. The individual who chooses to perceive meaning where others see happenstance becomes society's most feared subversive.

Therefore, the use of homeopathics requires cultural as well as individual changes. Certainly the medical and insurance industries must make room for a new way of thinking and working, one that is as firmly based in individuality as the present status quo is in uniformity. But perhaps more important, human culture must learn to express what has been suppressed and must replace its ongoing engine of denial with a society based on the kindergarten concerns of honesty, fairness, and interdependence.

The allopathic approach to medicine that is so based on denial, on the suppression of pain at all costs, is itself a symptom of the illness within our society. We are so busy with everyday crises that we have no time left for reflection, renewal, and change. In our culture, as in our own bodies, we have chosen the short-term goal of curing over the transformational goal of healing. Therefore, those people who turn their attention to homeopathy make a strong statement not just about their own bodies and how they choose to treat them but, more important, about how *we* should perceive our bodies, ourselves, and our communities. The change to homeopathy is a change of perception that goes far beyond sugar pills. As the individual is set free by the healing process, so, too, can this process, taken culturally, set our people free.

6

CARETAKING

At the 150th anniversary of the American Institute of Homeopaths, a young naturopathic physician asked homeopath and Jungian analyst Edward Whitmont how he treated difficult cases. Whitmont asked the man exactly what he meant. The younger man said that many patients in his practice could not be treated successfully with just one homeopathic remedy. He had had to treat them with multiple remedies given at once, and with a combination of herbs, remedies, and others modalities. Whitmont thought briefly and spoke quietly. He said, simply, "Luckily, this has not been my experience."

That short sentence spoke volumes. The practitioner who knows the remedies, and knows how to select the remedy most similar to the case, needs not to blend treatments or consult the Tarot. He or she simply gives the remedy and trusts the power of that remedy and of the vital force of the patient to do their work in bringing about healing.

One of the things I like best about homeopathy is its simplicity. The way a simple cold is treated is the same as the way a horrific and life-threatening condition is treated. As I said above, the principles are few, and the process, if done correctly, is, as Hahnemann promised, "rapid, gentle, and permanent." It is when the experimenters come to town that the process becomes complex and the situation, as the magic eight ball would say, becomes hazy.

Up until now I have dealt with the philosophy, as anyone should before he ever touches a remedy. But now is the time to become more practical and to look into the homeopathic kit and all its many uses.

THE PRINCIPLES OF HOMEOPATHIC TREATMENT

As a system of healing that stresses the uniquity of each person, homeopathy has few laws that govern its practice. Each case is dealt with as an individual situation, with the remedy selection as well as the potency and dosage selection made on the basis of this case alone.

But there are solid principles for procedure by which a practitioner can always practice a form of homeopathic medicine that is "rapid, gentle, and permanent." These are known as the Three Laws of Cure.

The first principle, the Law of Similars, is the single most important guiding principle of homeopathic practice. When we use this principle, we always know that we practice true homeopathy and that we always work in a manner that will help the patient to express his symptoms, removing them totally from his system.

The Law of Similars demands that we look not just at the symptoms of the illness that has caused the patient to consider homeopathy but also at the totality of the patient's symptoms. We consider all the information we have about that patient as a person, not just as a sick person. By stressing the symptoms' totality and working with the central motivational theme of the patient's life, we can help him to release the cause of the disease and not just its symptoms. We then give a remedy that *in a totally well person* would create the same symptom portrait that the patient is already presenting.

Perhaps the best way to understand the Law of Similars is to look at one of our basic laws of nature. We have all been taught in school that "for every action there is an equal and opposite reaction." Science affirms this principle and there is no longer any disagreement with it. The mistake we make is not applying this principle to all aspects of our lives. Matter is energy, and so all the physical laws of the universe apply equally to our matter—our flesh and bone, our energy, and our spirit. When working with the concept and practice of healing, we must also work with the laws of nature: For every action there is an equal and opposite reaction.

Allopathic medicine rewrites this principle. Take, for instance, the simple sleeping pill. If you can't sleep, you take a pill that knocks you off your feet. You sleep. That is the action of the pill. But the reaction of your body to that pill is wakefulness, as anyone who has ever taken a sleeping pill will tell you. When you have even more trouble sleeping the next night (because of your own reaction to the pill), you take another pill, which won't knock you quite so much off your feet but will still put you to sleep. Over time and with more doses of the medicine, you have trouble sleeping even using the pills, needing to take more and more of them to get to sleep. Sleep becomes quite impossible without the pill.

That is because the allopathic approach to sleeplessness is to set forth an action and try to ignore the equal and opposite reaction. The approach tries to suppress the symptom of sleeplessness at the moment and ignores the long-term reaction: increased sleeplessness.

The homeopathic approach to the same symptom is to increase the symptom, to give a remedy that in a sleepy person would create sleeplessness.

By working the Law of Similars, the homeopath uses the principle of equal and opposite reaction to bring about healing. Giving that patient the correct remedy causes sleeplessness—an action. The system meets this with an equal and opposite reaction—sleepiness.

That is how the Law of Similars works and why the action of homeopathic remedies are so very effective. They create a healing reaction.

Having said all this, you would think that this principle of practice would be agreed on by all those who practice homeopathy. But this is not the case. Because of the distorted laws that govern who may and may not practice homeopathy, which differ greatly from country to country and state to state, those who understand homeopathy least are those most free to practice it. Many medical doctors, whose education involved years of allopathic training and only a few weeks of homeopathic education, are licensed to use homeopathic remedies.

Many practitioners who either do not understand the core principles of homeopathy, or who ignore these principles for the overriding practice of allopathic medicine, simply take the homeopathic remedies and use them allopathically. They think of the remedies as headache medicines and trauma medicines, and, in doing so, they make homeopathy allopathic.

James Tyler Kent, who faced the same situation in his day, was constantly wary of allopaths who practiced homeopathy as an adjunct therapy.

He taught that homeopathic remedies are homeopathic in two ways: how they are made and how they are used. Kent believed that a perfectly created homeopathic remedy that is used allopathically—in other words, to combat disease and not to assist the person with the disease—becomes an allopathic drug.

And so it is today. Many practitioners, whose basic education was allopathic and whose basic thought is still allopathic in nature, use homeopathic remedies and wonder why they seem not to work very well. If homeopathic remedies are used in a suppressive manner—to treat disease and not the whole person—they act in a suppressive and palliative manner—for a while. But the disease reasserts itself, or, worse, moves deeper into the body to come back as an even more life-threatening situation.

Because the physician has forgotten or has not learned the most basic Law of Similars, the case is moving in the wrong direction. We must look at the whole person, and at the role that illness is playing in that person's life, and give the remedy that most closely corresponds to the totality of what is going on. Nothing else is homeopathy. Nothing else works in the total restoration of health.

The second principle is the Law of Simplex. It sounds simple, and it is. It states that we give one remedy at a time. Period.

Oh, how this simple little statement causes trouble. It brings homeopathic practitioners to blows as they argue over the necessity of using only one remedy at a time.

To use more than one remedy at a time is problematic because we can never be sure which remedy is doing what. I do not believe that homeopathic remedies are as benign as do many other people. They tell you that if you give the wrong remedy, nothing at all happens, that the energy of the remedy just vanishes from the patient's system. I don't believe this for a moment. Certainly one dose of a remedy should not overwhelm any patient, but repeated doses of the wrong remedy can have powerful and permanent effects.

Homeopathic remedies are energy. We, too, are made up of energy. And homeopathic remedies, in speaking to our energy bodies, have powerful effects in our beings. The power of the remedies should always be respected.

There is no respect in using more than one remedy at a time. The different remedy energies pull the system in more than one direction at once, confusing the case and perhaps over time making the case incurable. Say you have allergies and you buy a mixed allergy remedy at the health food store. This is easier and cheaper than going to a practitioner or working through the puzzle yourself. It also seems nicely holistic and better than taking an allopathic drug. But this may not be the case. Out of the twelve remedies mixed in the allergy combination there may be one that you need very badly. When you take the combination, you feel better immediately, even before the pellet dissolves on your tongue. You believe that homeopathy works and are happy that you tried it. But in time your allergies return. You take another dose, which takes longer to kick in and doesn't work as well. So you keep taking it. And as you keep taking it, you find that your allergies don't get better, they get worse.

Finally, you throw out that combination and get yourself a cortisone shot. Although you swell up something awful, your face looking a little like Humpty Dumpty, at least your allergies go away.

The problem here was in the combination. The combination had the one remedy you needed. If you had had a method of identifying it out of the twelve, you would be well and happy now, instead of swollen and miserable. The problem has to do with the other eleven remedies.

Homeopathic remedies are the only medicines that are tested on healthy human beings. They are tested by being taken repeatedly and seeing what they do to the whole system: body, mind, and spirit. These effects are noted in a number of people, and a map of the action of the remedy is set down. The process is known as "proving."

What you are doing in taking the twelve remedies over time is proving eleven out of the twelve remedies. You are seeing the combined effects of eleven extraneous remedies. The one correct remedy worked and helped you for as long as it could. But over time its action was overwhelmed by the other eleven. It wasn't a fair fight.

By the time you stop taking the combination remedy, your own symptom portrait has been so distorted that no one remedy can now clear the case. You have to suffer from the allergies for a period of time until the case again becomes clear. How long it will take until you are once again yourself in terms of your symptoms is anybody's guess. Months? Years?

That's why homeopathic remedies are given one remedy at a time and one dose at a time.

Many modern practitioners argue with this. They insist that in today's complicated world we have complicated diseases and need complicated remedies. That is the thinking behind all those "new and improved" products. Homeopathic remedies work as they have always worked. New situations may demand the creation of new remedies, often from the new poisons in our environment, but they in no way demand new methods of homeopathic practice.

Often those who say we need to combine remedies to combat our ills are caught up in doing just that: combating ills. The allopathic methodology has seeped into their homeopathic practice. These same practitioners would do well to go back to their materia medica in search of the one remedy that can bring about the cure in a given case. I equate combination remedies with allopathic drugs, as this is what they are.

If you are traveling to a foreign country and you want to use homeopathy, but have neither the education to know that you can select an appropriate remedy nor the room in your suitcase for seventy or eighty well-selected remedies that would prepare you for all events, you might well want to take along a small kit of combination remedies. Used in the short term for diarrhea or sunburn, these remedies will do no harm and may well be quite helpful. But know that what you are practicing is not homeopathy, efficacious as it may be. And know that for the long term, these combinations will do more harm than good.

The same is true of emergency situations. In emergencies—auto accidents and the like—remedies like Arnica and Aconite can and should be given in rapid alternation while waiting for the ambulance to arrive. But the use of more than one remedy like these should be restricted to the short-term preservation of life.

The third principle is the Law of Minimum. This Law of Cure is presented in two parts.

The first states that a remedy should always be given in the lowest possible effective potency. We want the remedy to have only slightly more power over the being than does the pain or issue presented. The patient who needs only a slight tap on the shoulder to make himself well should not instead be slapped across the face. The cure, while still rapid and permanent, above all else should be gentle.

When a remedy is given in too high a potency, it causes what is called an aggravation. An aggravation is a temporary increase in symptoms before these symptoms fall away. Although uncomfortable, this temporary bump on the road to healing is not dangerous. Some practitioners today practice by aggravations. They feel that if they are getting aggravations, they are choosing the right remedy. This is true, but it often means that they are choosing the wrong potency.

Hahnemann tells us in *The Organon* that aggravations are common and acceptable in the treatment of acute conditions like colds and flus. The symptoms increase for three or four hours before they go away for good.

But in cases involving chronic conditions, Hahnemann tells us that an aggravation is the sign that the potency is too high. The patient's system is being forced to express more than it can safely express. In chronic care the aggravation belongs only to the end of the case; after a period of correct treatment, the symptoms are likely suddenly and mysteriously to increase just before they disappear for good. He tells practitioners to watch this aggravation—it signals the completion of the action of the homeopathic remedy.

When we practice by aggravation, we cause unnecessary discomfort to patients. And when we practice by aggravation, we show our ignorance of homeopathic care.

As I have mentioned, homeopathic remedies come in three scales of potency. The X scale, created by a dilution of one part remedy to nine parts water, is the least powerful potency scale and is best used for situations in which the symptoms are held only in the physical body. The X scale remedies are appropriate for skin conditions, insect bites, and seasonal allergies such as hay fever.

The C scale, with its dilutions to the hundredths, is the medium potency scale. It is best selected for situations in which the symptoms blend the physical with the emotional, the visible with the invisible. It can be used in both acute and chronic situations and can be surprisingly powerful in long-term ailments. This is the potency scale most often used in homeopathic treatment.

The M scale is a continuation of the C scale and begins at the step of dilution just above 999C. The dilution here is to the thousandths, which, by the homeopathic concept of less being more, makes it the most powerful scale. The M scale remedies are most useful in situations in which the patient's symptom portrait largely involves mental and spiritual conditions. Ailments from grief, addictions, and emotional illness can all be well treated by remedies in the M potency.

The job of the practitioner, along with the actual case taking and selection of the appropriate remedy, is to select the potency of remedy to give and when to give it.

The Law of Minimum, by stating that we should always give the lowest effective potency of remedy, demands that we always err on the side of conservative thought when selecting a potency.

Kent tended, especially in the care of patients with chronic conditions, to begin with a very low potency, say a 9C or 12C, and slowly moved the potency up from there. He felt that the patient's energy should be stirred only very gently, and that, whereas you can always move up in potency to stir things up more rapidly, you cannot easily move the potency back down to calm the energy. Once you have started the expressive process, it is very difficult to stop it or slow it. If a practitioner finds himself faced with a patient whose symptoms blend the mental and physical and whose vital force is low, he would be wise to begin with that 9C potency and to watch and wait to see what happens next.

Paracelsus also gives us insight into the selection of potency. He likens the homeopathic potency to fire. He says that when you are chilly and need to build a fire, you do not sit and stare at the logs in the fireplace, trying to figure out how much fire you have to apply to the logs to cause them to burn. You simply strike a match, light a spark, and let that spark grow until the fire is raging.

Like Paracelsus, we need only give that patient a healing spark and trust the power of the remedy. That spark will spread, bringing healing to the whole being.

The understanding of this first aspect of the Law of Minimum comes with practice and with the actual use of the remedies. But the general trend toward conservative use of remedies always yields positive results.

The second part of the Law of Minimum tells us that we should use the fewest possible effective doses of a remedy.

This means that we can never use homeopathic remedies allopathically. We can never say that we should take a remedy once every three or four hours. Homeopathic remedies are the only medicines that should truly be taken only as needed.

When a remedy is taken, the first change that should take place is not a decrease in symptoms, but an increase in energy. The patient should simply "feel better." The migraine sufferer may still for a time have migraines, but he should be able to say, "I still get my headaches, but I can handle them better."

There is something of an arc to the energy increase. The remedy, by its potency, raises the patient's energy as high as it is able for as long as is possible. When the energy begins to fall and the illness again begins to take hold, a second dose should be given.

Many practitioners today simply give their patients a tube of 30C remedy and send them home, telling them to take the remedy three times a day for a month and then come back. This is a simple and easy way to practice, but it's not in any way homeopathic.

A great deal of what the patient comes to the practitioner for is education. The practitioner owes the patient an understanding of homeopathic philosophy and a treatment that adheres to that philosophy.

The patient should take the remedy as needed, with a clear definition of the maximum number of doses allowed in a given period of time. The patient should report back, by telephone if not in person, after a few days with how many doses he has had to take and how the remedy is acting in his system.

How often the remedy is needed is a guide to how high the potency should be. If the patient is taking 12C and the remedy is increasing his energy and improving his symptoms, but he needs to take it hourly to keep the process going, that is a clear sign that the remedy is correct but the potency is too low. The practitioner should move on to the next potency: 30C. (While remedies are, in theory, available and usable in all potencies, for simplicity's sake homeopathic pharmacies carry them in standard potencies: 6C, 9C, 12C, 30C, 200C, 1M, 10M, LM, and CM; the X scale potencies follow parallel to the C scale. Kent and other classic practitioners often started with the 9C and worked with a single remedy all the way up to the highest, the CM potency, before moving on to another remedy.)

In the same way, the potency also helps dictate the dosage. A patient who is given a 10M potency is very likely strongly warned against taking another dose of the remedy before some weeks or months have passed.

Through the guiding Laws of Similars, Simplex, and Minimum, homeopathy is practiced. All three principles are required for homeopathy to be practiced correctly.

Many modern practitioners differentiate between what they call modern homeopathy and classic homeopathy. With a wink they tell us that modern homeopaths, while clinging to the principle of Similar, have loosened their grip on Simplex and Minimum and that their methods have nearly miraculous results. With a second wink, they talk about classic homeopathy, which has to be allowed for those who do not accept the changes of the modern world. They conclude that, given the power of homeopathic remedies, even the uptight classic homeopaths can get some good results.

Unfortunately, classic practitioners cannot join their fellow practitioners in stating that there are two methods of homeopathic practice. Classic practitioners are most likely to follow the philosophical methods of either Hahnemann or Kent, both of whom would have been clear in their assessment of "modern" homeopathy: It may well work, but it certainly isn't homeopathy.

Remember, homeopathy isn't just remedies, it is a philosophy. And that philosophy, well understood and well practiced, is as vital to healing as are any of the remedies, no matter their potency or dosage. To throw out the philosophy, developed not just by Hahnemann but by Paracelsus and Hippocrates before him, is to join the allopaths in the belief that the principles by which we can become whole and well are constantly changing. But what the giants of homeopathy came to understand is that healing is healing is healing, and that the principles by which we can be healed are permanent and unchanging. Those who would kill these giants would also kill homeopathy.

THE SEARCH FOR THE SIMILLIMUM

A simillimum is, simply, the means by which the patient will be made well. It is the absolutely correct homeopathic remedy in the absolutely correct potency taken in the absolutely correct number of doses. Nothing else is a simillimum.

If any one part of the formula is in error, the simillimum, the total healing remedy, will not function as such. The patient may, for instance, be in need of the remedy Sulphur, but the practitioner has erred in his drug diagnosis and given Phosphorus, a remedy that is in many ways similar in its action to Sulphur. That remedy will certainly do the patient some good and cause some change for the better, but it will not be catalyst to a total healing.

The same is true for a correct remedy given in too low a potency. While some improvement of the case will surely take place, the healing will not be total. If the potency is too high, the healing process begins but with undue aggravations of the condition at hand.

Most often the distortion of the simillimum is in dosage. The appropriate number of doses of any remedy needed to open up any homeopathic case is one. Give the remedy once and see what happens. As with allopathy, more homeopathic cases are ruined by giving too much remedy than by giving too little.

When any one factor of the simillimum is incorrect, that remedy is said instead to be a similar. Homeopaths are human, so it is safe to say that more homeopathic cases are treated by the action of similar remedies than by any simillimum. That is why sometimes a homeopathic remedy brings about improvement without bringing a complete cure.

This makes the concept of the simillimum something of a Holy Grail of homeopathic practice. All practitioners seek perfection in treatment, but few attain it in any cases, and most attain it only in a few. But once you have witnessed the power of the simillimum to clear conditions that have been thought to be incurable—the power totally to transform the life of the patient and make him totally free of his illness—you become convinced that the practitioner must always painstakingly and prayerfully seek the simillimum.

Remember that the job of the practitioner is to free the patient not only from the illness at hand but also from the need to take any remedy. Homeopathic practitioners should be in the business of putting themselves out of business. The very principles by which they practice, especially the Law of Minimum, guide them to give only what remedy *must* be given in the potency in which it should be given and then to give no more.

If the very definition of health is freedom, both the freedom from illness and the freedom to live life completely in one's own body unrestricted from pain on the physical, mental, and emotional planes, then that definition must also include freedom from treatment. Homeopathic remedies used correctly are like the match striking the dry wood in the fireplace. They are catalysts, not crutches. They assist the human being in making the changes that need to be made to restore health and freedom, but they do not in and of themselves create health. They are the tools and not the finished product, the car and not the destination.

HANDLING THE REMEDIES

If you look at the tube of any homeopathic remedy you will find some information that will be troubling to you if you've been reading this book closely.

First, there are indications for the use of the remedy. For Phosphorus, you find "sore throat"; for Nux Vomica, "indigestion." There is no getting around the fact that listing the use of the remedy in this manner seems to make it a treatment of disease, not a treatment of persons with disease.

The remedy has directions for taking it, which usually read, "Take two or three pellets three times a day." This is, of course, a totally allopathic description of the use of a homeopathic remedy. It also has an expiration date.

The reason for all this is government standards. The rules set forth for product labeling by the FDA have no flexibility built in for products that do not work the way other products do. This labeling of homeopathic products is not only false but also counterproductive to their correct use.

A well-stored tube of homeopathic medicine will remain potent far longer than you will. It needs to be stored in a temperate place, out of bright sunlight and extreme temperatures either hot or cold. Store it away from strong smells, especially mothballs, as these smells can destroy the potency of any remedy. The remedies also should always be stored away from strong electromagnetic fields. Don't, for instance, keep the remedies by your computer, or on top of the television or refrigerator. Strong radiation of any sort (even airport X rays) can damage or destroy your remedies.

They are usually best stored on a closet shelf or under the bed. With their caps tightly on, homeopathic remedies will keep indefinitely.

Historically, homeopathic remedies were kept in glass vials topped with cork. Today, although some companies issue remedies in amber glass bottles, most sell them in plastic vials. In my experience, the remedies stored in plastic do not stay as potent as those stored in glass. I attribute this to the fact that glass is a natural product and plastic is synthetic.

TAKING THE REMEDIES

The label on the remedy tube tells you to take three or four pellets at a time. This would likely be necessary if the remedy were made from substance and not from energy. But the reality is that you receive the same energy if you take one pellet or if you take all of them. A dose of 30C is a dose of 30C is a dose of 30C, whether it is in the form of one pellet or ten. The power of multiple pellets comes from taking them over a period of time, in single doses, rather than in taking them all at once.

Some remedies tell you to take them all at once. Go ahead and do so, if you want to. You will only have to go out and buy more sooner, which will make that homeopathic retailer very happy indeed.

When taking the remedy, coat the tongue as best you can with the remedy. If your tongue is clean of any other flavors, most especially mint or coffee, all you need to take is one pellet. If, on the other hand, you have just brushed your teeth or eaten, you may want to use three or four pellets in order to coat the tongue. Anything beyond this offers no extra benefit.

Try to take the remedy either a good half hour before eating or at least an hour after. The taste you should have on your tongue is the taste of the tongue itself. Many people choose to take their remedy first thing in the morning, which is a great thing to do, if you don't follow the remedy with a cup of coffee or by brushing with a mint toothpaste.

It is important when taking a remedy—and especially when giving a remedy to someone else—that you do not touch the pellet. This is important for two reasons. First, you may have a chemical on your hands from soap, perfume, or lotion that ruins that dose of the remedy. Second, remember that your skin is you; through the contact of the remedy with your hand you have already dosed yourself. This is not so important if you are taking the remedy yourself, but if you are giving your kid a dose of Arsenicum, you could be creating trouble by taking that dose yourself.

This, however, can be a good thing to know if you want to give a loved one a remedy, but he thinks that homeopathy is crap. Ask him just to hold the remedy. Most people will, if only to shut you up. You'll know that he has been dosed, just as if he had swallowed it. This principle was proven by Hahnemann himself, who often dissolved the remedy in water and had the patient rub the water topically on the part of the body most affected by the ailment. Migraine sufferers, for example, would rub the remedy iris on their foreheads, sometimes taking the remedy orally as well. This turned out to be a very effective form of treatment. Some patients under care for chronic conditions also report that they feel better just by carrying their remedy in a pocket next to their body. They feel that having the remedy within their own energy field allows them to benefit continually from its potency.

The best way to take the remedy is to spill the pellet into the cap of the bottle and to drop that pellet onto the tongue. Let it dissolve there, either on or under the tongue, and then take no food or drink except water for a half hour while you give the remedy a chance to work.

ANTIDOTES TO TREATMENT

Many people panic over the idea of antidoting their homeopathic remedy. Some want to know that there are antidotes available and want to have them on hand when first taking their remedy, just in case they are not overwhelmed by health. Others fear the opposite, that they will accidentally antidote their remedy by something with which they have come into contact, through no fault of their own, making their chances of good health virtually over.

The reality is that homeopathic remedies are hearty energy packets. It is very difficult to stop their action once it has begun. Hahnemann kept a bottle of spirits of ammonia in his pocket while he was at the office. If a patient seemed to be going into aggravation from the remedy given, Hahnemann would hold the open bottle under the patient's nose. He said that the smell "blunted the action" of the remedy, making its continued action more tolerable for the patient.

In recent years we have become more and more interested in and frightened by the idea of antidoting homeopathic treatment. I ask my students what they have heard are antidotes to homeopathics, and the list of answers I receive gets longer and more ridiculous. Some people think that parsley undoes the work of their remedy; others refuse to get near a clove of garlic.

It is true that some substances and smells can interfere with homeopathic treatments, and the more allergic or sensitive you are, the more likely you are to be disrupted, especially by smells. But in general the things you have to look out for are very few.

Coffee is usually considered to be a sure antidote of homeopathics. But in fact coffee is, at most, problematic. It will disrupt most people in their treatment to the same extent that the coffee disrupted them before treatment. If one cup of coffee keeps someone up all night, then his homeopathic treatment will likely be disrupted by a small cup of coffee. On the other hand, the person who drinks twelve cups of coffee a day and sleeps at night will not be very disrupted by the beverage.

Some practitioners insist that their patients wean themselves off coffee before they can be treated. This seems unnecessary to me. First, homeopathic treatment always works from today backward, clearing away all that has been suppressed. If you demand that the patient first go off coffee, why don't you also demand that he first lose twenty pounds and finish his college degree? Then he won't need the practitioner's help at all.

Second, the use of coffee is a symptom, like anything else. We have to note it as such and note the impact of the bitter brew on the system. Then, with treatment begun, we have to note what changes are taking place with the coffee drinking, as with any other symptom, as the remedy takes hold.

It is seldom appropriate when beginning homeopathic treatment to take a patient off an allopathic drug that he is taking every day. Instead, the homeopathic remedy is given, and when the patient feels better and stronger, he will taper the use of the drug in his own time and his own way. (Certainly, drugs like insulin should never be removed without the full knowledge of the allopath who prescribed them. Indeed, it is of the highest importance that nothing be done in secret, that all doctors and practitioners know of each other's presence in the case, and if possible communicate their approach, philosophy, and practice.) The person addicted to coffee is addicted to a drug. So is the sugar addict. It is part of the healing process for them to free themselves from this addiction in their own good time. Those who insist on great personal changes and sacrifices up front before treatment begins do not really trust the power of homeopathy. Give the remedy to coffee drinkers, perhaps in a lower potency than you might ordinarily, with more doses than usual, to keep the remedy moving with the added weight of the coffee. Trust the remedy and watch what happens.

The other substance that is often considered a true antidote is mint. Although it can interfere with the power of the remedy, I am wary of using the word *antidote*. Instead, I simply caution those who take homeopathics to be aware that mint can disrupt the remedy and that the mint in toothpaste can be a problem in particular. Most homeopathic pharmaceutical firms make toothpastes that do not interfere with the remedy and are a good idea for those undergoing treatment to use. Candy mints, too, can be a problem and should be avoided. Again, this is largely an individual thing. The more sensitive the person to foods, drinks, smells, and environment, the more likely he is to be disrupted by mint.

Then there are smells. Perfumes and petrochemicals are the most troublesome. Some people are so sensitive that the briefest scent of a particular perfume gives them a headache for a day. These people find their homeopathic treatment disrupted by smells, perhaps to the point of total antidoting. People who are or have been environmentally ill must be very, very careful of the smells with which they come into contact when undergoing treatment. As the homeopathics strengthen the overall system, they will find themselves much more able to withstand such smells and environmental toxins in the future. But, for the duration of treatment, a trip to the local mall might undo a good deal of good work.

Perhaps the environment that is most difficult for successful homeopathic treatment is one that contains a great deal of electromagnetic interference. The person who spends all day in front of a computer screen may be setting up a very difficult healing situation, as is one who lives near high-tension wires. As seemingly benign an object as an electric blanket can make treatment very difficult as well as create major chronic conditions. Think about it. That blanket covers your body in a web of electricity for up to one third of your day. As your brain communicates with your body through bioelectricity, this can set up a very damaging situation.

So when you consider treatment, you need to consider your environment. Does your bedroom closet have a load of mothballs in it? Isn't it possible that what is poison to the moths is also poison to you? Mothballs, which leach into the wood of the closet or dresser drawers over time, making them impossible to get rid of, have been shown to be an environmental hazard in and of themselves. And they are a sure antidote to homeopathy and even destroy the remedies themselves.

In the same way, the bathroom, a hotbed of strong scents and perfumes, greatly disrupts the homeopathic treatment of the chronically ill. In fact, their presence in the household may well have created the problem to begin with. Add to this the cleaning products you have under the bathroom and kitchen sinks. All these strong smells can be toxic in the environment and can interfere with treatment.

Now consider the chemicals on the lawn and ask yourself why you feel ill every time you sit outdoors. And consider the radiation in your house. If you are in doubt, get yourself a battery-powered AM radio and walk around the house. Put it next to the microwave, the iron, the refrigerator, the television, the computer, and all your appliances. Whatever disrupts the radio signal is also disrupting your own bioelectric system.

Some of these toxins in and of themselves are not such a big deal. But put them together in one place, combine them in ways that their manufacturers never even considered, and you may find yourself in an environment that not only causes disease but also works to keep you ill, even when you undergo homeopathic treatment.

Again, it's like the coffee addict. We start treatment with today, using the current situation as the symptom portrait, seeking to strengthen the system in such a way that it's no longer affected by the environmental toxins. But in Aphorism 77 of *The Organon*, Hahnemann tells us that "those diseases are inappropriately named chronic which persons incur who expose themselves continually to *avoidable* noxious influences, who are in the habit of indulging in injurious liquors or ailments, are addicted to dissipation of many kinds that undermine the health, who undergo prolonged abstinence from things that are necessary for the support of life, who reside in unhealthy localities, especially marshy districts, who are housed in cellars or other confined dwellings, who are deprived of exercise or of open air, who ruin their health by overexertion of the body or mind, who live in a constant state of worry, etc. . . ."

In other words, people who live in damp houses shouldn't sling mud. Or, although practitioners certainly cannot demand change of the patient before change is begun by the remedy, we as patients must try to make what adjustments we can in our lives and lifestyles before we go looking for our solution in pills.

Another consideration is diet. And, again, there is no one simple answer for a world that is made up of unique individuals.

One thing is sure, though. No one diet is suitable for all of us. Each of us is nourished by some foods and poisoned by others. Paracelsus tells us that *all* things are poison; it is just a matter of amount that makes it toxic. This means that even a food as wonderful as carrots can become toxic if they are all you eat. The same for meat and spinach and sugar. *Any* food will become the cause of an allergic reaction over time if it is overeaten. Just look at how many of us are now allergic to wheat and to dairy products, which was not the case a century ago. Why? These two foods were not eaten in such large quantities; consumed in moderation they do not become the poison that Paracelsus warned against.

Food allergies can be tricky things during homeopathic treatment. It is best to try and put aside, temporarily, the foods that you know are problematic for you. That may mean no pizza for a few months, but it also means that ultimately you'll get to eat a pizza every now and then without the stomach cramps that the wheat and cheese combination now gives you. As with environmental poisons, foods that are toxic become less and less toxic as the overall system is strengthened by homeopathic treatment.

The first step is to identify what foods are nourishing to you.

There are a number of good nutrition books and books of food allergies on the market. Most of these include a rotation diet that allows the patient to identify which food or foods are most problematic. Those foods should be avoided during the homeopathic treatment.

While undergoing treatment, Hahnemann always tried to convince his patients that a somewhat bland, well-balanced diet is best. In the footnote to Aphorism 260 of *The Organon*, Hahnemann writes that those undergoing treatment should avoid: "highly spiced dishes and sauces; spiced cakes and ices; crude medicinal vegetable for soups; dishes of herbs, roots and stalks of plants possessing medicinal qualities; asparagus with long green tips, hops, and all vegetables possessing medicinal properties, celery, onions; old cheese, and meats that are in a state of decomposition, or that possess medicinal properties (as the flesh and fat of pork, ducks and geese, or veal that is too young and sour viands), ought just as certainly to be kept from the patients as they should avoid all excesses in food, and in the use of sugar and salt, as also spirituous drinks, undiluted with water, heated rooms, woolen clothing next to the skin, a sedentary life in close apartments, or the frequent indulgence in mere passive exercise. . . ."

Certainly, we remember that homeopathic treatment always begins with today, and with the lifestyle and habits that we have today, but the patient should also remember that if his lifestyle were perfect, if it were not in need of some change, he would not be sick to begin with. The changes for the better that the patient can make on a conscious level speed the cure and make the healing process easier.

Hahnemann was something of a stoic when he insisted that his patients get up and exercise just as much and as soon as possible. But in making this demand, far from displaying a heartless character, he was showing his patients just how he cared for them. Look at the Gospels, specifically at the passages in which Jesus brings healing to individuals. Without exception he tells them to arise. He says, "Get up and walk."

This is another area in which modern medicine seems to have missed the boat. All too often, doctors and nurses use medicines to soothe pain and to knock the patient unconscious, when what is needed is to keep the patient moving. It is of great importance to healing that the patient move and exercise as much as he is able.

Certainly, we cannot expect people to change more than they can change. We should not give a remedy in a potency so high that it seeks to make them express more than they can safely express. In the same way, the caffeine addict needs to be allowed to hold on to his coffee for a bit longer. And those who love spicy foods should be allowed to continue with these foods if they feel that they need to.

But it is important that at every stage of homeopathic treatment, from the first step to the last, the practitioner remind the patient that change is always possible. That change can be a form of spontaneous combustion. He can let go of his need for toxic habits and, in doing so, bring himself a step or two closer to being a totally whole person who is free from illness, who is free altogether. While the practitioner should never require change of the patient, because that almost ensures a continuation of his "noxious habits," the practitioner owes the patient a reminder that change can and will occur.

SIGNS OF IMPROVEMENT

As has been mentioned, the immediate end of symptoms is not the usual response to homeopathic treatment. Most often, the first sign of improvement is simply a sense of well-being, a feeling that the burden of a patient's symptoms is not as great and heavy as it has been.

Another clear sign of improvement is increased clarity of mind. Many people when they are sick feel as if they have lost a part of themselves. Their memory is now confused, and their mind is clouded. Allopathic drugs only add to the mental confusion. But homeopathic remedies increase clarity of mind. Patients on homeopathics need not fear driving or using heavy equipment as they have to when they take Nyquil.

Another very important sign of improvement is an increased sense of freedom. Patients with colitis, for example, no longer feel that they have to know the location of every restroom between their home and their destination. Instead, they feel that they can simply get in the car and drive. In the same way, phobics find themselves somewhat mysteriously able to do things that before were impossible, when their life was defined by fear and not by freedom.

In some cases, however, the physical condition grows worse before it gets better. A phobic is a perfect example of this. As others who suffer from mental and emotional conditions discover, a phobic often finds that, as his mind clears and his emotions calm, he suffers the brief reemergence of some physical condition that he had some years before and was suppressed into the system.

As the mind is more important to the being than is the body, it follows that as the symptoms of the mind become balanced and clear, the deeply suppressed symptoms of the body that had affected the mind and the emotions have to be brought forth again. These must flow down from the mind into the body before they can be fully expressed and removed from the system. It can be difficult indeed for the practitioner to explain to the patient that the reappearance of asthma, a condition that the patient thought was cured many years ago, is not a sign that he is growing sicker and weaker but is really a sign that all that has been suppressed is now being brought again to the surface and will soon be washed away.

Homeopathic treatment is all about letting go. The grief that the widow has clung to since the death of her husband has to be let go if she is to be well. The rage that powers and kills the violent man has to be let go if he is to be well.

The same is true on the physical level. Whatever conditions have been suppressed by powerful allopathic treatments have to be brought to the surface before they can be let go.

In this way, homeopathic treatment is about removing layers. As each suppressed layer is removed, the layer below is exposed, and symptoms that the patient has not had for twenty years are likely to reappear. It is the job of the practitioner to educate and, in some cases, warn the patient about this process.

The patient who, at age forty, suddenly experiences symptoms that he has not experienced since age thirteen, has simply cleared his system of all suppression dating back to that thirteenth year. As the homeopathic process continues, he may find himself again with symptoms dating from earlier and earlier years.

As these symptoms from past suppressions reappear, it is vital that they *not* be treated. As homeopaths never treat specific diseases, this should be a simple concept, but many patients panic over the recurrence of some pain that they hoped they would never have to face again. The sheer force of this fear can influence the practitioner, who might make the mistake of treating that recurring symptom instead of continuing the present treatment and simply waiting as the past condition reappears and then disappears for all time.

It is important that the patient know that the suppressed condition will never recur with the same violence that it once contained, that its appearance will be brief, and that once gone again, it is gone for good.

Homeopathic literature is full of cases of gonorrheal flow that begins again when the patient undergoes treatment. Certainly in a case like this it can be quite difficult for the practitioner to keep the patient on course, but after the recurrence of one or two old ailments, the patient will be calm in the knowledge that this is how the remedies work and how he or she will ultimately become well.

Everything that is suppressed must be expressed. This is the method by which we are made well.

THE SECOND PRESCRIPTION

Based on his many years of practice, Kent tells us that "the first prescription is easy, the second prescription is hard."

This may be daunting to the overburdened homeopathic practitioner. On top of the need to find the simillimum in the first place, he must be knowledgeable and skillful enough to determine when that first remedy has done all that it will do and when to go on to another remedy.

With acute cases, it can be fairly simple. Most common colds need two or three remedies to clear up. You can judge most easily when to shift remedies by when the quality and amount of the mucus changes. A remedy that worked well for watery discharge is of little help when the nasal flow is yellow and thick. In the same way, modalities, especially body temperature, hunger, and thirst, can be of great help in determining the second remedy.

Also important are the mental symptoms. The person who has become angry with his cold is not helped by a remedy that produces a gentle and even tearful persona in a healthy person.

In chronic cases, the same blend of mental symptoms and modalities is of great help, but even the finest practitioner may be puzzled as to whether to raise the potency but keep the remedy the same, or to go on to the next suggested remedy.

A great sign of needed change is what I call the "pentimento effect." If one paints a picture over a previous picture, in time the first painting begins to blend in with the second. So, too, do the symptoms of a remedy type that a patient is moving into begin to bleed into the present picture. But not until the new image replaces the old should the practitioner move on to the new remedy.

Here the practitioner must remember always to treat the symptoms as they are presented today and try not to guess what tomorrow will bring. (This may well be more difficult for practitioners with a strong sense of materia medica, who are more likely to have a case suggest multiple remedies to them than are those less versed in the different remedy types. These practitioners are likely to think in terms of the entire flow of different remedies that make up the entire treatment program, rather than simply to choose the remedy needed today. This skill can be very helpful, but it can also color the practitioner's judgment process as to just when to move on to that next remedy.) When the symptom picture today matches the remedy portrait of a new remedy, then it is time to give that remedy. Up until that moment, when the second remedy may be bleeding in, but the overall picture is still clearly the first treated, it is appropriate to continue the same remedy, perhaps increasing its potency in order to continue the healing process.

But, as all patients are individuals, it always comes down to a judgment call. If the practitioner is wise, he is once again conservative in his actions, knowing that, should he choose to continue with the same remedy, he can always move on to the next one in the future. But if he moves on too quickly to the next remedy, he may hamper or even disrupt the case.

For this reason, when in doubt, the wise practitioner waits. This may take more patience on the part of the patients than they are happy to give, but ultimately it brings about a swifter and gentler cure.

MIXING MODALITIES OF TREATMENTS

A friend of mine once sought relief from her seasonal allergies. The homeopathic remedy she was taking had been given to her on a constitutional basis—treatment for her whole being and not just for the allergies—and she was struggling through that particular season. Even though she knew that the treatment would help prevent future seasons, she was still suffering and still in need of relief.

She had heard that acupuncture acts on the human system in a manner very similar to homeopathy. She went to a very fine acupuncturist and received several treatments in rapid succession. She found that not only did her allergies get no better, but they got a great deal worse.

Because acupuncture works in a manner that is so similar to homeopathy, the blending of these two modalities at the same time has an action in the human system that is very similar to taking two homeopathic remedies concurrently or, even worse, to taking combination remedies.

Combining any form of energy treatment with homeopathy sets up the same sort of situation that you find when taking multiple remedies. The symptoms shift here and there in the system, and the system as a whole is asked to respond to several messages at once. The result is that the overall case becomes muddled and confused. And the patient may find the symptoms shifting wildly and the old, familiar patterns being distorted, the symptoms themselves growing worse and worse.

The way homeopathy and acupuncture work best together is to use one modality at a time. Start, for instance, with acupuncture and continue the treatments until the improvement plateaus, until the symptoms reach some form of balance. Then move on to homeopathy, taking the remedy until the symptoms once again improve to the next plateau.

This method of alternating modalities of treatment works well with any form of energy treatment, from reiki to Bach flower remedies. Bach's remedies are in their way homeopathic; they are mother tinctures, or zero-potency remedies, that while homeopathically prepared have yet to be fully potentized. They are also similar enough to Hahnemann's remedies in their actions to be used successfully with the standard homeopathic pharmacy. The way Bach's remedies may be used with Hahnemann's is by giving the patient a single dose of a high-potency Hahnemannian remedy, usually in a potency of 1M or above. After a period of time, a week or several weeks, this dose can be followed by the Bach remedies as a supplement to the single dose. But using Bach remedies with a lower potency of homeopathic remedy once again totally confuses the case and possibly worsens the entire situation.

Direct energy work, from polarity therapy to faith healing, also works directly with the system's energy body and interferes with homeopathic remedies, confusing the case and disrupting the patient's symptom portrait.

On the other hand, because of their similarity, these other modalities of healing are useful in clearing a muddled case. If, for whatever reason, the practitioner cannot discover one clear symptom portrait, it is often helpful for that patient to have a treatment or two from a good acupuncturist *before* he is given any homeopathic remedy. As sorbet clears the palate between dinner courses, so too does acupuncture clear the muddled symptom portrait and place the patient more clearly with the symptom portrait of the remedy needed.

My friend with the seasonal allergies faced the question that many other patients undergoing constitutional treatments for chronic conditions do. Constitutional treatment allows patients to work through all their various suppressions and denials and work backward to health and freedom. But having come face to face with an acute situation, should patients step away from their constitutional remedy and deal directly with the acute situation, or should they stay the course with the remedy that is already working and get through the acute as best they can?

As always seems to be the case in the world of homeopathy, there is no one clear answer to that question. Instead, we must answer that question on a case-by-case, situation-by-situation basis. The rule of thumb here is that, if the patient can deal with the acute situation, if it is not so powerful or violent that it creates its own loss of freedom on the part of the patient, it is far better to stay with the remedy that is already working and to let the acute situation resolve itself. Certainly in the case of a simple headache or cold, the patient should just go forward, knowing that the acute situation at hand will not in any way truly challenge his ability to live life fully. But say you trip and fall, and manage to scratch your cornea in the fall. In a situation as painful as this, even if the cornea is one of the fastest and most effectively self-healing parts of the body, some consideration must be given to the acute situation.

If you go on to use another remedy for the sake of an acute situation, it is very important not simply to go back to the old remedy when the acute situation is cleared. Certainly with a physical trauma like a scratched cornea, it is highly unlikely that the acute remedy will in any way change the patient's need for the deeper-acting constitutional remedy. It may be that the acute situation, such as a simple cold, is actually the expression of a previously suppressed disease. In fact, one of the healthiest responses the system can make to first undergoing homeopathic treatment is to come down with a cold. This represents the detoxification of the system and should under no circumstances be treated with a different remedy. It is a clear sign that the remedy selected is doing exactly what it needs to do.

So the best course of action in this situation is once again to wait—and, if necessary, take the case once again, to see if the acute ailment and its treatment have in any way changed the overall symptom portrait. Wait and do not give any remedy until a specific remedy is called for.

Without a doubt the best medical modalities for use in combination with homeopathic treatment are those that center their action primarily on the physical body. Massage therapy, physical therapy, the Alexander technique, and chiropractic medicine all are holistic modalities that seek to stimulate the physical body in much the same way that homeopathics do the energy system. For this reason, a combined treatment of homeopathics and especially chiropractics often moves a situation along much more quickly and easily.

Homeopathics also work extremely well with the insights and techniques that a psychologist brings to a case. The remedy, used in conjunction with psychotherapy, stimulates expression, both verbal and systemic, and supports the patient's vital force through the rigors of psychological treatment.

In general, those therapeutics that work best alongside homeopathy are those that share the holistic viewpoint but seek to come at the patient's motivating issue from another angle. Vision therapy, which can tackle a patient's chronic complaints through the avenue of eyesight, also work very well with homeopathic treatment.

Finally, there are times when combining homeopathic and allopathic modalities can be not only acceptable but actually helpful.

Take, for example, a headache. You are on a homeopathic remedy, and that remedy is bringing about great changes in your system. Body, mind, and spirit, you are feeling increased clarity, improved energy, and a sense of well-being. On Sunday morning, you awaken with a headache. You do not get them often, and this one seems related to the stress of your last work week. I believe that you are better off taking a Tylenol than you are seeking a homeopathic alternative remedy or just sitting in pain all day. But know what you are doing: You are simply suppressing the symptoms of that headache. Unless you work with the cause on some deeper level, it will recur. So take the Tylenol, it won't kill you, but also go for a walk or get a massage—deal with the stress at hand. A little suppression in an acute situation is far less damaging in the long run than is being a homeopathic martyr.

Allopathic medicine, which basically functions from crisis to crisis, is excellent in emergency situations. If I broke my leg, I would go to the emergency room and have that leg set. At the same time, of course, I would take Arnica to promote healing, and follow up with Symphytum to help speed that bone's reconstruction after being set.

The same is true in life-threatening situations. There is nothing wrong with taking an antibiotic when a life-and-death crisis is at hand. I believe that we must save the life by any means necessary before we can promote total health and freedom by undertaking homeopathic treatment.

But we have to face the reality that allopathy and homeopathy each work in a very different manner and do not work very well together. In a life-threatening crisis, we may have to blend these two modalities of treatment to preserve life at that moment, but for long-range treatments, suppressive medicines and expressive remedies together only further stress an already weakened system. There are those practitioners, both homeopathic and allopathic, who seek an "interface" between these opposite healing philosophies. But such an interface cannot exist. An individual cannot both suppress and express symptoms at the same time. Our desire to be well ultimately demands that we choose the path of our healing.

CONSIDERING THE REMEDIES THEMSELVES

The literally thousands of remedies on the market are made from many substances, animal, vegetable, and mineral. About 60 percent of the remedies are taken from vegetable substances, with about 20 percent each made from animal substances and minerals.

It is important to remember that the homeopathic pharmacy is taken from the ancient herbal tradition, the same tradition that was the basis for allopathic medicine. It is simply a matter of what is done with these substances, whether they are diluted and potentized as in homeopathic medicine, or processed, and often synthesized, as in allopathics, that determines their different actions.

Examples of remedies that are made from vegetable matter are Pulsatilla, which is created from the anemone, also known as the windflower. The plant was called the pasqueflower by our ancestors because it blooms at Easter and was used in the dyeing of Easter eggs. The whole plant, just at the flowering stage, is used to create the remedy. The remedy Thuja is made from the arbor vitae, a plant that in ancient Greece was considered sacred and from which the incense that was burned in the religious temples was made.

Remedies taken from mineral substances include Natrum Muriaticum, which is taken from regular table salt, Aurum, which is made from gold, and Argentum, which is made from the metal silver.

Many remedies are made from animal substances as well. Bee venom is used to create the remedy Apis, and snake venom is used in the creation of Lachesis.

Of the animal remedies, perhaps the story of Sepia's creation is the most interesting. Samuel Hahnemann had a patient come to him who was in chronic pain. This pain was such that it literally made him weep to talk about it, yet he was curiously stoic and uncaring when it came to his own family and their ills. Hahnemann, as was his habit whenever possible, spent time with the man and followed him as he went through his day. The man was an artist. Hahnemann watched the man at work and noticed that he was using a brown liquid in his painting. The man would touch his brush in the liquid, then touch it to his tongue to dilute the color, then brush it on his canvas. Hahnemann asked what the liquid was and learned that it was cuttlefish ink, which the artist was using in a process of tinting called sepia tone. Hahnemann asked if he could have some of the liquid, which he diluted and succussed and made into a homeopathic remedy that he called Sepia. To his amazement, the remedy not only cured the man of all his ills but over time became known as one of the most powerful and important homeopathic remedies.

Any natural substance can be made into a homeopathic remedy because all things natural to creation have the same spark of creation in them, the same vital force.

Another way to look at it is to remember Paracelsus's statement that all things are poison and it is just a matter of dosage that determines toxicity. Match this with Hering's pronouncement that "the stronger the poison, the stronger the cure" and you have the basis for the creation of the entire homeopathic pharmacy.

If all things are toxic at some level, then nothing is truly inert. Everything, in some amount or other, is a catalyst for change. What the potentization process does is release the energy that is the catalyst while leaving the physical toxin behind with the remaining substance.

Given that "the stronger the poison, the stronger the cure," those homeopathic remedies made from very toxic substances, commonly called poisons, such as arsenic from which Arsenicum is made, are the more powerful tools for change and are very often more powerful remedies than are those created from more benign substances.

It is important to note however, that a patient need never worry that a remedy such as Arsenicum will cause arsenic poisoning. By the action of potentization, the substance of the remedy has been left behind, with only the energy remaining. In other words, while the substances from which homeopathic remedies are made are often very toxic, the remedies themselves are not. Quite the opposite. Remedies made from toxins are very healing to the system.

Today, many homeopathic remedies are made not from natural substances but from artificial toxins. They are created most often from the chemicals that poison our environment. An example of this is the remedy Naphthalene, which is taken from the chemical of the same name that is used in the process of dry cleaning and in the making of mothballs. Many people have been made sensitive to the chemical by years of constant exposure, and the remedy was created specifically to combat that poisoning.

The remedies made from artificial toxins that have invaded our lives are thought of as acute remedies. They are used in a manner that is almost allopathic, that is, to combat a specific poisoning or disease. They seldom speak to the totality of a person's symptom portrait, but rather are used in the short term to clear away a specific weakness in that system and to build a foundation of strength on which the healing process may stand. Some practitioners use these remedies taken from specific allergens; some do not, instead standing by the "classical" approach to homeopathy and selecting one remedy that best matches the overall symptom portrait. While I certainly prefer the second approach, both are effective forms of treatment, and the use of remedies taken from specific allergens does no harm.

Another method by which homeopathic remedies are classified has to do with the quality of the source materials from which the remedy has been made.

Remedies that are made from healthy plant and animal tissue or from pure mineral substances are known as sarcodes. This category includes most of our homeopathic remedies, like Natrum Muriaticum, which are taken from natural substances that are in no way tainted. The action of the remedy, therefore, reflects the vital force of the substance itself in its natural state. For example, Natrum Muriaticum reflects salt's natural ability to absorb and retain. The person who needs Natrum Mur, as the remedy is usually called, follows a similar theme in his own life, absorbing and retaining (while usually also denying that he is either absorbing or retaining) all of life's insults and injuries on the physical, mental, and emotional levels. Sarcodes are remedies with clear signals, reflecting the vital force of the substance from which they have been taken.

Some remedies, however, are taken from tainted substances such as diseased tissue, as in the case of Tuberculinum, which is made from tubercular lung tissue of sheep or cattle, or Pyrogenium, which is made from rotted and putrid beef and/or pork. These remedies speak with a deeper message, not only of the substance from which they have been taken but also of the disease that infected that substance. Therefore, the remedy Tuberculinum speaks not only of the substance of that tubercular tissue but also of the deeper causes of the disease itself. It should not surprise that these are our most potent homeopathic remedies. They can carry the system toward healing with the deepest and most permanent result. They are called nosodes.

The final grouping in this classification is controversial. It is also the fastest growing group of remedies in the modern practice of homeopathy. Known as isodes, these remedies are made from your own tissues in order to treat your own diseases. The most common tissue from which a remedy can be made is blood, and remedies are also commonly created from saliva and urine. Any part of the body, like any other natural substance, can be made into a homeopathic remedy.

For many practitioners and patients alike, the use of isodes seems to be the most homeopathic application of homeopathic philosophy. What poison, they ask, can speak more specifically to your own than your own?

My own experience with a remedy made from my own blood, a fad in the homeopathic world for the past few years, is that it doesn't work very well. I believe that isodes palliate symptoms for a time, but they do not bring about any sort of permanent transformation.

I took my blood remedy in order to clear seasonal allergies. When I first took it, I found that I was filled with energy—four hours of sleep a night was more than enough. And, as if I were taking speed, I seemed to be moving faster than everyone else around me. The impatience that has clung to my nature for many years now seemed to be racing out of control; it seemed to have taken over my whole being. In other words, the remedy made from my own blood made me act even more like myself than I usually do. I feel sorry for those around me, who had to deal with me when I was taking this remedy. All my virtues and flaws were still in place, except magnified in their aspect. I was myself, cubed.

My allergies disappeared immediately, only to return slowly over a period of weeks. And after a couple of weeks of experiencing my intensified nature, I began to collapse inward, as if I had finally tired of being myself. After a time, the remedy stopped working altogether.

I have heard it explained that the reason isodes do not work very well is that they really aren't homeopathic in their use. The Law of Similars states that "like cures like," not "exactly the same cures exactly the same."

The way I see it, no one can ever be his own simillimum. If our vital force knew how to heal itself, it would have already done so. So a remedy taken from our own vital force simply does not have the power to begin and end a healing process.

Besides, there is a great problem in the using of isodes. They are not thoroughly tested and proved as remedies, and until a remedy is completely proved, we cannot know its actions. Therefore, while you may be walking around with my cure for cancer in your blood, there is no way of predicting that your own blood will be your own solution to anything.

HOMEOPATHIC SCHOOLS OF THOUGHT

Homeopathic remedies represent not aches and pains, but persons with bodies, minds, and spirits who are themselves experiencing some form of ache or pain. So there are as many ways of classifying the remedies as there are methods of classifying persons. But basically the classification of homeopathic remedies follows one of two schools of thought. These schools of thought determine the method by which the remedies are used.

The first school, made up largely of those who reject the work of Samuel Hahnemann in his Paris years, is known as biochemical homeopathy. This school is rational in its approach, and its treatment emphasizes the physical body. Like a French rationalist, the biochemical homeopath is likely to find that the patient's unsettled emotions and troubled spirit are the creation of a chemical imbalance in the physical body. Much emphasis is given to the development of the embryo in biochemical homeopathy, and much credence is given to the results of any number of tests performed on the physical body.

The second school of thought is largely filled with those who follow Kent and who also approve of Hahnemann's writings in his final years. These are the anthropomorphic homeopaths, and they stress the invisible parts of the human system, the emotions and the spirit, over the tangible and visible body. For them, as for Kent, the disease diagnosis takes on less and less importance the more the practitioner works with the remedies, and these remedies are increasingly prescribed in response to the patient's basic motivations. The anthropomorphic homeopath believes that if you give the right remedy to the patient, that remedy acts on the entirety of that patient's system, improving the quality of his entire life, including the group of specific symptoms that we call disease. This, of course, is irrational medicine, in that it believes that disease is conceptual in nature, caused by thoughts and emotions and not by viruses and bacteria. Practitioners of this school believe that if they can change the concept that is creating the illness, then they can shift the patient from disease toward wellness.

Like the high-potency versus the low-potency prescribers, the biochemical and anthropomorphic practitioners are divided by a schism wide enough to seem unbridgeable. Instead of offering a solution to the problem, I can only acknowledge that it exists. I believe, though, that as long as one practices homeopathy following the Three Laws of Cure and trusts the action of the remedies, it really matters very little where one goes from there. High-potency or low, single dose or many, anthropomorphic or biochemical—no matter the philosophy behind the treatment, it will work, just so long as it is given a chance to work homeopathically, which is to say by the principle of expression.

The best homeopathy is now and always will be the simplest homeopathy. Nothing, no machine or fad application of homeopathic principles, will ever take the place of solid case taking to select the needed remedy. Along with this, a good practitioner needs a complete understanding of materia medica.

With thousands of remedies available, it has become more and more difficult for the modern practitioner to keep up with his materia medica study. But perhaps another classification of remedies is most useful here. Out of the thousands of remedies great and small, constitutional and acute, a small group have been identified and called polycrests.

Like everything else in homeopathy, the exact number of remedies that can be called polycrests is largely left up to the training and experience of the individual practitioner. But all agree that the polycrest remedies are those that are most important in the practice of homeopathy. This is because polycrests are those remedies that speak to the widest range of symptoms and to the basic motivations, like fear and grief, that are most common to the human condition.

Many students of homeopathy overlook the polycrests in treatment, in the mistaken belief that an individual needs to have all the listed symptoms of a remedy present in his system for that remedy to be helpful. This is not the case. Think of a polycrest remedy like Sulphur as being a big house. For you to need Sulphur, you need only be in that house, to be living out some aspect of this remedy type. You don't have to be that whole house yourself. The important thing is that all the symptoms you are now experiencing are part of Sulphur's remedy portrait, not that all of Sulphur's symptoms are a part of your own experience.

We use the polycrests in all forms of treatment. That is why it is most important that we study and understand them above and beyond all other remedies. Beyond this, we need to know how to repertorize and to select the smaller remedies when they are needed, as they sometimes are. But the practitioner who seeks to wow the homeopathic world by coming to a great understanding of tiny remedies like Heckla Lava will be of little help in actually removing disease.

Kent tells us that the beginning practitioner uses only about a dozen remedies, because those are all the remedies he knows, and that he does good work about half the time. Practitioners who are in their middle years of practice, who have read many books and taken many classes, make use of dozens and dozens of remedies and do the patient some good only about a third of the time. Practitioners who have a lifetime of experience in homeopathy use pretty much the same dozen remedies they started with, but because they now understand the remedies and human nature, they are successful in their treatments about 90 percent of the time.

In the next section, I explore some individual remedies, all of which are polycrests. These remedies are essential in the practice of homeopathy and represent archetypes of the human condition.

Part Three

EXPERIENCING

The patient of tomorrow must understand that he and he alone can bring himself relief from suffering, though he may obtain advice and help from an elder brother who will assist him in his effort. In the future there will be no pride in being ill: on the contrary, people will be as ashamed of sickness as they should be of crime.

—*Edward Bach*

7

CONSIDERING EMERGENCIES: ACUTE TREATMENTS

The Bible tells us that "faith without works is dead." Even if we have the deepest and most abiding faith in God, unless we somehow activate that faith and do something to show God's creativity in our own lives, all we have in our faith is an empty promise. The same is true in homeopathy. At some point, we must handle the remedies themselves. We have to use our faith that if we follow the philosophy of homeopathy in using the remedies, we not only will do no harm to anyone, including ourselves, but we may do a great deal of good.

It has been my experience as a homeopathic educator that those who do not bother to learn the philosophy first just cannot wait to go out and buy a kit and a book that distills all the remedies to a sentence each and start handing out the remedies like candy on Halloween. The fact that they might be practicing incorrectly, might even be practicing allopathy by their misuse of the remedies, doesn't bother them one bit.

Even at best, it has been my experience that those who go about learning homeopathy by starting with emergency treatments and not by learning the guiding philosophy never seem to progress in their understanding beyond acute treatments. Their thinking seems to stay mired in the treatment of disease and never in the transformation of the person. This is true of professional practitioners as well as laypeople—their patients never seem to get totally well.

Acute homeopathy seeks only to restore status quo and is at once the simplest form of homeopathic practice and the most similar to allopathic medicine. If someone has fallen and hurt himself, or has a cold or the flu, you don't particularly care about what his total health has been like up until that moment. You just want to end the discomfort and restore his health as best you can.

This makes for an easier form of case taking. What the prescriber needs to know is not the entire medical history of the patient but simply what has changed about the patient—the total patient, body, mind, and spirit— since the emergency began. In other words, for the homeopath dealing with an acute situation, it is less important to know about the moment you were hit by the truck than to know what you did after you were hit by that truck. Are you now afraid of trucks? Are you angry at the driver? What happened since the event took place and how did you, as an individual, deal with the shock of the injury? The point of the case taking is to individualize the case out of the standard. Often, in emergency situations, the prescriber has to know even more about the materia medica of the situation than does a constitutional prescriber, because the patient may not be able to give any information at all. He may be unconscious, or in such great discomfort that he cannot cooperate with the case taking. So the prescriber needs to know what to look for, how to differentiate this case as an individual event.

If the prescriber does this, if he puts the time and energy into a solid knowledge of the handful of remedies that are most often used in emergency situations, and if he takes the time to learn to receive information in ways other than verbal, then he is able to do a great deal of good in situations that otherwise are painful at best.

In working with acute situations, one quickly learns that in most instances, instead of choosing a simillimum from thousands of remedies, as in constitutional cases, one selects a remedy from perhaps six or seven that the situation suggests.

In terms of that remedy's potency, the course of treatment is also simplified. Most often in acute homeopathy, there are only low potencies and high. And for most acute remedies, one need have only the most basic potencies—usually 30C and 1M—on hand. Whether a bump or bruise or a common cold, as long as the patient seems basically himself, but with aches and pains, the 30C clears things nicely. If the pain has overwhelmed the situation, until the patient seems changed on the mental and/or emotional plane as well as the physical, then the 1M is called for. You can do only good with the homeopathic remedies that you actually have on hand,

and it will save you a good deal of money to follow the idea of just the two potencies of basic remedies. In time, and with practice, you will come to recognize the sorts of remedies than any given person is likely to need. The child who is accident-prone may require you to have several different potencies of Arnica, as well as a topical Arnica balm. The child who is severely allergic to bee sting may require you to have the remedy Apis in potencies above 1M.

The philosophy that guides the given doses of the remedy remains the same: The remedy is given as needed. As long as the patient's energy remains improved, and the symptoms lessened, refrain from giving the remedy again, even if the patient wants more and your own allopathic background tempts you to give it again. More acute cases are ruined by giving the remedy too often than by any other mistake in treatment.

Emergency care often calls for the mantra, "Do no harm, but do what you can." There will be times when, after the acute case has been taken, you do not have the needed remedy at hand. If you have the remedy that is the second on the list of needed remedies, give it. It will do some good until you can get the remedy you need.

The key to acute treatment is to know your limits. Some situations dictate that we take actions beyond our usual comfort range. Most often medical help is just a phone call or car ride away. When in doubt, get help. And if allopathic help is the only help available, get allopathic help. A lifesaving allopathic treatment is far better than a life-ending homeopathic treatment.

But with this warning in place, remember that acute homeopathics in the usual range of household emergencies—skinned knees and the like— are not only fairly simple but are also almost miraculous in their power to cure. Centuries ago, the acute homeopathic prescriber would have likely been burned as a witch, as the remedies often work even before the pellet dissolves on the patient's tongue. Those whose backs are out often sit up without pain in seconds. Sneezing ends, as does bleeding. Toothache is soothed until the tooth can be filled. Bones knit at amazing speed. Patients recover almost too quickly from surgery.

Remember, homeopathy has been kept alive for years by the tradition of lay practice in emergency situations. Lay practitioners, from the European herbalists who turned to homeopathy to the New England housewives who knew a good thing when they saw it, often know more about the remedies and their uses than the professionals do. And even though acute treatments often can be thought of as "homeopathy lite," there is no excuse for any serious student of homeopathy not knowing at least the basics of acute treatment. And as long as health food stores sell both the remedies and the

LET LIKE CURE LIKE

basic texts required for case taking, there is no reason not to reach for the Arnica when next you experience discomfort, instead of taking a Tylenol.

On the pages that follow, I list the twelve essential acute remedies. This list is biased by my own experiences and by my own needs as far as acute homeopathics are concerned. There is no real line separating the remedies into the categories "acute" and "constitutional." Any acute remedy may be needed on a constitutional basis in the treatment of a chronic situation, and a so-called constitutional remedy may be called for in an acute situation. But for simplicity's sake, we divide the remedies in our thinking, much as we divide the North and the South by the imaginary Mason-Dixon line.

The remedies listed here cover the general topic of pain and the ways a symptom portrait containing pain of any sort can be dealt with homeopathically. The remedy Rhus Tox, which is listed among the constitutional remedies in the next chapter, in that it speaks to so many types of physical pain, could well be considered the thirteenth pain remedy.

The remedies included here, while they are all important to the issue of pain in the human system, do not tell the whole story. Literally hundreds of remedies speak to pain of one sort or another. But listed here are some of the first remedies to consider in situations involving pain.

Twelve Essential Acute Remedies
ARNICA

Remedy Source: Arnica is taken from the plant of the same name, which is common to the mountainous areas of Europe. It is also known as leopard's bane and mountain tobacco. The name arnica was given to the plant from *arnakis*, meaning "lamb's skin," referring to the woolly appearance of the plant's leaves. The Germans call the plant *Fallkraut*, or "fall herb," and say that these plants, commonly found on mountaintops, grow just where they are needed to help tend injuries from falling, tripping, skiing, and so on. The use of the plant as a medicinal predates history, and the Roman legion carried the plant along on military maneuvers to treat those who were struck down in battle. Arnica, as an herbal remedy, is used both as a poultice and brewed as a tea.

The whole plant is used in the preparation of the remedy, with the roots, leaves, and flowers collected for potentization at the flowering stage. As a homeopathic remedy, Arnica was created by Hahnemann.

Situations That Suggest Arnica: Physical trauma, blows and bruises, head injuries, concussion, arthritis after physical trauma, rheumatism, nosebleed, vertigo, strains and sprains, pains associated with childbirth, post-surgical pain, dental procedures. A very valuable remedy for the period of recovery after heart attack or stroke. Also influenza, pneumonia, gastritis, headaches, eczema and boils, nightmares and emotional trauma.

Remedy Portrait: While it is often considered only an acute remedy, Arnica is a deep-acting remedy that can often bring about healing in even long-lasting conditions, most especially in situations in which the chronic pain began with physical trauma, no matter how much time has passed since that initial trauma.

Often Arnica is the first homeopathic remedy that a person new to homeopathy encounters, and it is probably by witnessing the power of Arnica alone that most go on to learn more about homeopathic healing.

Patients who need Arnica are in shock. They are, like live radio talk shows, on a seven-second delay. You ask them how they are and there is a pause before they answer. It is as if the physical blow that put them in an Arnica state has somehow driven the spirit a bit out of the body. You have someone who may be struggling to give you any information at all.

It is also typical of Arnica that patients insist that there is nothing wrong with them. They are, after all, in shock and may be disconnected from their pain and even from any memory of the events that put them into shock.

Classic homeopaths insist that the shock of Arnica can be emotional as well as physical, and that the remedy is as effective for the child who has awakened screaming from a nightmare as for the woman who has just learned that her husband is dead as for the person who tripped and fell down the stairs or who has received a black eye.

A way to tell if the patient needs Arnica is by gently attempting to touch the injury. The Arnica person is terrified of being touched and is terrified by even the idea of pain. Kent says, "You will see the old grandfather sit off in a corner of the room, and, if he sees little Johnny running toward him, he will say, 'Oh, do keep away.' Give him a dose of Arnica and he will let Johnny run all over him." The patient's head is very hot and his body, especially the extremities, feels very cold. An unusual symptom of Arnica is that the tip of the nose feels very cold after injury.

The patient says that he feels bruised. The sensation of the pain is bruising, even if the situation does not have to do with physical trauma. For instance, headaches that can be helped by a dose of Arnica have the same bruising pain as does a head injury. But don't give Arnica as soon as you see any bruise. Arnica is certainly considered the premiere blow and bruise remedy in the homeopathic pharmacy, but it is by no means the only one. For instance, Calcarea Carbonica, one of the most prescribed constitutional remedies, is very useful in old bruises that have yet to fade away. One dose of the remedy helps the body to reabsorb the blood and clears away the bruise. For Arnica to be useful, there must also be the hesitation, the fear of pain, and the shock.

Extreme sensitivity runs through the remedy portrait. The patient complains that he cannot get into a comfortable position, that the chair or bed is too hard. To picture the Arnica prototype, think of "the Princess and the Pea." Like that royal daughter, the Arnica person will find that, if you put one uncooked pea at the bottom of a pile of twenty mattresses, she will not be able to sleep because the mattress is just too hard. Like the princess, the Arnica person is too sensitive to touch. The touch of a human hand, or a mattress, a chair, or even clothing can be too hard to bear.

Of particular sensitivity for the Arnica person is the region of the abdomen, particularly the pelvis and uterus. Pregnant women who feel the movement of the fetus and feel sore and bruised find great comfort in Arnica. Because of the particular sensitivity in the abdomen, Arnica is also a major remedy for appendicitis that has been brought on after a blow to the abdomen. It is also useful in cases of abdominal gas and bloating.

Arnica is very helpful for sprains and for general injuries, bruises, and shocks, particularly injuries to joints. A sprained ankle, for instance, can be cured almost miraculously with Arnica, a dose of which may allow the patient to put his full weight back on the ankle instantly.

Arnica can also be used preventatively, and it is always a good idea to take a dose before visiting your dentist. Arnica used after dental procedures and surgery aids in the quick healing of that physical trauma. And, as Arnica is a very useful remedy when the patient has overexerted, it is useful when returning to aerobics class after an absence of several years. In fact, the middle-aged among us who are trying to get back in shape after a decade of ignoring their physical condition need to keep Arnica on hand to deal with the traumas they are likely to face—emotional and physical—as they work their way back to a physical peak.

It is, of course, possible for a patient to be constitutionally Arnica and to need the remedy long-term. These patients are most often those in whom an original injury slowly deepened and overwhelmed the patient's vital force, developing into chronic conditions like migraine, rheumatism, or arthritis. These people especially insist that nothing is wrong with them. They refuse to see the doctor, although they are in obvious pain. Those who are accident-prone may also be in need of the remedy on a long-term basis, as are those who, like the princess, are too sensitive to their physical surroundings ever to be able to relax and feel both comfortable and safe. They are always wary, always on guard, and need an extremely large personal space, wanting everyone to approach them only very slowly and gently. The patient may have a deep fear of being touched and actually act like a cornered animal when approached by someone he does not trust.

Arnica is an important chronic remedy when a patient is recovering from either a heart attack or stroke, especially in situations in which the left side of the body has some paralysis but there is a full and strong pulse. The patient sighs often and mutters quietly. He has a red face.

In general, the modalities of Arnica are as follows: The patient is worse after any motion, after being shaken or touched, after any form of exertion, in a damp environment, when cold, after lying in one position too long, after blowing his nose.

The Arnica patient feels better in the open air and lying down with his head low, with no pillow.

Arnica may be taken orally or used topically, and most health food stores sell the remedy both ways. If all you have is the pellet form, you can dissolve the remedy in water and apply it topically to the injured part of the body, giving the remedy orally at the same time. But please note that Arnica should never be used topically on any injury that involves broken skin. While Arnica will do no lasting harm, it will hurt like hell. Instead, the remedy Calendula can be very helpful topically to scratches, scrapes, cuts, and the like. Arnica works only on blows, bruises, sprains, and other injuries in which the skin is whole and healthy, although in either case the remedy may be taken internally to speed healing. Arnica is an effective remedy in any potency, from topical rub to highest potency. It may be repeated as often as needed.

ACONITE

Remedy Source: Aconite is created from the roots and stems of the plant *Aconitum napellus*, also known as wolfsbane and monkshood. The plant is native to Europe and must be gathered in the flowering stage in order to be made into the remedy Aconite. It was first created as a homeopathic remedy by Hahnemann in 1805.

Situations That Suggest Aconite: Shock. Also angina, arrhythmia, cerebral accidents, headache, injury and trauma, neuralgia, vertigo. Also upper respiratory infections, colds and flu, conjunctivitis, croup, otitis media, pneumonia, tonsillitis. Also panic attacks.

Remedy Portrait: Aconite is among the most "restless" remedies. The person needing Aconite is very restless, pacing the floor, changing positions almost constantly, thrashing about. In the same way, almost everything about this person suggests haste. He does everything in a hurry, everything in a panic. The person cannot become calm; everything startles him.

The symptoms of Aconite come on very quickly. It is, for instance, effective for colds that come on suddenly, with the patient starting to sneeze and an hour or two later having a full-blown cold. Ailments whose symptoms come on slowly counterindicate this remedy. Symptoms have extreme intensity. The pain of the symptoms spikes rapidly to overwhelm the patient's vital force. In the same way, if recovery comes on, it, too, is quick. The pain in Aconite disappears as quickly as it appeared.

The symptoms of Aconite are often triggered by exposure to cold, most especially to cold, dry winds. A child goes out to play on a cold winter's day, becomes chilled, and has a sore throat in a very short time.

The symptoms of Aconite often seem to overwhelm the patient's senses. Sight, smell, and especially hearing become distorted and may even disappear altogether. In that Aconite disorders hearing, it is a major remedy for tinnitus, or ringing in the ears.

The pains in an Aconite patient tend to be numbing, with tingling and pricking sensations also very common. The muscles, especially the leg muscles, become very relaxed, and every attempt to move is difficult and painful. Because of this aspect, Aconite is a major remedy for sciatica that comes on and leaves very suddenly, with brief violent attacks that are worse in cold, dry weather.

Aconite is a remedy common to inflammatory diseases of all sorts and can be very useful in aphonia, tonsillitis, croup, laryngitis, bronchitis, pneumonia, pleurisy, and otitis, all of which come on during or are made worse by cold, dry weather or exposure to cold wind. It is also the first remedy to consider in conditions of quick onset in which the pain is unbearable: facial neuralgia, toothache, orchitis, and pericarditis. Aconite is a helpful remedy in cases of asthma that follow the general remedy portrait.

Aconite is a major remedy for conditions that involve fevers characterized by a red face, or a face that alternates between red and pale. The skin is dry and hot. The patient has a great thirst for large quantities of cold water. The whole body seems burning hot. The patient is restless, refusing to lie still.

Aconite is a quick-acting remedy and needs to be repeated often. Also, it usually is effective only if used soon after the onset of symptoms. This is especially true of respiratory infections. If Aconite is not given early on, it no longer has an impact in the case. If there is a truly acute remedy, it is Aconite. Because of the brief nature of the remedy's action, it is never given long term and is seldom useful in chronic cases.

Very important to the understanding of this remedy are its emotional symptoms. The patient is frantic and filled with fear, especially the fear of death. The patient also commonly predicts the time of his death. Fear, like the pain in Aconite, is worse at night. Patients have the irrational fear of having their hair cut. Some even seem afraid of having their hair touched. Ailments come on after fear and anger, or from hearing shocking news.

As a shock remedy, Aconite is often used in alternation with Arnica. In cases such as car accidents, in which the patient has received both physical injury and shock, the two remedies, depending on the potency on hand, may have to be repeated in alternation as frequently as every five minutes.

The color red is common in Aconite. The face is red with fever. The ears are red at the onset of the illness. All blood is bright red in color.

The general modalities of the remedy find the Aconite patient worse at night, when lying on the painful side, on rising, and when hearing music, which most Aconites cannot bear. The patient is better in the open air, which he often feels he can breathe although unable to get heated air into the lungs. He often feels better after sweating.

Aconite is effective in all potencies and can be repeated as needed. In fact, it usually needs to be repeated often in acute conditions. Where there is great fear, consider using 1M and higher as needed. One dose of the remedy can be effective only for from six to forty-eight hours.

APIS

Remedy Source: Apis is created from the whole honeybee, and the remedy is created in an inhumane fashion. Live honeybees are put in a bottle, and the bees are irritated by shaking the bottle. For eight days, the bottle is opened just long enough to pour in diluted alcohol. The bottle is shaken some more to anger the bees and get them to emit venom. When the bees die, the alcohol is poured out, strained, and filtered, and that liquid becomes the mother tincture for the remedy.

The other way the remedy can be created is from a drop of bee venom that the bee secretes when it is held in forceps. This drop of venom is then poured into a tube and diluted alcohol is added.

The remedy is a sarcode because it is prepared from healthy animal products. It was created in 1852 by Dr. Fredrick Humphries.

Situations That Suggest Apis: Allergies (especially to bee stings). Also asthma, arthritis, herpes, headache, shingles. Also sore throat, colds, scarlet fever, pleurisy, pneumonia, meningitis, chicken pox. Apis may also be useful for ovarian cysts, endometriosis, miscarriage, urinary incontinence.

Remedy Portrait: To understand the actions of the remedy Apis, just think for a moment about the symptoms of a bee sting. The remedy is filled with burning, stinging, redness, and swelling. No matter the cause, from infections to arthritis, these are the symptoms that guide the use of the remedy. Affected parts of the body have a red glossy look to them—for example, the sore throat not only looks red but has a shine to it as well. The swollen parts of the body are so swollen that they resemble a water balloon about to burst.

Look for the Apis patient's personality to follow the physical symptoms. Because of the swelling and the heat, the patient often feels that a portion of his body, or the whole body, will burst. Like a bee, he may seem to be overly intense, "busy as a bee." Constitutionally speaking (Apis may be considered a constitutional as well as an acute or emergency remedy), Apis is a remedy for workaholics who are so caught up in the task at hand that they ignore the needs of everyone around them. They are also jealous and easily angered, leading people to be intimidated by them, afraid of their sting.

In the same way, patients with an acute need for Apis are angry and very controlling. They demand drinks when they are thirsty and become aggressive if their needs are not met.

Apis is a strong remedy for allergies of all sorts, especially food allergies. The patient experiences swelling, most commonly swelling of the eyes, as a reaction to allergy. Apis is a major remedy for hives and for allergic reaction to puncture wounds.

As an acute remedy, Apis is often used for punctures. In terms of homeopathy, an insect bite is considered as much a puncture wound as is a wound made from stepping on a nail. The Apis puncture wound has the typical symptoms of Apis: It is red and swollen, and it feels hot. The patient wants to put cold things on the wound in order to soothe it. In fact, this desire for cold, from cold applications on wounds to cold water for a sore throat, is so common a symptom of Apis that if the patient does not want cold, it is likely not an Apis situation.

Apis is a good general pain remedy when the totality of the patient's symptoms follow the remedy's symptom portrait. The pains of Apis usually move from right to left in the body; a sore throat, for example, begins on the right and moves toward the left. Symptoms migrate suddenly from one part of the body to another, apparently without rhyme or reason.

Apis is a remedy in which red rashes cover various parts of the body in combination with other symptoms. The red skin of scarlet fever is a typical example. Apis is also a common remedy for measles and is very effective if the patient's symptoms follow the remedy portrait. The patient wants to have cold applications placed on the skin and is much worse under warm coverings.

Warmth in general is the greatest aggravation for the Apis person; a warm or stuffy room causes all symptoms to get worse, including mental symptoms. The typical mental symptoms include deep sadness, with the Apis patient often crying constantly for no apparent reason, and ongoing worry, which keeps the patient from sleeping. Anger is also typical, as is childishness. The Apis adult may speak baby talk, most especially when in pain or when dealing with fever.

Apis is also a strong remedy for the eyes, and for problems with vision. Kent tells us that Apis should be the first remedy considered when dealing with inflammations of the eye, especially inflammations that include enlarged blood vessels and swelling of the eyelids. The eyes burn and sting. The patient feels not only pain in the eyes but also a decrease of vision when looking at any flame, from a fireplace to candlelight. The patient also is worse when looking at anything that is white and when moving the eyes from right to left.

The sore throats of Apis can be dangerous because they involve swelling, often enough to cause choking. The patient typically is unable to swallow any solid food at all and may not even be able to swallow water. Either there is great thirst for cold water or no thirst at all. The pain extends into the patient's ears on swallowing. The throat may be ulcerated; there may or may not be swelling of the tonsils.

Apis is also a useful remedy in cases of joint pain and swelling caused by arthritis or by injury. The joint is worse with applications of heat and better with cold. The pain is stinging. Note that the heat of the joint is internal; the joint does not feel hot to the touch. (If the joint feels hot to the touch—or, indeed, any other affected part feels hot to the touch—consider the remedy Belladonna instead of Apis.)

Certainly Apis is the first remedy to consider in cases of bee sting, especially for someone who is allergic to bee stings. In all cases of anaphylaxis, Apis is the first remedy to consider.

In general, the modalities of the remedy include a general aggravation of all symptoms at 3 P.M., at which time the patient may experience fever with chills. If the patient becomes thirsty at all, it is most usual during this period of chill. The patient is worse in the heat and in a stuffy room. The patient may even faint entering a sauna. The patient is also worse for the heat of the bed and worse for lying down, worse for sleeping, worse for being touched, or when experiencing any pressure, especially on swollen parts of the body.

The Apis patient feels better after a cold bath, in the cool open air, sitting up erect. He usually is eager to move around and exercise and feels better afterward.

The remedy is usually given in low potencies, from 9 to 200C, although someone who is allergic to bee stings requires potencies of 1M and above to counter shock. Apis may be repeated as needed, especially in low potencies.

BELLADONNA

Remedy Source: Belladonna, a remedy taken from the deadly nightshade plant, has a long history as a medicinal herb. The plant is native to Greece and Italy, where it was first used due to the wide range of its actions. Belladonna is highly toxic, although somehow it is not poisonous to rabbits and goats, and is not as poisonous to any other carnivorous animals as it is to humans. Ingesting the plant creates symptoms similar to those that the remedy removes: high fever, fears, throbbing pain, and rage. The remedy is created from the whole plant, picked at the flowering stage. The remedy was created by Hahnemann.

Situations That Suggest Belladonna: Fever, migraine, appendicitis, convulsions. Also constipation, hemorrhoids, influenza, low back pain, sinusitis, tonsillitis, vertigo. Also Ménière's disease and otitis media. Consider for hallucinations, delirium, mania. Also sunburn, sciatica.

Remedy Portrait: As a household remedy, Belladonna is most often used for fever. Fevers in very young patients often come on suddenly and spike to become dangerously high. The patient may have hallucinations with the fever and may see ghosts, insects, and black animals, especially dogs or wolves. The patient fears the things he thinks he sees and wants to run away. Belladonna is suggested for fevers with convulsions that come on suddenly, fevers during teething, and fevers with hot head and cold feet.

The symptoms in Belladonna come on suddenly and leave just as suddenly. During a fever, or during the violent pain that is common to this remedy, the patient acts violently, breaks into fits of laughter, tries to bite those who attend him, gnashes his teeth, and tries to escape.

Belladonna is also an important acute remedy for headaches. The headache symptoms follow the general symptom portrait of Belladonna: They are congestive in nature, and the patient has a red face. In fact, once again the red face is a common symptom that suggests the remedy, no matter the specific symptoms of the ailment. The patient is unable to deal with noise or light during the pain, another common symptom of the remedy. Whether the patient needs the remedy for headache, sunburn, or a scratched cornea, he is unable to bear light from any source, specifically sunlight. Belladonna is the primary remedy for photophobia. The patient's headache is worse after any exertion. It is better after wrapping the head tightly; this, too, is a general symptom of Belladonna. The patient is commonly worse when moving around and feels better when lying down in a quiet, dark place, tightly covered or wrapped. Even with a fever, the patient wants to be "tucked in."

Belladonna patients are given to vertigo, especially when rising from stooping. Vertigo can come on with any change of position.

A Belladonna patient's eyes alone often suggest the remedy. Look for glassy eyes with dilated pupils. The patient's hands and feet feel cold, but the rest of the body feels almost too hot to touch.

Think of sunburn and the heat that the patient gives off and you have some notion of the feeling of Belladonna symptoms: disorientation, exhaustion. And just as the last thing someone with a sunburn wants to see is the sun, the Belladonna patient is unable to bear the heat or the light of the sun.

The patient has no thirst, even with the highest fever (although some patients crave lemonade). The illness, as do illnesses suggesting Aconite, comes on suddenly, like a freight train, and like that train rages loudly while it passes, only to leave as suddenly as it came on. Ailments of long standing, especially long-term fevers, seldom yield to Belladonna. Like Aconite, it is a short-term remedy.

This is not to say that Belladonna is not and could never be a constitutional remedy. But those needing Belladonna on a chronic basis are fairly rare, and the true power of the remedy is in its acute uses. In chronic cases, note that the symptoms come on very slowly, often taking several years to develop fully.

In general, Belladonna patients feel worse in sunshine and in heat in any form, but also in cold winds or drafts. They are much worse when subjected to light and noise. They are worse when their heads are uncovered, when lying on the painful side, and when drinking. All the symptoms are typically worse at 3 P.M. and after midnight. Patients are worse when stooping and bending forward.

Belladonna patients are better when resting in a dark and quiet place. They are also better when sitting quietly, with their heads covered, in a warm place.

The remedy is most often used in the 200C potency and below. When delirium and other mental symptoms are part of the picture, higher potencies are needed. For inflammatory disease, lower potencies are often the most effective. Belladonna can be repeated as often as needed. Each dose, however, can be effective for up to seven days.

BRYONIA

Remedy Source: Bryonia is created from wild hops, a high-climbing perennial plant native to Germany and France. It's also known as white bryony.

The mother tincture is made from the roots of the plant, which must be picked just before the first flowering. This is a remedy of Hahnemann, although it was re-proved as a remedy by the Austrian Society of Homeopaths.

Situations That Suggest Bryonia: Appendicitis, rheumatoid arthritis, physical trauma, tendonitis, connective tissue disease, low back pain, sciatica, bursitis, gout. Also influenza, bronchitis, pneumonia, pharyngitis, cough. Consider strongly for constipation, diarrhea, gastritis. Also toothache, nosebleed, headache, migraine, coma, vertigo.

Remedy Portrait: Bryonia is a very important remedy that has been used in the treatment of serious disease, including typhoid and tuberculosis. It belongs in every home kit. While it can be and often is a constitutional remedy, used to clear a wide range of troublesome chronic conditions, Bryonia is one of the most important acute remedies.

Perhaps the most important symptom of a person needing this remedy is that he does not want to move. If the back aches, he wants to lie very still. (Bryonia is, in fact, the most important remedy for cracked ribs, a circumstance in which movement of any sort can bring on intense pain.) A patient with a Bryonia headache does not want to move his eyes; even this small movement causes pain. Some of those needing Bryonia, however, are driven to restlessness by their pain and move about a bit, although every motion causes great pain. If the Bryonia patient is restless, the motion is specifically of the left arm and leg.

Another characteristic of Bryonia pain is its splinterlike nature. The patient lies on the painful side, because the pressure of the weight of the body lessens the pain.

A second important feature of Bryonia patients is that they are angry and irritable. Classic literature suggests that the ailments of Bryonia are those brought on by "anger, mortification, fright, and chagrin." They are angry. They want to be left alone. Often, they simply refuse to speak, even to answer the simplest question about their condition. In refusing to answer questions about themselves, their wants and desires, or their aches and pains, patients quite often clearly reveal themselves as needing Bryonia.

Third, Bryonia patients reveal themselves through a symptom of unique thirst. Bryonia is a very thirsty remedy, and yet patients seldom drink. As they do not want to move, they wait and wait before drinking and then drink great quantities of cold water all at once. Like camels, they drink to store the liquid until they drink again.

Bryonia patients have a fever, sometimes as high as Belladonna or Aconite. But here the fever is slow in coming and slow in building.

When they are in pain, and especially when they have a fever, Bryonia patients may keep saying that they "want to go home." A need for home and for security is a core issue for the Bryonia. They also often are very work oriented, wanting to work or fearful of losing their jobs because of illness.

During the illness, a Bryonia patient's tongue may be coated with a brownish or white film, the coating being most distinct in the center of the tongue. The mouth may be very dry; dryness of the mucous membranes throughout the body is common.

The typical Bryonia headache comes on either as the patient first opens his eyes in the morning, while he is still in bed, or shortly after rising. The headache increases in severity throughout the day, gradually disappearing as the sun sets. The headache is usually accompanied by constipation. In fact, for Bryonia patients, constipation usually accompanies just about any other symptom. The worst position that any Bryonia person with a headache can be in is stooping. This not only worsens the severity of the head pain but also brings on vertigo.

Bryonia can be a very healing remedy for those with irritable bowel syndrome, in that it speaks to both constipation and diarrhea. The constipation involves a totally inactive rectum, with no desire whatsoever to move the bowels. What stool does come is large, hard, dark, and black. It appears burnt. The diarrhea is so acrid that it causes soreness and burning of the anus. It contains undigested food and comes on with motion of the body. Often first thing in the morning, the smallest motion of a hand or foot forces the patient to run for the bathroom.

For all rheumatic pains, the symptoms are similar. The joints are red, hot, and swollen. They are painful during the least motion and aggravated by any touch or pressure. The pains are stitching or tearing in nature. If the patient sweats, the pain feels better. The Bryonia patient is, in general, improved by sweating.

As an acute remedy, Bryonia is probably most often used for flu. The symptoms mirror the general portrait of this remedy. The patient has a deep-down feeling of pain that is made much worse by motion. He wants to lie perfectly still in his own bedroom (it is very important that he is *home*) and wants to be left totally alone. There is usually a cough with the flu, and the motion involved in coughing is very painful. Constipation also accompanies this flu. The tongue is coated brown or white. The patient is almost totally impossible, making demands that, when carried out, he then refuses. One minute the patient wants soup. When you make it, he doesn't want it anymore, and he is rude about it.

In general, the person needing Bryonia is worse when moving, coughing or sneezing, and during sleep. Not eating makes him worse, as does warmth and summer weather. Bryonia is the best choice for summer diarrhea. The patient suffers from any motion of the eyes, even closing the eyes, which can bring on vertigo.

Bryonia patients are improved by being left alone and being quiet. They want cool open air, a dark room, and cool food and drink. Most important, Bryonia patients are improved by lying on the painful side and by gentle pressure on virtually all their painful body parts.

Bryonia is used in all potencies, although the lower potencies tend to be most effective, especially when treating chronic constipation. It is a quick-acting remedy, and its actions tend to be somewhat short lasting. One dose is effective often for as few as seven days. Bryonia tends to work most on the physical plane—which is perhaps why the lower potencies are most effective—and is usually not useful for deep psychological conditions.

CALENDULA

Remedy Source: This remedy is created from the marigold flower or *Calendula officinalis*. The mother tincture is created from the leaves and flowers. A similar remedy, Calendula Succus, is created from the fresh juice of the same plant. The plant belongs to the family of flowers that gives us our other two most effective healing agents: Arnica and Bellis Perennis, a remedy for persons who are experiencing deep bruising pain that even Arnica cannot clear. Bellis is created from the daisy.

Situations That Suggest Calendula: Wounds, abrasions, cuts, scrapes. Also recovery after surgery, infected wounds and sores, burns.

Remedy Portrait: As Calendula is a natural antiseptic as well as an astringent, it is one of our most important acute remedies. Many people purchase the remedy as a part of a homeopathic kit and come to believe that it is only a topical remedy. But Calendula, while most readily available as an ointment, has been potentized at every level and is very useful both topically and orally.

In today's world, we think of Calendula first (with Hypericum a close second) for gunshot wounds or any other form of lacerating wound, especially if the wound has become infected. In such a case, Calendula should be used both topically and internally, or in combination with Hypericum and/or Arnica in emergency situations. This remedy helps knit broken skin and helps prevent infection as it does so.

Topically, it is also a very important remedy for stopping bleeding and is therefore useful for healing any sort of cut or incision. It is also an important remedy to use after dental surgery. Where Arnica may not be used with broken skin, and is therefore not helpful topically for cuts and the like, Calendula soothes the situation and promotes quick healing. In the case of dental surgery, the patient may dissolve Calendula pellets in water and swish the water around in his mouth to soothe pain, stop bleeding, and promote healing.

Although Calendula is available in a petroleum salve and an alcohol-based liquid, I find that it works best by simply dissolving the pellets in water and using this liquid both topically and internally. Although the salve is very gentle and soothing for scrapes, it should never be used for burns because the petroleum jelly base seals in the pain of the burn and increases pain and slows the healing process. For burns, Aqua Calendula—the remedy dissolved in pure water—is the best bet. The alcohol-based liquid should never be used for dry skin or eczema; the alcohol itself further dries the skin. Aqua Calendula is once more the best option for these conditions.

Calendula may be of great comfort in all sorts of joint pain and in arthritis of any sort. The salve, liquid, or water-base may all be used very effectively and may allow the patient to avoid the use of topical cortisone, which itself can be highly suppressive and toxic to the whole system.

Calendula patients, who are likely to be in great pain, are very irritable. They are usually easily frightened and very nervous, although some may be so overcome in their vital force that they become disconnected from reality and appear sleepy. They tend to feel very chilly, which causes them to become worried; they are sure that something terrible is about to happen.

In general, the Calendula patient needs reassurance and is improved with warmth, attention, and the reassurance that things will be all right.

Although Calendula is most often used in very low potency as a topical ointment, it can be used internally as well. When taken as an internal remedy, Calendula should be selected in potency with regard to the patient's vital force. It may be used in all potencies.

CHAMOMILLA

Remedy Source: Chamomilla is taken from the German chamomile, a flowering plant native to Europe. The plant is picked while in full flower, and the whole plant is used in the creation of the remedy. The remedy was created by Hahnemann.

Situations That Suggest Chamomilla: Pain, especially pain associated with teething and toothache; PMS. Also coughs, colic and fever, otitis media. The remedy is also useful for the hot flushes that accompany menopause. It is a great remedy for behavioral problems. Consider also for neuralgia. Excellent remedy for cases involving diarrhea that follow general pain pattern.

Remedy Portrait: There is perhaps no finer pain remedy than Chamomilla. And there is no patient in greater pain and more sensitive to pain than is the Chamomilla. The patient is so hypersensitive to pain that he even becomes angry, violent, and abusive.

Chamomilla helps heal pain that is unbearable in nature. The boring pain of an ear infection, the relentless pain of toothache. When in a Chamomilla state, the patient's whole life is defined by this kind of pain.

As the physical often reflects the emotional, patients feel that they are not only in crisis but that their entire life is pain. They feel that no one in the world, historically or at present, has ever experienced this much pain. As no one can understand their pain, they become angry when told that someone knows how they feel.

The interesting thing here is that the effect of the pain seems out of whack with the pain itself. No one could be in *that* much pain from an earache. The Chamomilla patient cries out, "OWW!" if you just touch his arm.

Characteristically, no other patient is quite as angry and mean as Chamomilla. Nux Vomica may be angry, but as long as he feels that you might be able to help, he cooperates. Nitric Acid is unpleasant, to be sure, and negative in all ways and about all things, but for a sheer feeling that at any moment you might have to duck to avoid flying things, there is no remedy type that equals the Chamomilla patient.

They become angry if they are looked at. They become angry if you cannot bring about an instant end to their pain. They throw things. They are verbally abusive.

Patients have diarrhea. Twitching may develop in various parts of their body, even convulsions.

The patient also feels hot. There is likely to be hot sweat on the forehead; night sweats are very common to this remedy. Any warm application or environment makes the patient much worse—and much angrier. Yet the patient doesn't want open air and feels worse in the wind or any moving air. Many are even afraid of the wind, thinking that it will increase their pain. Wind in the ears is worst of all. The patient's feet are hot, too, in particular the soles. They likely stick their feet out from under the covers of the bed at night.

The Chamomilla patient is contrary. He is sleepy and yet he cannot sleep. He wants things until he gets them, then he no longer wants them. Even his face reveals this contrary nature: one cheek red and the other pale.

The patient sweats after eating and is hot and very thirsty. In adults, the Chamomilla state comes on especially in those addicted to coffee and narcotics.

Chamomilla patients cannot be consoled, no matter what you do or how hard you try. They are impatient—they feel that they cannot get well soon enough, and yet, contrary as they are, they do not cooperate with any measures that are likely to get them well. They are restless, often driven by their pain. In that they cannot be consoled, they tend to weep in despair of their condition, even in their sleep.

An odd but telling symptom of Chamomilla patients is that they want to be carried. Chamomilla children have tantrums, strike out or kick, every time they are put down. They must be carried in a rhythmic way, walked up and down the hall over and over again, in order for them to be quiet.

Think of a toothache and you have the core idea of the remedy. Toothache here can come on just from entering a warm room or by drinking coffee. The toothache hurts not only in the tooth and jaw but in the whole body. Patients become nauseated from the tooth pain. There is a bitter taste in the mouth, and they have bad breath. The tongue has a yellow coating, which is characteristic of the remedy. Diarrhea may accompany the pain, as may twitching or convulsions.

Chamomilla is a wonderful remedy for the child who is an ongoing behavior problem, who kicks his mother, who demands constant attention, and who always wants to be carried. This child may be given to convulsions and to violent rage. With several doses of this remedy, he may seem to be another child altogether.

In general, Chamomilla patients cannot bear to have anyone near them. They don't even want anyone to look at them. They are averse to talking and answer with anger. Patients are worse in any heat, after their angry outbursts, and in the evening before midnight.

Chamomilla patients are improved by being carried when they are in pain. They feel better if they don't eat. And they feel much better in warm, wet weather.

Hahnemann commented that Chamomilla works best in the 12C potency. It assists in all general aches and pains that follow the Chamomilla pattern. Higher potencies are useful in more long-term situations and in behavior disorders. One dose of this remedy remains effective for up to thirty days.

HYPERICUM

Remedy Source: The remedy Hypericum Perforatum is taken from Saint-John's-wort, an herb known for its yellow star-shaped flowers. It is native to Europe, Asia, and Africa. Often the flowers cover whole fields. The mother tincture from which the remedy is taken is made from the whole plant, which is picked while at full bloom. The remedy was proved by German homeopath George F. Mueller.

Situations That Suggest Hypericum: Punctures, lacerations, or contusions involving any part of the body dense with nerves, especially the fingers, tongue, teeth, eyes, and genitalia. Also for injuries to the spine, from sprains to fractures; injuries to the coccyx; phantom pains of all sorts.

Remedy Portrait: You will not need this remedy often, but when you do, you will thank God for it. Like other remedies, Hypericum is most associated with the physical body and is a true acute remedy.

Like Aconite and Arnica, it is something of a remedy for persons in shock. It's for those who have received bad news, those who are afraid. Classically, the remedy has been given to those who, upon being given bad news, respond by becoming very nervous. This remedy is also very helpful for those who, during a long illness or after surgery, fall into a deep depression.

Think of how it feels to slam your finger in a car door and you have a basic understanding of the action of this remedy. The pain experienced by the Hypericum patient runs along the nerves in the body, as the pain experienced by the fingertip runs all the way up the arm and into the neck and shoulder. Think also of the pain of some toothaches, or following dental surgery, in which the pain seems to follow along your whole jaw and into the ear, and you have another example of the Hypericum situation.

The remedy Hypericum soothes nerve pain. (It should be alternated in its use with Arnica if there is nerve pain following surgery of any sort, particularly dental surgery.) Hypericum is also an important acute remedy when it is alternated with Calendula in the treatment of lacerated wounds, gunshot wounds, or knife wounds. Hypericum has been known to bring about healing and to restore the skin in cases in which skin has been all but cut away from the body in an accident or attack.

It is also the major homeopathic remedy to be used after amputation, in that it not only soothes the pain but removes all traces of phantom pain in the removed limb.

Consider the remedy also in cases of concussion. Hypericum removes headache after a blow to the head or after a fall in which the occiput has been traumatized.

Hypericum is also one of several homeopathic remedies to be considered for rabies. It has been shown to prevent tetanus after traumatic injuries. Classically it is considered the major remedy for use after a rat bite.

Similar to Arnica patients, Hypericum patients often seem to drift away. They stop speaking in the middle of a sentence, just sort of drifting off to quiet. They forget what they were going to say. Their handwriting changes.

Because they are in a fog, Hypericum patients are much worse during foggy weather. They experience asthma during fog and are unable to breathe. To stimulate themselves, they usually crave tea, but tea disagrees with their system, making all the symptoms worse.

In general, patients are worse when touched; when their wounds are exposed, and when uncovered. They are worse in cold and damp. They do not want to move and feel pain if their body is in any way jarred.

The patients feel better lying down on their stomach. They also feel better if they bend their head backward.

Like Calendula, many persons know only Hypericum as a topical remedy, as it is often sold in liquid tincture. And of course this topical application can be very effective, both in soothing nerve pain and in inducing the healing of lacerated skin. But also like Calendula, Hypericum is available in all potencies and can and should be taken internally. This is a very short-acting remedy that needs to be repeated often until improvement in the condition begins.

IGNATIA

Remedy Source: Ignatia Amara is taken from the Saint-Ignatius's-bean, a large shrub or climbing tree native to the islands of the South Pacific. The shrub has fragrant white flowers. The mother tincture is made from the seeds of the shrub. The remedy was proved as a homeopathic by Hahnemann.

Situations That Suggest Ignatia: Hysteria, anxiety disorder, compulsive behavior. Also asthma, chronic fatigue, environmental illness, chronic headaches and migraine. Also spasms and tics of all sorts; depression, sometimes clinical depression. Physical ailments include low back pain, obesity, rectal ailments, and encephalitis. Hirsuitism.

Remedy Portrait: While Ignatia is similar to the other remedies gathered here, in that it speaks to the general topic of pain, the pain experienced for the Ignatia patient is largely emotional and spiritual, with physical pain being a minor part of the overall Ignatia picture. Ignatia may, at times, be considered a constitutional remedy, but it is much more important as an acute treatment. The Ignatia profile attaches itself, through a series of circumstances, on top of the true constitution, and the remedy works best in the short term, to break through the wall of pain that the patient creates around himself. (The Ignatia pattern, by its very intensity, often moves into the constitutional type Natrum Muriaticum, which replaces the raw wound of Ignatia with the placid face of denial.)

Ignatia is, first and always, a remedy for persons in a deep state of grief. And, as a so-called grief remedy, Ignatia is largely misunderstood. Many give Ignatia automatically to any patient who has experienced some emotional loss. Grief is a natural and necessary process after loss. Ignatia fails to work on those who are grieving naturally, who are working through their loss, and who, in time, will move on in their lives. The grief of Ignatia is one that traps the patient, that does not at any time let go of him or let him move on. Like Miss Havisham in *Great Expectations*, the Ignatia type stays frozen in time and space, still trapped in the time of the loss or betrayal. Miss Havisham still sits, years later, in her tattered wedding dress, by her rotted and rat-eaten wedding cake, refusing to change her clothes and open the windows to let in light and air. And, most important, Miss Havisham, who was betrayed and deserted on the day of her wedding, still plans her revenge.

The Ignatia patient not only is in grief but has interpreted the loss as a form of betrayal. The widow, while she knows logically that her husband did not choose to die, still feels in her heart that he betrayed her by leaving her. There is always this aspect of betrayal and desertion in the Ignatia picture.

Because of this feeling of betrayal and loss, Ignatia types are often jealous. Not only can they not bear to watch others go about their lives in happy relationships, but they also often do everything in their power to ruin these relationships. Literature and, especially, soap operas are filled with Ignatia characters, who are usually written as women, although in the real world there are as many men in need of this remedy as there are women. Those who are old enough to remember the night time soap *Dy-*

nasty can understand the remedy through the actions of Alexis Carrington Colby Dexter Dexter, who, having been divorced by her beloved husband Blake, seeks not only to destroy Blake but to disrupt his happy second marriage to Krystle.

In their hearts, Ignatia types are true romantics who love the idea of love. They believe in soul mates and in the perfection of their own mate. Pity the poor mate, however, who turns out to be merely human and who behaves in any manner that the Ignatia type can interpret as betrayal.

This pattern occurs again and again until the Ignatia issues are resolved. The Ignatia sets impossible standards for each new person, each new cause, only to be disappointed again and again, until it seems that life itself is against him.

Often they are most easily recognized by their crying. Like the character Lucy on *I Love Lucy*, Ignatias will cry out loud, with that typical Lucy "Whaaa . . ."

Since they are themselves off balance, the Ignatias keep everyone else off balance. Take the characteristic crying. The other people in the room when Ignatia bursts into tears and runs out the door are left to wonder what was said, what happened to so hurt his feelings. And this is just as Ignatias would have it. They do not want to cry in front of others, but they want others to know that they are crying, that they are in real emotional pain. So they run from the room, up the stairs, stomping all the way, and into their bedroom, slamming the door. Then they throw themselves on their bed and sob loudly.

Other times, the Ignatia laughs hysterically, still leaving the others in the room to wonder just what is going on. Sometimes, the Ignatia moves from laughter to tears in a matter of moments, for no apparent reason.

The most typical physical disorders that Ignatia is given to often reveal the need for the remedy in and of themselves. Ignatia patients are given to fits of hiccups, or to hysterical vomiting. Just as the tears come bursting out of them, so do their hiccups, which are loud, loud, loud, or their vomit, which gives them another excuse to run from the room.

Ignatia patients are also given to tics and spasms of all sorts. They cannot bear the smell of tobacco and refuse to enter any smoky rooms. They are usually improved by traveling and feel much better and happier when they are away from home.

The headaches in Ignatias reveal a sensation common to their physical pains. The headache feels as if a nail were being driven into the head, sometimes as if the nail were passing in one side of the skull and out of the other. The patient wants to lie on the painful part of the head in order to soothe the pain.

Ignatia is a major remedy for constipation. The pain of the constipation is usually felt in the upper abdomen. He dreads the attempt to pass the stool, fearing pain. The same sensation of a nail being driven into the body that the Ignatia experienced with headache may also be present with constipation, with great pain in the rectum.

Ignatias are often addicted to coffee, which instead of stimulating the bowels seems only to increase the constipation. They crave the coffee even though it disagrees with them, making their stomach feel acid.

Ignatias have two odd symptoms to watch for: They are afraid of birds, and they sweat only on the face. In fact, the face of Ignatias is often very telling. They grow a good deal of hair on the face but not on any other unusual part of the body.

As Ignatia patients can be hysterical and feel betrayed and out of control, they are often given to eating disorders, especially bulimia, which allows them to make use of their hysterical vomiting.

And, in that Ignatias use virtually all their vital force on the emotional level, they often fall prey to nonspecific physical ailments. Ignatias are given both to chronic fatigue and to environmental illness. In both cases, although no scientific tests can spot any problem, the patients are exhausted and unable to attempt even the simplest task.

In general, Ignatias feel worse after eating, especially fruit, which they may crave, and sweets. They are worse when using tobacco in any form, even just smelling it. They are worse when it is raining. Most important, Ignatia patients are made worse by consolation. When they run to their room and cry, they do not want to be held or comforted. They will return at some time in the future and act as if nothing happened. What they want is that everyone else act that way as well. In general, Ignatias are very loud when crying, laughing, or screaming obscenities. They are much quieter when they are dealing with the aftermath of their actions and their words. They have a great deal of trouble apologizing for what they have done, although they are well aware of just what it is that they did. (This is particularly true when Ignatias succeed in ruining someone else's happy relationship. While they quietly grieve over the terrible thing that they have done, they never ever apologize for it.)

Ignatia patients are also worse during the winter. They are worse in the presence of strong smells and strong emotions. They are worse when touched. And they feel terrible when they have to walk too fast.

Ignatia patients feel better when they are warm. They like hard pressure, as well as hard chairs and other hard surfaces. They feel better when walking slowly and if they change their physical position often.

When the remedy Ignatia is given to those who exhibit symptoms brought on from a sense of betrayal and disappointment with an underlying foundation of unresolved grief, the Ignatia layer quickly yields, uncovering the patient's true constitutional condition.

In its action, Ignatia is similar to another homeopathic remedy, Staphysagria, which is created from the herb stavesacre, also know as larkspur. Like Ignatia, Staphysagria is an acute remedy that often mirrors a constitutional in that the patient can for a very long time be trapped in an emotional prison. Staphysagria is the remedy for people who have been harmed, who have, through no fault of their own, been mistreated. They know that they have been wronged and they feel angry about it—righteously indignant—but they do not know what to do about their anger. Some are always angry, totally motivated in life by their anger and rage. Others deny their anger and hold it deep within, seeming to be the calmest and nicest people possible. Either way, the righteous indignation is the key. Staphysagria is a useful remedy for victims of child abuse and rape. (Some homeopaths feel that Hahnemann himself could have used the remedy, in that he was treated most unfairly by the medical establishment of his day.) Like Ignatia, Staphysagria can resolve this issue, releasing patients from this emotional prison and unveiling their true homeopathic constitution.

Both Ignatia and Staphysagria speak to the emotional and spiritual parts of the patient. While both remedies can be effective in lower potencies and repeated doses, they are most effective in a single high-potency dose of 1M and above. Both remedies are fairly brief in their action, lasting only days at a time, but both can usually complete their healing action with just one dose.

LEDUM

Remedy Source: The remedy Ledum Palustre is taken from the wild rosemary, also called marsh tea, which grows in damp regions throughout Europe and North America. The remedy is made from the whole plant, which is gathered just after flowering has begun. The plant has long been considered a medicinal herb. In northern Europe, a tea made from marsh tea was used to remove lice from humans and animals alike. This same tea, taken internally, was considered a powerful headache remedy. The Swedes use the plant in making beer, and the leaves of the plant have been a part of the tanning process.

Because the plant was known to remove parasites, Teste, a noted homeopath, began to consider the remedy in situations involving bites. Later, he enlarged the remedy's circle of action to include all puncture wounds. Ledum is a remedy created by Hahnemann. Dr. Teste later re-proved the remedy's actions.

Situations That Suggest Ledum: Puncture wounds from stings and bites, bruises. Also abscesses of all sorts. Also headaches, sprains, rheumatic pains, nosebleed, alcoholism.

Remedy Portrait: Patients who need Ledum first and foremost are chilly. They are cold all the time. There is a constant lack of vital heat. The parts of the body affected by injury are cold to the touch, yet the patients want only cold applications to the wound.

The patient has a red face, yet the face may be cold to the touch. Kent says that the face will look "mottled, puffy, and bloated." Often the red face is accompanied by a congestive headache, the pain of which is improved by cold air.

The patient bleeds easily. Often there are nosebleeds accompanying the chilliness and the wound.

Most often, Ledum is called for in situations that involve puncture wounds of any sort: wounds made by a needle, nail, or any sharp instrument. Wounds may also be made by an insect sting or animal bite, especially cat bite and the stings of bees, wasps, and scorpions. Mosquito bites can also cause the Ledum range of symptoms.

Look for the puncture wound to be cold to the touch and to feel cold internally to the patient. The wound looks bruised and seems "squishy" to the touch. The wound remains discolored for a long time, purplish or blue in color. The area of the wound swells and seems swollen with liquid. The wound is greatly aggravated by heat and ameliorated by cold. The patient may want to take a cool bath to soothe his aches and pains.

Ledum is also the best choice for a black eye. Think about it. A black eye most often follows the pattern of Ledum: the purple discoloration, the squishy feeling. The black eye also most often feels cold to the touch, and yet the remedy is to put something cold—a piece of raw meat—on the wound. The black eye also stays discolored for a long time. A dose or two of Ledum quickly clears the black eye of both its discoloration and its discomfort.

Ledum is a major remedy for sprained ankles. The remedy has an affinity for the lower limbs of the body and quickly soothes the ankle that has been twisted or sprained, in which the general symptoms of the remedy are present. Ledum is also a good remedy for physical trauma that crosses the body in its impact. The pains in Ledum often flow from the left shoulder down to the right hip.

Ledum is a wonderful rheumatic remedy and can act curatively for a wide range of rheumatic pains. Rheumatic situations that respond to Ledum, however, tend to follow a common pattern: The pain is located in the lower limbs of the body; the pain rises from the feet upward, often starting in the balls of the toes, and, over time and with increased severity, travels upward to the hips. The rheumatic condition is improved by cold bathing of painful parts. The pain is sticking in nature and tends to throb as well. It is worse when the patient moves, and at night, especially from the heat of the bed. The patient does not want to be covered and is greatly relieved by having his feet in cold water. Ledum is very helpful for cases of elephantiasis, in which feet and ankles are inflamed and swollen, if the patient wants to put his feet into cold water.

General swelling in Ledum is common, with a sensation of coldness running all through the swollen parts. Like the rheumatic pain, the swelling begins with the feet and travels upward to the ankles, which usually makes walking painful if not impossible, and finally up to the knees.

The chronic Ledum condition most often makes the patient reluctant to walk. Ledum patients do not trust their next step and feel as if their ankles will give way at any time. They do not want to put their full body weight on their ankles. Ledum can be particularly valuable as a remedy for those who have repeatedly injured their ankles and who feel that the joint is permanently weakened.

Finally, Ledum should not be discounted as a remedy for the alcoholic who has all but ruined his health. The vital force is very low, as is the vital heat. The alcoholic patient who can be helped by Ledum follows the general pattern of Ledum, the flow of its pain, and the amelioration of symptoms with external applications of cold water.

In general, Ledum patients are aggravated by heat, motion, alcohol in any form, and scratching the wound. They are worse lying down.

Ledum patients feel better bathing in cold water, in cool air, and after eating.

This remedy is most effective in a single dose. The potency 200C tends to be the most effective, although all levels of potency should be considered in a given case.

RUTA

Remedy Source: Ruta is created from the common garden plant rue, also called bitterwort. It is native to southern Europe. For centuries, rue has been considered an important herbal medicine. It was used in the treatment of such diverse diseases as hysteria, rabies, and blurred vision. Most important, the ancients considered rue to be antidotal in action to nearly every form of poison. The flowers of the plant were often held up to the face to ward off toxic smells. The remedy is created from the whole plant. The remedy Ruta was proved by Hahnemann.

Situations That Suggest Ruta: Injuries, specifically to the muscles and connective tissue. Also colds and coughs, allergies, asthma. Also eye pain and strain, strabismus, amblyopia. Consider for constipation and worms.

Remedy Portrait: Ruta is a small remedy but a wonderful treatment for acute aches and pains.

The central issue of the remedy is one of stiffness. While there may be pain involved in the situation, the patient complains most of stiffness. This issue is involved on all planes of being, body, mind, and spirit. The patient is mentally and emotionally stiff, certainly nonemotional and noncaring, if complaining and somewhat angry. He sometimes exhibits fears and may have a good deal of anxiety, especially around the idea that he can't think, that he can't easily recall, that he may be losing his mind. Ruta has been used successfully in the treatment of anxiety disorder where the characteristic stiffness is displayed throughout the entire constitution.

The stiffness is perhaps more noticeable on the physical plane. Any part of the body affected exhibits the characteristic stiffness. The eyes, for instance, if part of the symptom portrait, not only feel pain and strain but feel stiff. And no matter the muscle or joint affected, in addition to any other sort of pain present, it feels both stiff and numb.

Ruta is particularly helpful in situations that involve pain in the area of the hips. Look for the patient to have trouble getting up out of a chair or out of a car, as this rising motion is the most difficult.

Ruta is also a helpful remedy for situations in which the patient is experiencing lameness after strains or sprains of the wrists or ankles. It is characteristic of the remedy that the pains experienced in these parts of the body blend a bruised sensation with numbness and tingling.

Look for patients to have trouble climbing stairs. Ruta can be helpful in situations in which patients feel as if their knees will give out under them. Ruta can also be helpful for lower back pain, in situations in which the patient feels better lying down on something hard and applying pressure to the pain. After a rest, the patient suffering lower back pain wants to rise up and feels better slowly walking outside.

Those suffering with sciatica also may find relief with this remedy. The patient feels better in the day and worse at night. He feels better when slowly moving, worse when lying or sitting still.

Ruta also works well with the pain remedy Arnica, often completing the healing action of Arnica, especially in situations involving injured and bruised bones.

Ruta has a particular affinity to the eyes and to vision. It is one of the first remedies to consider when the eyes have been overexerted. This can be brought on from close work like sewing or by overworking the eyes reading in too little light. Vision is blurred, and there is aching in and over the eyes, spasms of the lower lids, and a feeling of weakness in the eyes and of paralysis. The eyes may physically turn in or out. One eye may develop a chronic weakness of vision.

In general, Ruta patients feel weak as well as stiff. They want to rest, but after lying down for a brief period, they feel that they must get up and walk. Patients feel worse in damp and/or cold weather. They are worse when stooping or when sitting up.

Ruta patients feel better in the morning. They are better when slowly moving about and lying still, when in a warm room, and when applying warm things to their pain.

Ruta is a helpful acute remedy, one dose of which may be effective for up to thirty days, although it may be repeated as needed. It is usually most effective when used in low potency, running from the lowest 6X up to 200C.

URTICA URENS

Remedy Source: Urtica Urens is created from the stinging nettle, a plant native to northern Europe. The stinging nettle is similar to the common nettle; both plants have been considered medicinal herbs and both are ingested and brewed into teas. The stinging nettle has for centuries been considered a remedy for inflammatory diseases of all sorts, particularly whooping cough. In addition, it is considered an antidote to any number of poisons. Dioscorides considered it a tonic for the system and felt that it had the power to cleanse the entire body. The whole plant is used in the creation of the remedy. It was popularized as a remedy through the work of Burnett.

Situations That Suggest Urtica: Burns and fevers, sore throat, whooping cough, rheumatism, gout, kidney stones, puncture wounds such as insect bites and stings, chicken pox, worms.

Remedy Portrait: Urtica Urens is a small but very important homeopathic remedy for situations that involve pain. The sensation of pain unique to Urtica is burning. This is the first remedy to think of in situations that involve physical burns, especially first-degree burns.

It is characteristic of the remedy that patients feel as if they have sand in their eyes. It is also characteristic that the right arm feels sore and the muscles of that limb feel bruised.

Along with the burning sensation, patients complain of itching—of the burned area as well as other parts of the body. The skin of the affected area has raised red patches. This makes Urtica a solid remedy for hives and for allergies that affect the skin with the set of symptoms listed above. The same applies to cases of chicken pox, for which Urtica is one of the chief remedies if the other symptoms follow the remedy portrait.

The remedy is effective for burns of all sorts, including sunburn when other symptoms follow suit.

Urtica patients are somewhat disconnected from their pain. They tend to feel drowsy and may fall asleep.

Urtica is a cleansing remedy. Suppressed eruptions appear on the skin when the remedy is given. Again, these are raised and itching red patches.

With its cleansing action, Urtica also often removes toxins from the system. It has long been considered a remedy specific to the kidneys and can help remove kidney stones from the system.

Utica is a remedy of a rheumatic type, like Arnica or Bryonia. The pain always includes the right shoulder. The pain may be continuous and increase when moving the shoulder inward and from any action like that of putting on a coat.

A useful part of Urtica's action is its ability to act as an antidote to various poisons. This is the first remedy to consider when the patient becomes ill from eating tainted shellfish, or for those who are in general allergic to shellfish. Further, Urtica is considered a fine antidote to ingesting poison mushrooms.

In general, patients want to lie down and may fall asleep soon after doing so. They are worse, however, lying on the right side; the right shoulder becomes stiff and painful.

Patients are worse when it is snowing, damp, or cold. They are worse if they overtax their muscles and joints and if they apply water, no matter what temperature.

Like Calendula and Hypericum, Urtica is available in both topical and pellet form. And, like these other remedies, I have found that most often the best topical application is made by simply dissolving Urtica in water and then applying this water to the burn. The remedy may be taken orally and topically at the same time. Expect patients with burns to be worse after sleep and much worse after the application of water to the area of the burn.

This remedy bears repetition well and may be given in any potency. In cases of burns, the remedy may be repeated often and may have to be increased in potency until improvement begins.

8

CONSIDERING CONSTITUTIONS: CONSTITUTIONAL TREATMENTS

When it comes to constitutional treatments, even some serious students of homeopathy find themselves confused. They have come to think that when we treat constitutionally, we are somehow using a different set of rules from those that apply to acute conditions. And this is sometimes true. In a true emergency, we sometimes use more than one remedy. But this is the only exception. In all other ways, the constitutional and the acute treatments are very much the same; both proceed from case taking to remedy giving by unchanging principles.

In both cases, we are trying to match the symptom portrait that the patient is already experiencing with a remedy portrait that most closely parallels the situation at hand. And in both cases, we may well be making use of the same remedies. The polycrests—those remedies that speak to the largest number of people and to the largest number of symptoms—are the most likely candidates for use in either case.

The difference between the two methods of treatment is largely the goal of each treatment. In acute situations, we seek only to restore that status quo that the patient calls good health. In constitutional treatment, we are seeking to raise that patient's standard of health above and beyond anything that he experienced before. We are attempting to increase his level of freedom and to decrease the amount of his life and energy that has been given over to circumstances that can be identified as disease.

The idea of constitutional treatment versus acute is somewhat new to homeopathy. For Hahnemann, there was truly no such thing as an acute treatment. There were certainly emergency situations and long-term patterns, there were acute and chronic diseases, but for him all treatment was constitutional. Hahnemann always had as his goal the total health and freedom of his patient, no matter the circumstances of the illness.

It is part of the bastardization of homeopathy that we even consider as our goal a return to the status quo. This goal is in its very nature allopathic and shows how the philosophy of allopathy is blending its way into homeopathic philosophy. And by allowing this to become the goal of even the lightest and slightest of homeopathic treatments, we are undermining all that Hahnemann set forth for us to accomplish.

We can be easily confused about constitutional treatment if we equate it with disease. Many people, even some long-term students of homeopathy, still think that when we have completed our homeopathic treatment, we are no longer a constitutional type.

Like we all have astrological signs, we all have constitutional types. Just as no person on Earth has managed to be born at a moment for which there is no sun sign, so, too, each of us is born a constitutional type. What that type is is largely determined by genetics. From the moment of birth, we are unique individuals, but at the same time we are examples of homeopathic types. Well or sick, strong or weak, from the moment of birth until the moment of death, we belong to one or another homeopathic type. I call this the birth remedy or core constitution.

Instead of thinking of constitutions as diseases, start to think of them as people. While we are all, to be sure, whole beings and unique unto ourselves, we are also from the moment of birth gifted with certain strengths of body, mind, and spirit and cursed with certain thorns in the flesh and in the soul. By grouping together individual people in terms of their similar weaknesses and strengths, we are able to ascertain certain types. They may all, for example, have a tendency toward diabetes. This doesn't mean that they have the disease, or ever will, only that the tendency is present. One symptom such as this, along with others in the remedy portrait, may help to determine a constitutional type.

Think of each type as a continuum of health and illness. Within every type we can find individuals who are so ill that they are barely alive, individuals who are totally and perfectly healthy, and everything in between. So the notion that if you treat a Sulphur type with Sulphur he will automatically cease to be a Sulphur type is just not true. What you may end up with is a totally healthy Sulphur whose system is balanced and whose life has been freed. While still holding the talents and tendencies that are common to Sulphur, he is no longer held in check by its weaknesses.

Many of us may shift from one constitutional type to another while undergoing treatment. Those of us who were healthy enough not to have received much suppressive medical treatment in the course of our lives usually still are the same constitutional type that we were at birth. But most of us are not. Life gets to us. For example, many children shift constitutions if their parents divorce. Others do so if the family moves, or if a beloved person or even pet suddenly dies. Many of us shift constitutions during puberty, or during menopause or pregnancy, when the hormone balance in the body dramatically shifts. And certainly most of us shift type if ailments of any deep sort are suppressed deeper into the system through allopathic treatments, especially through treatments with antibiotics or steroids.

Since most of us have had multiple allopathic treatments—after all, most of us were given antibiotics for ridiculous reasons like earaches and acne—and since life has given most of us our full share of tragedy, we have developed several levels of constitution.

This shifting of constitutional type during life is a defense mechanism geared to the survival of the being. The body is doing its best to find its highest level of health and its strongest level of vital force. In order to do this, it may move into a profound level of denial (common to the Natrum type) or toward anger or rage (as with the Nux type). These adaptations, while necessary in the moment for the sake of survival, can become more and more toxic to the system over time. All that was suppressed is still suppressed, which, given time, overwhelms the vital force, weakens the whole being, and drives the patient either to a deeper, weaker constitution, or into deeper disease conditions within its original type.

It is the goal of the constitutional treatment, therefore, to work through these levels of pain and suppression and, ultimately, to bring healing to the core constitution. This is the process, finally, in which the sick Sulphur becomes the healthy Sulphur. And, for the practitioner, it is the observation that the patient's being is no longer shifting from one constitution to another, but is rather becoming stronger and clearer within one set type, that confirms that the healing is near completion.

When we work our way back through the layers of built-up constitutional debris, it is important that we always work from today. This is where we remember that Hahnemann considered all treatment—for so-called acute conditions as well as for chronic ones—to be constitutional. If, after the patient first takes the constitutional remedy most similar to his type, he suddenly gets a cold, you have to consider what to do. Better still, you have to ask yourself: What would Hahnemann do?

The answer is to assume that, because the condition has changed in some way, the remedy is working. If the energy of the remedy brings about a change, any change, the best thing to do is wait and see what happens next. The practitioner who is still segregating his treatment into acute and constitutional is forever tempted to stop what has already been begun and to treat the cold, since the cold is what is happening today. The practitioner who sees only constitutions and can recognize the shift within constitutions from disease toward health understands that the cold, while it may be unpleasant, was on some level necessary—most often to detoxify the system— and waits. The remedy is doing what the remedy should be doing.

Working in this way, if we can learn to not examine each small change or each expression of a suppressed symptom, we can begin to see the patterns of our illnesses emerge. In revisiting suppressed symptoms, as they are expressed and released forever, we begin to see the causes of those symptoms and to release those causes—anger, fear, loneliness, and the like—as well.

In always working from today backward, we allow ourselves to explore our lives fully, and we slowly learn to forgive and release all that we have held within. In always working from today backward, we unwrite the past and allow ourselves to become free to explore our future.

The practitioner who divides treatments between the acute and the contitutional is always changing gears between curing and healing, between allopathy and homeopathy. The practitioner who sees healing on a more profound level gets to live by the Law of Similars.

Homeopathic remedies are effective even for those who are not conscious of taking the remedies when they are given. If you give remedies to animals and to plants, both respond quite nicely, although neither filled out an intake form. Still, it is important to the constitutional practitioner to work hand in hand with the patient. Both must be equal partners in the healing process. Both must be open to change, as change is involved in all healing.

It is always amazing to me that so many so-called healers are themselves unwilling to change. It seems to me that the chief blessing in working with the principle of healing is that, in working as a partner in another's healing process, the practitioner, if he is also willing to undergo change, may also be healed. Again, many think that it is mere coincidence that this patient with so many issues and problems so similar to his own has wandered into his office. I say, let like cure like. Use the similarity and get started on healing. In refusing to let the patient be a full partner in the medical process, the allopathic doctor gives up the possibility of a healing taking place all around, leaving only the hope that something can be cured.

In the pages that follow, I present what I call the Twelve Essential Constitutions. The number twelve is arbitrary, and the word *essential* may have been selected more out of a need to be dramatic than out of actual fact. But I want to put forth some of the central issues of our most important homeopathic remedies and to present these remedies as people and not as disease. I believe with all my heart that the anthropomorphized form of homeopathy, which stresses the mind and spirit over the body, is the method by which homeopathics can be used most effectively. Therefore, I stress the emotions and the situations that motivate each type, both in their relationships and career and in their creation of disease.

There are more than fifty remedies that could have been put on this list. And, for those already versed in homeopathic materia medica, the selections that I have made for the "essential" constitutions likely say more about me than they do about homeopathy. But, having given a quick sketch of some acute remedies that can be of great help in household emergencies, I want to go deeper, because I believe that homeopathy can work on a level so much deeper than merely curing a bee sting. (Although, as a homeopath once pointed out to me, even a beginning student of homeopathy can, with the help of some very common and well-known remedies, cure a cold— something that all the money and time thrown into allopathic medicine have never allowed their practitioners to do. So perhaps I shouldn't underrate these acute treatments.) I want to show that, with the proper constitutional treatment, the patient can change fundamentally and change for the better, that we don't have to spend our lives collecting new diseases and putting them next to the old.

Twelve Essential Constitutions
SULPHUR
The Egoist

Remedy Source: The remedy Sulphur is created from the element sulfur. The substance occurs naturally as a brittle, crystalline substance. Sulphur was known to the ancients as brimstone and has been used therapeutically for thousands of years. As a substance, it has traditionally been considered a tonic and has been used specifically for the treatment of various skin conditions. Animals as well as humans have been treated with the substance; for example, dissolving sulfur in a dog's drinking water was once considered a method for protecting the health of the animal's skin and fur. In India, sulfur is called *gandhak*, a word that refers to the substance's unpleasant smell. Even before sulfur became a staple of Western medicine, the Ayurvedic practitioners of India used the drug constitutionally.

Hahnemann, who first proved the drug as a homeopathic remedy, notes that the substance was used curatively for at least 2,000 years.

Situations That Suggest Sulphur: Skin conditions of all sorts: acne, eczema, rash, herpes, measles, chicken pox, psoriasis, ringworm, worms; allergies, particularly food allergies; asthma; low blood sugar; diabetes; digestive disorders: irritable bowel syndrome, constipation, diarrhea, ulcer, rectal fissure. Also mental disorders: depression, mania, dementia, anxiety; functional disorders of all sorts: chronic fatigue syndrome, arthritis, rheumatoid arthritis, multiple sclerosis. Also pregnancy and menopause, menstrual troubles. Also headaches; migraines; inflammatory conditions; alcoholism; sleep disorders, especially sleeplessness; vertigo.

Remedy Overview: Kent tells us, "When I prescribe, I prescribe Sulphur." Other classical homeopaths refer to the remedy as "the fuse to the bomb," in that the remedy, as a constitutional, often opens a case, uncovering what has been suppressed, while not acting as a completely curative remedy.

Sulphur is the most used of all homeopathic remedies. It is an essential tool of all three levels of homeopathic care: acute, constitutional, and transformational. It is considered that the vast majority of humans, perhaps as many as 90 percent, would have some sort of curative reaction with a dose of the remedy, whether on a superficial or profound level.

Remedy Theme: Itch, restlessness, malfunction.

Remedy Motivation: Curiosity.

Emotional Portrait: When we think of the Sulphur personality, we think of the adage "Jack of all trades, master of none." No one is more interested in more topics than is a Sulphur, and no one is less willing to put forth the effort really to come to understand any of those topics. Classes in homeopathy are filled with Sulphurs, who come to hear about it because it's new to them and therefore exciting. Anything that is new is exciting to Sulphurs; they want constant entertainment, constant excitement. This is due to the restlessness they always feel. Like a little child, the adult Sulphur has to be entertained if you want to get his attention.

Some Sulphurs want to own anything new—they are the first with a satellite dish, the first one on the Internet. They love new technology, new ways of doing old things. In fact, if there's something they hate, it is something old, something familiar, something that offers no new excitement. That's what brings on the itch.

Itch is the core feature of this remedy on all levels of being. From a physical allergy to wool, which causes Sulphur unbearable itching, to the clichéd seven-year itch, an itchy Sulphur is a miserable Sulphur. Mental, physical, and emotional itching is perhaps his main sensation and motivation in life. Beware the itchy Sulphur—he will do anything to scratch that itch.

So Sulphurs come to classes in homeopathy because, if they can learn a whole lot about something in a very short time, their itch gets scratched. And they eat foods that shock their systems and stop the itch. They want really, really spicy foods; the heat of the food (particularly Mexican) makes the physical itch in their throat stop for a while. And they want a quick sexual fling to stop the emotional and physical itch. But none of this lasts for a very long time before the itch starts up again, in another part of the body, another part of the mind, and they are off looking to scratch.

So the Sulphurs who come to learn homeopathy soon walk away, saying that it's just too complicated. Or they leave that relationship saying that they don't know what they saw in him or her. Or they end up with a garage full of gadgets that looked like so much fun but turned out to be boring.

If there is a fear that Sulphurs all share, it is the fear of boredom, of tedium. This can make them very dramatic in their lifestyles, especially as, over time, the itch gets worse and they have to do more and more to scratch it. They dress in brighter and brighter colors, dye their hair red, talk in a more and more baroque manner.

The words they choose are very important to Sulphurs. Some speak in only scientific, medical, or mathematical jargon. Others are psychics, speaking only to the dead or interpreting the universe for others. Here, too, no matter how they embody it, they have one thing in common: Sulphurs have a deep need to have some sort of knowledge that no one else possesses. That's another reason they are running out to learn homeopathy, because they can still be the first one on the block to learn it, and they can then make pronouncements about everyone else's constitutionality, both to their face and behind their back.

Sulphurs want to be the center of attention. This satisfies their itch for approval. They are the class clowns and the happy drunks who tell the same old jokes at every party. Sulphur is one of the major remedies for this alcoholic type, the happy drunk, who can get a bit abusive at a party. Like Sulphur Homer Simpson, they will drink too much, eat too much, and end up passed out on the carpet, drooling.

In that they crave foods and drinks that take their mind off the itch, Sulphurs love alcohol. They love sugar and salt, especially salt, and fats of all sorts. The American diet, especially the diet of teens (who often go through a Sulphur stage with the onset of puberty: look for the greasy skin and hair, the messy room, the dirty clothes, the junk food habit and the characteristic Sulphur slouch), namely pizza, hamburgers and fries, and extra large ice-cold sodas of all sorts, reflects the cravings of Sulphur and prove the large numbers of Sulphur persons lurking in our lives.

Sulphurs are also perhaps the most thirsty of all the constitutional types, or at least the least choosy about what they drink. They like cold things best, cold water especially, but thirsty Sulphurs will drink anything. They tend to need a lot of liquids and to need them quite often. This is particularly interesting in that just as the substance Sulphur and water do not mix, those who follow the Sulphur remedy type hate water and do not want to get wet. But while Sulphurs do not want to take a bath, they will almost drink water from a puddle like a dog if they have to.

Along with wanting new and exciting things, Sulphurs are collectors. Some collect knowledge, rushing from class to class without ever managing to declare a major. Others collect objects, any objects. Some are busy rebuying the comic books their mothers threw out when they left for college—and paying premium prices to repurchase their past. Others are unable to pass a garage sale without buying several things that no one else could possibly want.

Another way to scratch that itch is by sheer volume. It is as if they are playing the game "the one who dies with the most stuff wins" with the entire planet. Their closets, garages, car trunks, and office desks are loaded with stuff they couldn't pass up. Some of it stays in its original box for a few years before someone else in the family makes it disappear. (You do have to make things disappear to get Sulphurs to let go of things. They tend to love certain shirts or to have a pair of "lucky socks" that they wear although they are stained and ripped beyond repair. Noble spouses have to burn these things to get the Sulphur to let go of them.)

A perfect example of the Sulphur's need to possess can be seen in an incident with a friend of mine. When I moved into my present apartment, one with a large fireplace, she invited me to her home. When I arrived, she told me that she wanted to give me a pair of andirons. With that, she took me into the basement and opened the door to her andiron room. I swear to God, it was as if she had cornered the market on andirons. There were dozens of pairs, large and small. She must have been collecting them for years. After I picked a pair, she showed me the rest of the house: the cut glass room filled with hundreds of pieces of unmatching cut glass; the furniture room stacked to the ceiling with every sort of furniture, none matching; the library, which was not a real library, just a large room stacked to the ceiling with every sort of book, none organized so that you could find anything or even remove anything without being killed by falling books. The whole house was a maze of collections.

This need to collect is typical of Sulphur. Along with this is also Sulphur generosity. Sulphur types are the most generous and the most stingy. They pour forth gifts and give you their last dollar—but only when they want to. In other words, when you need nothing you may be overwhelmed with their generosity, but when you really are in need, your best friend the Sulphur may give you nothing. You cannot predict the flow of generosity with Sulphurs; you can only realize that, because they work from their ego, which is usually wounded, they need to get something back for their giving. If they feel that someone does not make a big enough fuss about their giving, they close off to that person in every way.

This principle of generosity ties in to Sulphur's eternal itch. Sulphurs give anything to anyone who can bring them relief. Therefore, they are incredibly generous with those who make them laugh or who excite them. But this flow of generosity is brief; the excitement soon ends and the itch returns.

The itch can drive Sulphur from relationship to relationship, career to career. It can also, however, drive the Sulphur deeper and deeper into a philosophical nature. Many Sulphurs relentlessly search for meaning. They want to know the Truth. They want to know God. Beyond that, they seek to learn the name of God's father.

Mentally, Sulphurs are given to anxiety. They can be very future directed, often not wanting anything to do with their past. They do not tend to be particularly nostalgic; no Sulphur wants to have the family photos, for example, unless such things are on his mental list of things that need collecting.

Anxiety can play a large part in their lives. They become anxious that they have not achieved all the things in life that they feel they should achieve. Some feel that they should be more famous, others that they should have won more academic acclaim. This anxiety plays off the Sulphur's ego issues and need to be noticed.

They tend to be extroverted and are usually quite willing to share their private tragedies with anyone who is willing to listen. Some Sulphurs, those who are more shy by nature, may use alcohol or drugs as a method by which they can become louder and be noticed.

In that they are future directed, some Sulphurs are made anxious by the idea that something bad is about to happen. They tend to project this anxiety onto others. If their child is ten minutes late, the Sulphur is sure that she is lying in a ditch by the side of the road and may even rush to the car to search.

Sulphurs can be very critical. God protect you if they find you less intelligent than they are, or, worse, boring. If it connects with whatever they are collecting, the criticism can get out of hand. If the Sulphur is collecting all knowledge about diet, for instance, the fat among us had better cross the road to avoid him. He lectures and even verbally abuses the offenders, more out of a need for center stage and the need to possess secret knowledge than for any real concern for our health.

Sulphurs often start sentences with, "What's wrong with you is . . ." They walk into a room and say, "It's too hot in here." This comment actually is pretty common—Sulphurs are among the hottest people. They crave open air, usually wear less clothing than do other people, and drink cold liquids as an attempt at keeping cool. When they become too warm, they begin to itch, and you'll remember that this is a very bad thing.

The fact that Sulphur works out of his ego cannot be overstated. Whether the Sulphur is a college professor or a cashier at Walmart, he needs to feel good about himself. Sulphurs need to feel that others envy them on some level or other. This leads them to spend more than they can afford to have a swimming pool to invite their neighbors to swim in (even if they themselves do not swim), or to wear outrageous things, or simply to talk very loudly with great authority about books that they know only through Cliff Notes.

In acting in this way, they are largely harmless, needing only a momentary boost to their flagging ego. In terms of their ego, they are for the most part creatures of the moment, needing a brief massage, and unwilling to put forth the planning and effort required to make their desire for fame a reality. Many, given their love for salt and grease, turn to food to comfort their damaged ego and end up, by their middle years, with a girth that matches that ego.

Our poster child for Sulphur, the person who best and most embodies the nature of this constitutional remedy, is Albert Einstein, whose need for truth led him to discoveries that changed our understanding of our universe and who redefined our relationship with the cosmos.

Picture Einstein and you picture Sulphur: the wrinkled suit and the stained tie; the hair a white nest sitting on his head; the sloppy mustache; an office filled with books, papers, and blackboards covered with equations. No one else could find anything in that office, but he knew if you touched a single piece of paper or smudged a number on the blackboard. This is Sulphur: sloppy, somewhat dirty, and always a little confused. He may not know what day it is, and he may always be at least an hour late, but he can, with his cluttered, muddled mind, almost literally know God.

Physical Portrait: The physical ailments of Sulphur tend to run from two grand themes: itch and malfunction.

Itching runs through all the aches and pains of Sulphur, as does burning. A headache burns, and the pain sensation has itching as well. The sore throat burns and itches, relieved only by cold liquids and salty things.

Almost all these ailments respond well to cool things, to anything that can counteract the burn. This is particularly true of two areas of the body that are especially problematic for the Sulphur, the skin and the digestive tract. The skin is given to any sort of rash—acne, eczema, psoriasis, etc.—and is very red and very itchy. As for the digestive tract, the characteristic itching and burning run through all the various ailments, from diarrhea to hemorrhoids to ulcers.

Allergies are common enough to the type, perhaps to be considered essential. They regularly involve the skin, the digestion, or both. Sulphur allergies manifest most frequently on the skin, with redness, itching, and burning. Food allergies are also very common, and the Sulphur is likely to crave the very foods to which he or she is most sensitive.

The Sulphur type has red skin. This is displayed especially in what is called the "Sulphur Mask," a patch of red skin that goes from one cheek across the bridge of the nose to the other cheek. It's like Santa Claus, who also shows his Sulphur nature by being very generous with you at Christmas, but only if he considers you to have been "nice."

Sulphur alcoholics also have red skin, usually with large, red bulbous noses, like W. C. Fields, who was a Sulphur if there ever was one.

Sulphur is given to headaches. They come on periodically, sometimes with a cyclical regularity. Every weekend is a common time for headaches, as the Sulphur is letting down his guard and stopping his need to appear very busy.

In general, the Sulphur is aggravated by heat and better in cool. Sulphurs cannot bear to get too hot in bed. They stick their feet out from under the covers in order to keep cool.

They are also aggravated by standing. They rock, lean, slump. No Sulphur wants to stand up straight. (Think of a sixteen-year-old boy.)

And then there is the typical Sulphur smell. The remedy is made from brimstone, which is known for its unpleasant smell, so the remedy type follows suit. Sulphurs' sweat, urine, and stool all have a strong smell, and their clothing has a strong, unpleasant smell.

It is an interesting feature of the remedy that, even though Sulphurs do not like heat, they like the sun. Sulphurs feel better while the sun is out and tend to feel worse in the evening and on cloudy or rainy days. They also tend to prefer summer—heat, allergies, and all—to winter.

Another interesting feature of the remedy is Sulfurs' aggravation at 11 A.M. Like clockwork. Often this manifests in hunger, an aspect of the low blood sugar that runs all through this type. They need a doughnut or a candy bar in the late morning. Usually they say that it is an early lunch or that they skipped breakfast, and usually this is a lie. But they do tend to feel weak and dizzy in the late morning and tend to feel better after eating. It is important that they are allowed a snack at this time—try, though, to get them to eat an apple. If they are not allowed to eat, they can get a headache or vertigo and become downright unpleasant. Note that some Sulphurs show this trait at 11 P.M. instead and are unable to sleep if they do not first have something to eat. They, too, must be allowed their snack, as it is a true symptom of the type and not a mere whim.

Many a constitutional Sulphur is created and not born. The type can be artificially created by the suppression of diseases, especially diseases involving a flow from the body. As simple a suppression as the regular use of an antiperspirant can create the Sulphur symptom portrait, as suppression of sweat is key to the creation of ailments in Sulphur. Any other continuing suppressions, from diarrhea, vertigo, measles, asthma, and rash, can lead a person to become a Sulphur type.

This is particularly true of rash. Consider diaper rash. So many chronic conditions begin with a simple thing like diaper rash. The baby has the rash and the mother spreads antibiotic ointment all over the affected area. The rash disappears, but the mother notices that the child's ears are starting to turn red and are burning to the touch. The child cries and cries and the doctor says that the child has an ear infection. He gives the child more antibiotic. Over time, the recurring ear infections disappear. The doctor says that the child is cured, but the mother notices that the child is now starting to be allergic to things. The allergies are treated with an antihistamine, which suppresses the allergies. If they become really bad, the child is given steroids, either in injection or by inhaler. The allergies go away, but the child starts to have troubles with an irritable bowel. And so on and so on.

The problem is that we do not look at the price we pay for suppression. And the greater problem is that we take what is essentially so simple a situation and ultimately make it life threatening. A little thing like rash can become multiple chronic conditions if we do not work with it correctly, if we do not learn to think about it correctly. This is especially important when dealing with the Sulphur types, who tend to get so many rashes. If they don't learn very quickly not to suppress those rashes in any way, they are likely to develop chronic conditions and greatly complicate their case.

Chronic conditions are common to the Sulphur type—conditions created by suppression, that are functional in nature, like allergy and chronic fatigue. You can give every test in the book to discover the cause of the disorder, but you will not find it. The cause is invisible—it is the suppression of physical and emotional symptoms, the suppression of the vital force.

Because Sulphur, by the nature of its action, pushes forth whatever has been suppressed, it is perhaps the homeopath's most powerful tool. Consider the action of the remedy to be similar to that of a volcano, which again mirrors the substance from which the remedy is made, in that it is most often to be found near volcanoes.

This is what makes Sulphur so helpful: It uncovers what is really going on in a given case and brings to the surface what has been shoved down. Now, if the total cause of illness and of disease in the person has to do with this suppression, then Sulphur acts curatively. But most often Sulphur is a layer or layers created by allopathic medicines. The remedy removes these layers but does not create total health in the person. Instead, the true nature of the patient is uncovered, which then can be properly treated.

The first Sulphur was likely created when a certain caveman discovered that a particular leaf made the rash on his arm feel less itchy. He covered his arm with more and more leaves and noticed that the rash seemed to go away. The last Sulphur will likely be created when we stop putting leaves on our itches at some postapocalyptic future time. Until then, given our lives, our diets, our egos, and our need to stop the itch at any cost, we will likely all need Sulphur at some time or other in our lives.

Poster Children: Albert Einstein, Homer Simpson, Santa Claus.

ARSENICUM
The Controller

Remedy Source: More than one remedy may be described as Arsenicum. The two most important are Arsenicum Album, which is the remedy that I use for an explanation of the type, and Arsenicum Iodatum, which is a blend of Arsenicum and Iodine. Arsenicum is also used in blended remedies as Natrum and Kali in the creation of hybrid remedies.

Arsenicum Album is created from a chemical compound of arsenic and oxygen. It was created as a homeopathic remedy by Samuel Hahnemann.

We have all read mystery novels in which the victim is slipped a deadly dose of arsenic. In these works of fiction, the poison is usually mixed with sugar, which, as another white powdery substance, tends nicely to hide the arsenic. In considering the remedy, consider the symptoms of the poison: extreme pain with anxiety about death, wasting effect, vomiting, and diarrhea.

Situations That Suggest Arsenicum: Mental disorders: anxiety, neurosis, obsessive behavior, compulsive behavior, depression, panic attacks; allergy: shingles, rhinitis, hay fever, food allergies, environmental allergies; immune dysfunction: AIDS; respiratory infections of all sorts: bronchitis, influenza, pneumonia, pharyngitis, isophagitis, colds. Also fever; eating disorders; chronic fatigue; digestive disorders: colitis, food poisoning, irritable bowel, chronic diarrhea; heart disease; congestive heart failure; insomnia.

Remedy Overview: If there is a constitutional type that is easy to identify, it is Arsenicum. And if there is one that the average person thinks of as being easily made fun of, it is Arsenicum. The Arsenicum is controlling, critical, fearful, irritable, sure that he is dying of an incurable disease.

Like the other polycrests, Arsenicum speaks to many different people and the different sets of symptoms they inhabit. For this reason, all of us will happily take our arsenic at some time or other of our lives, either for an acute flu that has us wondering which end of our spine to stick in the toilet first, or for a deeper, constitutional action, one that can free us from a lifetime of fear.

Remedy Theme: Order, control, criticism, hypochondria.

Remedy Motivation: Fear.

Emotional Portrait: There is no homeopathic type that is quite so organized or so fearful as Arsenicum. By day, they keep a clean house and a perfectly organized office. By night, they pace the floor, sure that if they let their guard down even for a moment, robbers will break in and kill them in their sleep.

These people spend their lives always a little insecure, a little worried, sure that something bad will happen, sure that if they trust other people to do their jobs that all hell will break loose: The wallpaper will be the wrong pattern; their dog will be run over by a car; by evening, there will be a ring marring the surface of the coffee table.

And, as they manage to keep everyone around them off balance, their prophecies of disaster have a way of coming true. In this way, the Arsenicum feed into their own neuroses. They see again and again that if they let their guard down for a moment, things just go wrong. What they fail to see is that they fill their lives with these situations by manipulating people and facts so that they can be right. Of all constitutional types, Arsenicum, given the choice, would much rather be right than happy.

Arsenicum people tend to be somewhat conservative: the librarian who spends her life whispering for people to be quiet. They tend to be small and thin, with a great deal of nervous energy that they use in creating order and enforcing the rules. They tend to give off the aura of "wound up" and excitable, instead of the aura of rigidity that belongs to Silica (a remedy type that is the natural butler or expert in manners).

Arsenicum types also tend to be irritable and peevish. They can have sharp tongues, but they are not abusive. The Arsenicum would have a person who offends him removed from further contact rather than ever confront that person or argue with him.

Arsenicum types are restless. They amaze their friends and confound their enemies with their energy. They never stop. The Arsenicum mother who visits her son in his new apartment has the dishes done, the laundry in the wash, and the whole place dusted within minutes of her arrival.

They are fastidiously neat. Our popular entertainment is filled with them, both as characters and as performers. Felix Unger of *The Odd Couple* is an example of a fictional Arsenicum. Certainly Joan Crawford, with her tight and even abusive control over her adopted children and her demand that there be "no wire hangers," is an example of a very sick Arsenicum. And when they are very deep in the type, they spend more and more time and energy cleaning. It is as if by cleaning they are keeping the world safe.

Arsenicums' favorite smell and taste tends to be lemon. They tell you that lemon smells so fresh, so clean. It is not for nothing that so many of our household cleaners are lemon scented. The Arsenicums, and there are millions of them, snap them up the way the Sulphurs buy used clothing and french fries.

They are attracted to order. If you want to impress them, invite them to your home and have just a hint of Comet cleanser in the air. Have the magazines perfectly organized, alphabetical even, and the house dust free. Cook them a complicated dinner and make sure that everything is timed perfectly and that the kitchen stays spotless while you cook. By dessert, they will be putty in your hands.

Arsenicum types live in their heads. While they certainly have the emotion fear down pat, they tend to back away from other emotions and to stay a little cerebral. Some consider Arsenicum to be one of the most intelligent constitutional types. My experience has been that, while they are certainly intellectual, they are not particularly smart. They come to class on time and have all their pencils sharpened. They learn what is put forth for them to learn, but their thinking tends to be as controlled as the rest of them, and they have difficulty applying what they have learned to new situations. In fact, they have trouble with new situations in general and can be very challenged by the changes that life imposes on them.

The worst thing that can happen to an Arsenicum is being left alone. All their symptoms of any sort increase. Especially after midnight, they become convinced that they will die during the night if they are left alone (and, indeed, seriously ill Arsenicum types most often die during the hours just after midnight). They can be quite desperate in their need to have others physically with them, or can spend the entire night on the telephone in order to have some sort of human contact.

The homeopath who takes on an Arsenicum patient has to be willing to allow that patient to stay in almost constant contact. He calls at any hour of the day or night, always insisting that it is an emergency and that he needs attention right now. The Arsenicum who feels that he is not receiving the attention due him becomes very angry and can be almost impossible to deal with.

As a person enters more deeply into the Arsenicum type, his fears manifest increasingly around the idea of poverty. He becomes sure that he will die penniless and alone. He becomes increasingly stingy because of this fear and soon has a reputation everywhere for both poverty-focused thinking and a willingness to do just about anything to save a penny. When he goes out to lunch, he sighs and moans over the cost of every item on the menu. Having had the salmon to your cobb salad, he wants just to divide the check down the middle. If, however, you had the meatloaf and he had the soup, he calculates the amounts due down to the tip. And he calculates it in his head, just as he does crossword puzzles in ink.

Another sign that the patient is moving deeper into the remedy and that its symptoms are becoming more pronounced and further inhibiting the patient's freedom is that he moves on to more of a spiritual level and becomes increasingly compulsive. Where once he had worked out a system of cleaning the kitchen that worked for him, he now develops a ritual. He counts the exact number of wipes that he makes with the sponge on the countertop. He memorizes and counts the number of steps from the back door to the garage. And he begins to save things, which combines the fear of poverty with compulsiveness: grocery bags, rubber bands, and twist ties are all placed in an orderly fashion against future need.

Food is a big issue with an Arsenicum, and it gets bigger and bigger over time. Even the Arsenicum who has not studied some form of medicine (this is rare) has strong opinions as to what should and should not be eaten. As he has put more of his time and energy into his health than any other type, the Arsenicum often has done a ritualized and exhaustive study of nutrition and knows precisely what he will and will not eat and rigidly holds onto that list. Over time, the number and types of food that he feels he can and should eat shrinks. As with the rest of his life, the allowable foods list gets shorter and shorter.

Another way Arsenicums use food as a control issue is through eating disorders. Since they are usually naturally thin, you wouldn't expect them to become concerned with their weight, yet many Arsenicum types, men and women, consider themselves to be fat. The male Arsenicum then usually goes to the gym and develops a ritual through which he can exercise to lose the weight. Arsenicum women often turn to anorexia as a method of weight loss, feeling that if all the rest of their life seems out of control, they can at least control their eating and their weight.

This idea of control is very, very important to Arsenicums. If they can only control this or that aspect of their life, or of the world, if they can only bring order out of the frightening chaos, then everything will at last be all right and they can at last feel secure.

As the Arsenicum's illness intensifies, he makes his world smaller and smaller in order to feel safe. He tends over time literally to withdraw from the world that scares him so much into a small space that he can control and keep clean. For this reason, Arsenicum is a major remedy for agoraphobics, allowing them to rejoin the world around them.

The method most often used to withdraw from the world is illness. Arsenicums keep developing new allergies. They love to come upon new allergies.

Allergies can be as vague and general as environmental illness, which allows them to avoid any crowd in which someone might be wearing perfume, or as specific as allergy to dairy, which allows them to avoid the cheesecake that you made in a kitchen that they are sure is not clean enough.

Arsenicum, more than any other type, looks upon those with illness as victims, particularly themselves. And illness can bring about some surprising changes in their personality.

First, understand that no matter what illness they have, even if it's just a cold or the flu, the illness intensifies their need to have people around them. They cannot be left alone for a second when they are ill. And second, realize that no matter what the illness, they are quite sure that they are going to die from it. They do their best to instill this notion in everyone who hovers around them, and they keep those people on their toes, doing their best to make the Arsenicum's last moments peaceful and happy.

But something surprising happens. When Arsenicum gets ill, he loses all his energy. He just goes to bed and stays there. The person who used to drive you crazy running around and cleaning, fixing, adjusting, looks like a cadaver in bed. The key word now is *cozy*. The Arsenicum, who tends to be chillier than everyone else at the best of times, now becomes very cold. Aches and pains come on with the chill. But if you wrap him in a warm blanket and build a nice fire in the fireplace and give him some tea with lemon to sip, he feels much better. When he is sick it is as if his worst fears have been realized. That you are there with him and he is warm and safe and cozy allows him to morph into a different person, one who is calm and quiet and very nice to be around.

In the same way, Arsenicums can be wonderful to have on hand when you are sick. Since they live their lives expecting the worst, they are great in an emergency. When you have a terrible cold, they see to it that the refrigerator is filled, the house is clean, and you have someone by your side to make you laugh and help you get through the bad time.

In emergencies other than illness, Arsenicum types tend to be analytical and organized, but dispassionate. In emergencies that have to do with poverty and with your needing their money, they would rather not even hear about it.

In the 1950s, we let the Arsenicum types take charge of our lives. The notion spread that there was better living to be had by chemistry, and that if we could just kill all the germs, we would be so very healthy. At the same time, we began withdrawing from all the things in life that were untidy and uncontrollable. Sex, dancing, and the like were to be avoided.

During this same time, doctors and scientists were greatly revered. It was felt that they should earn more money than anyone else, because they were doing more important work than anyone else. What could be more important than spending your life making people well by stamping out the disease germs that lurk waiting around every corner and on the doorknob of every public lavatory? The only thing that comes close is research, and a government that is controlled by Arsenicum types pours millions into scientific research, because it is so orderly and so likely to yield more weapons against disease. Arsenicum types worship doctors just as Lycopodium types worship lawyers and Phosphorus types want a back rub.

With all this, it is interesting to note that Arsenicum types often have a wonderful sense of humor. They tend toward insightful humor that is highly verbal, twisting and turning on the clever comment. Many successful comedians are clear Arsenicum types. Male Arsenicums tend to choose much younger women as mates. This is perhaps an example of their control issues; they can shape a younger woman into the mate of their dreams much more easily than they can a peer. Arsenicum men also tend to use money as a method of controlling their mates and their children. They, like Lycopodium, constantly threaten to take the offending person out of their will.

In general, Arsenicums are chilly, restless, fearful, demanding, and controlling. They take on illnesses from fright, from grief, and from shock. They tend to get ill when they get bad news.

Arsenicum is a very thirsty remedy type. They want to drink all the time, but the way they drink drives all but other Arsenicums crazy. They like warm drinks, and they like to sip. An Arsenicum will fill a mug with tea and sip it for an hour. Sip sip sip. Put it down. Sip sip sip. Put it down. They walk around the house with the mug, just sipping away.

This sipping is a metaphor for their lives. It's how they experience life. Sip sip sip. In the same way, they want warm foods. They want to feel cozy. They want lemon. They also tend to like fats, especially olive oil. They like alcohol, especially wine and often most especially brandy, and alcohol that is drunk warm.

They are at their best in the morning, clear minded and ready, and at their worst at midnight. Just after midnight can be a daily crisis for an Arsenicum; all symptoms are worse and the fear all but uncontrollable.

The person who best sums up the concept of Arsenicum is Nancy Reagan. Picture her in her little red coat and little red hat at the inauguration, and you have a portrait of Arsenicum. They love the color red. This little sparrow of a woman with the strength of an eagle, who treated our entire nation as a misbehaving child, is the archetype of the remedy.

Physical Portrait: Like Sulphur, Arsenicum is a burn remedy. All the symptoms that suggest this remedy are burning in nature, no matter what part of the body is affected. Skin conditions in the remedy type also have itching, much like Sulphur, and often the practitioner has to look to the emotional symptoms to select the appropriate remedy.

It is important to note that even though the symptoms of Arsenicum have a burning quality, they are in general improved by heat. Coldness is the great enemy of Arsenicum. He becomes worse in every way by becoming cold or by applications of cold compresses. Instead, even if his throat throbs and burns, it is the warm drink that soothes.

The general symptoms, including the burning symptoms, come and go with organized regularity. Allergies that return each year on Memorial Day often yield to Arsenicum, as does the flu that hits each year just before Thanksgiving.

Respiratory weakness is common. Arsenicums tend to take cold easily, and their colds go deep into their system, moving into deeper and more threatening illness. In the same way, they tend toward seasonal allergy. Just as with food allergy, they often know exactly what they are allergic to, exactly when it blooms and for how long. (In fact, Arsenicums can be very easy to treat. Of all the various types of patients, they tend to have the most complete and best-organized information concerning their symptoms. Often, within moments of meeting the person, you can be quite sure that he is Arsenicum when he takes out a typed transcript of his case and hands you a Xerox so that you can read along.)

Arsenicums have particular issues with milk and milk products. Some have their digestive problems relieved by milk, but in most Arsenicum types, milk and dairy products cause them not only digestive distress but also greatly enhance their body's natural ability to create mucus.

The mucus of Arsenicum is clear and watery. With a cold or with allergies, the right nostril tends to flow much more than does the left. In fact, in general, Arsenicums experience symptoms of pain either first or more deeply on the right side. Whether right- or left-handed, the right side of the body is weaker and more given to illness.

With respiratory weakness, breathing can be a great problem. Asthma can be very common, as are bronchitis, pneumonia, and emphysema.

The other area of great weakness in the Arsenicum system is the digestive system. Vomiting and diarrhea are common, sometimes at the same time, and both can be caused either by emotional distress or physical illness. Gastritis, colitis, and peptic ulcers are common, as are malignancies of the organs of digestion and elimination. Hemorrhoids are very common as well.

And Arsenicum should be the first remedy considered in cases of food poisoning that involve general chilliness and anxiety.

Arsenicum is a common remedy for liver disease, particularly for hepatitis and cirrhosis. It is also the first remedy to be considered for all wasting diseases and for all situations in which there is a rapid weight loss.

While one dose of Arsenicum remains active in the system for a month, this remedy usually has to be repeated often, particularly in emergency situations. In emergencies, Arsenicum can be repeated as often as every fifteen minutes. The remedy is effective in all potencies. But it must be noted that high potencies of Arsenicum should be avoided at all costs in situations in which the patient's vital force is weak. It is best to start with a potency that is lower than the one that we feel we will ultimately need; Arsenicum, for the classic practitioner, is the remedy of peaceful euthanasia.

Poster Children: Nancy Reagan, Jerry Seinfeld, Woody Allen, Felix Unger, Joan Crawford.

CALCAREA
The Laborer

Remedy Source: Calcarea is part of a group of remedies that share calcium as their basis. The most important remedy of the group and the one that I consider here is Calcarea Carbonica, taken from calcium carbonate, which Hahnemann prepared from the middle layers of oyster shells. As a homeopathic remedy, Calcarea Carbonica is known for its wide range of healing action and for the depth of its curative power.

Sulphur, Lycopodium, and Calcarea Carbonica form a triad of remedies that are vital in the treatment of persons with long-term ailments.

Situations That Suggest Calcarea: Digestive disorders and malnutrition; heartburn; constipation; functional disorders and immune dysfunctions: multiple sclerosis, chronic fatigue, environmental poisonings, night sweats; allergies: rhinitis, food allergies, sinusitis, asthma; respiratory disorders and inflammations: colds, flu, bronchitis, otitis media, pharyngitis; obesity; PMS; connective tissue disorders: low back pain, sciatica, rheumatoid pain and rheumatoid arthritis; skin diseases: acne, eczema, rash; anxiety and related disorders: phobia, depression; malignancies of all sorts.

Remedy Overview: Calcarea Carbonica is perhaps most often required in young children, and certainly a large number of children need the remedy in their youth as their bones and teeth develop. But most of these children soon move on to other remedy types. In fact, it is a sign of an extraordinarily strong system if a person remains a Calcarea for a lifetime. Most older Calcareas have many layers of constitutional types below the surface Calcarea.

As the remedy is created from one of the basic substances that are both so common and so essential in our own bodies, it speaks to our spirit in the same way: directly and simply. The Calcarea type is a person without subtext, one who faces the world if not easily at least honestly.

The Calcarea child tends to be heavy. The infant has a large head and has difficulty holding the head up. Look for the infant's head to flop about to the left and right, to the front and back. At all stages of childhood, the Calcarea child tires easily and seems to have little resistance to coughs and colds. While attending school, he seems to come down with any illness that any other child has.

Calcarea children seem to be a little slow in learning as well, even though they are curious and want to know about things. And the method they use to learn in infancy is key to Calcarea: They put things in their mouths. Throughout their lives, Calcareas tend to be guided by the sense of taste particularly, and when stressed, threatened, and interested, they tend to put things in their mouths. This alone may account for the fact that they are usually overweight.

Calcareas tend to be followers as children. Although very strong willed, they do not like confrontation and spend a good deal of time trying to keep up and fit in.

Finally, Calcareas are clammy children, with damp hands and feet. Expect them to sweat on the top of their heads and their perspiration to be sour smelling.

Remedy Theme: Work and responsibility.

Remedy Motivation: The need for security.

Emotional Portrait: Think of the oyster. The oyster lives on a functional level. To be alive is to function, and to function is to be alive. It is just simple, both for the oyster and for the Calcarea.

The oyster lives in its shell and attaches that shell to a rock and just stays there. Instead of moving about and seeing the world, the oyster lets the world flow through it. The oyster sees its function as filtering water. To do this, it has to open its shell a crack, just enough so that the water can flow through but not enough that anything else can get in, and certainly not enough that too much water gets in and tears the oyster off its rock or rips open its shell. If the shell is forced open, the oyster is washed away, and that is the end of the oyster.

In the same way, Calcarea people want to find their life's work as early as possible. Often these are the students who prefer vocational training. They need to find their life's work and they need to think that they are good at it. Then they need to be left alone to work and to finish whatever task they have been assigned to the best of their ability. When faced with a new task, Calcareas may seem to go inert. They look almost as if they are in a coma. But internally they are working hard. They are planning the methods by which they can accomplish this task. When they are secure in their methods, they begin. They work long and hard in accomplishing this task, thinking nothing of working late or starting early. In fact, it could be argued that there is no one who is happier than a Calcarea who is in the middle of a task.

If that task is ever assigned again, Calcareas follow exactly the methods previously used. They do not see each situation as unique; instead they look for similarities between current work and past tasks. This not only feeds their need for security, in that the assignment instantly becomes familiar, but it also allows them access to the information they need to complete their work.

Calcareas love the familiar. They also tend to love the past. Their desks are covered with pictures of those they love and souvenirs of both work and personal events. They also want to be familiar with coworkers, needing to be on a first-name basis with everyone and wanting to share both personal information and favorite recipes.

Bosses tend to love Calcareas, because they apparently give their full loyalty to their work. But employers often make the same mistake concerning Calcareas that teachers do. Since they must go through their apparently inert period when faced with anything new, the employers think that they are not smart. But this process has nothing to do with native intelligence, or IQ. It merely reflects the process that they must go through to access information.

At home and in their family relationships, Calcareas tend to follow the same pattern: They equate their family with work and function. They see child-rearing as a responsibility and find their joy not in the personal relationship with their child but in a job well done.

They see their homes as their shells. They buy a house, buy some good solid furniture, and then just get on with their work. The idea of redecorating or moving the furniture around for the sake of change never occurs to them. The home is the safe place, the center of security in their lives. And, because of this, beauty is not the issue; calm simplicity is. In the way that Arsenicum types want to create order out of chaos, often leaving total chaos in their wake, Calcareas have a way of simply putting things right. As Arsenicums fuss at you for not making your bed, clicking their tongues at you all the time they are doing it for you against your objections, Calcareas sweetly make your bed, telling you that you shouldn't work so hard. They wander into your kitchen and make you dinner, without Arsenicum's sermon, and organize a joint effort after studying your refrigerator's contents, and with a good time being had by all.

Calcareas are perhaps the ultimate team players. They have the ability to bring people together, not under their orders but instead around the completion of a specific task. Their focus is not on personal power or credit but on simple completion. Because of this, Calcareas are as emotionally important to society as calcium is to the formation of bones. Without these worker bees, our society would cease to function.

Again, in a way that is very different from Arsenicum, Calcarea types take great pride in their mind. Arsenicums are proud of their wit and of their unerring insight into the weak spot of just about anyone they meet. Lycopodiums are incredibly proud of their own sheer intellect and feel that all others should acknowledge it as well. Calcareas, on the other hand, take pride in their ability to create order and function and structure. They consider their ability to map out a project mentally from start to finish to be the pearl in the oyster's shell.

For Calcareas who are moving from health to illness, you begin to see the battle between order and confusion. If they become confused by any part of the task at hand, they begin to be confused by all of it. In order to solve the situation, they must return into their shell. As the work becomes harder, the confusion builds, and Calcareas must spend more and more time with their shells slammed shut.

Confusion, for the Calcarea, leads directly into weakness, which leads directly into illness. Calcareas take on illness from overwork and from confusion. One feeds the other. When Calcareas become confused, they have only one method to bring clarity: work harder. They let anything suffer for the sake of working harder when that is what they perceive as being necessary in a given situation. They happily sacrifice their own health in order to complete their task.

Overwork is the very heart of Calcareas. When they are able to complete the task, all is well. But when life gives them a task they cannot handle, they apply a vise of work around the task. They not only want to work harder themselves, but they also want others to do so. The Calcarea who once was so gifted at motivating others can become demanding, not understanding why everyone else wants to go home just because it is 10 P.M., when there are still hundreds of envelopes to be stuffed. The Calcarea stays on, stuffing those envelopes himself, wondering how everyone else can be such slackers.

What fear is to Arsenicum, worry is to Calcarea. If the work environment is changed in any way, especially if their way of doing their job is threatened, they give way to worry. They do not have flexibility, and their only protection is a rigid shell, so they worry that their shell will be cracked open and they will be washed away and killed.

This can be true when their old boss, the one who understood them, is replaced with a new one who wants all the old files reorganized. Or when a new coworker is brought in, one who plays music at his desk. Or especially when the Calcarea who always worked from an office ten miles from home is suddenly required to travel for work. Calcareas don't travel well; they want to stay stuck to their rocks. They especially do not want to be taken from their homes, which represent security and the oyster shell to them. Calcareas are given to great homesickness when they are required to spend any time away from home. (Also, in that they tend to love to cook, they do not want to be eating the hotel food, but want their own kitchen, which is the center not only of their evening meal but also the happiness and harmony in their lives.)

Calcareas cannot bear to have their control over their lives disrupted. Unlike other types, Calcareas don't particularly want to control anyone else, but they demand total control over their own lives and their own methods of completing their work. For anyone else to take that control is intolerable.

When their personal control is threatened by anything as small as a new company policy that requires all personal possessions to be removed from the top of workers' desks, Calcareas begin to worry. And worry makes them want to slam their shells shut and close down until the change goes away. Worry, if not corrected on this level, moves on to stress, and stress of any sort opens the Calcarea up to all sorts of physical illness.

The Calcarea type tends to fall prey at first to all sorts of little illnesses instead of saving up for one major crisis. They start to have colds, sore throats, headaches, bouts of vertigo, all seemingly unrelated. This is the "beginning of the end" for Calcarea.

With the added stress of illness and missed work, the Calcarea moves into fear. One fear is that he will not be able to keep up. It all comes back to him how, as a child he was always the slowest in the neighborhood, both physically and mentally. He panics at the notion that he is falling behind and that his mind, his wonderful mind that once could figure out the solution to just about any problem, is now failing him when he needs it most.

At this point, the Calcarea's gentle nurturing nature shifts, and his sense of humor fails him. He begins to have longer and longer illnesses and to have trouble sleeping.

Finally, the Calcarea has a major break in health, either a deep chronic physical condition setting in or an emotional breakdown. Either way, from this moment onward the Calcarea never again is able to work the way he once worked, and his joy in life seems lost forever.

Calcareas take on many other fears: of losing control, of losing their mind, of accidents, of dying. They have a tremendous fear of anything or anyone unknown. They can become agoraphobic. They become controlled by their fears: of dogs, mice, or rats; of earthquakes and storms.

In treating Calcareas, remember that it is often not enough just to give the remedy; you must also give Calcareas a plan. They are eager to follow the plan to the letter, a map they can follow back to health. Calcareas, in that they are too practical ever really to buy into the homeopathic mumbo-jumbo, also want to know what vitamins to take and what foods to eat. If they have a plan to follow, and if they have a basis of security to work from, their return to health can be complete.

Physical Portrait: The classical homeopaths sum up Calcarea Carbonica with three words: fair, fat, and flabby. From birth, they are lacking in skin and muscle tone, sometimes seeming to be heavier than they really are, due to their large heads and solid skeletons. It was for Calcareas that the term "big boned" was invented.

Calcarea children are given to late closure of the fontanels. In fact, they tend to be late in talking, walking, and other milestones. Again, this is more likely to be due to their need to understand before doing than to any lack of intellect.

Calcarea children tend to have large heavy heads and to sweat from their heads. They have wet pillows in the morning. They also have large abdomens, curved legs, and pale skin. Curvature of the spine can be a difficulty for Calcarea children. They are slow to teethe and have difficulty while teething. As they grow, they often grind their teeth, a habit that remains through adulthood.

Calcarea children attempt to eat indigestible things: paste, dirt, pencil erasers; sometimes it seems that they want anything but food. In terms of food, they crave eggs and cannot get enough of them.

In general, Calcareas of all ages are chilly people. They are worse in the winter and hate cold air. They do not ever want to get cold. And they tend to take illnesses on when it is cold out.

They take illness also from physical exertion. If they are forced to work past their physical ability, they get diarrhea or pains in the hips, back, or limbs. They also become ill from fright and have a terrible fear of having to speak in front of others, which can bring on diarrhea.

Along with diarrhea, constipation, even chronic constipation, is common to Calcarea. This constipation is almost completely without urging. The patient has little or no desire to produce a stool and moves the bowels far less than does the average person. They do not feel ill during their bouts of constipation and sometimes seem almost happier when constipated.

They may have very weak assimilation of foods and may have many food allergies. But unlike Arsenicum, which actively avoids all foods that disagree, Calcarea seems drawn to the very foods that he cannot digest, craving them wildly. This mirrors the childhood desire to eat things like dirt that cannot be digested.

As part of these digestive disorders, Calcareas, particularly children, are given to worms and parasites of all sorts. Their digestive tract and their system as a whole have little ability to defeat these intruders.

Another area of great weakness for Calcareas is the musculoskeletal system. They are given to chronic low back pain and often to arthritis of the spine. Arthritis of all sorts and in all parts of the body is common.

They are rheumatic types and are worse in cold or damp. They have pain throughout their body and feel general weakness in their entire system in cold, damp, weather.

They have poor muscle tone. Even the Calcarea who makes the gym part of his life does not have the results that other constitutions do. In fact, the Calcarea who exercises often opens himself up to cramps, most especially cramps in the thighs, calves, or foot muscles, all areas of weakness for the Calcarea.

And once the Calcarea has injured his system in a particular area, most especially in the ankles, the injury seems to weaken the system permanently. That ankle gets injured again and again, each time seemingly with less trauma required.

The Calcarea's feet are worthy of special note. They tend to be both damp and smelly at all times. Also, the Calcarea tends to feel that he has to protect his feet. His feet feel very vulnerable when they are uncovered. He cannot bear his feet to become cold, let alone cold and wet, which creates the worst circumstances possible for both physical and emotional health. He wears socks to bed. He wears thick, warm slippers long after everyone else has gone barefoot. Yet he cannot bear his feet to get too hot or sweaty either. So a good deal of time and energy goes into the comfort of his feet. No Calcarea ever buys shoes for the way they look. The way they feel is all-important.

In general, Calcareas are the first to cry at the movies. They feel stiff in the morning and are a little slow getting started. They often feel as if gravity increased during the night.

Further, Calcareas have a low threshold for pain. They will do anything to avoid pain and happily take any medication to block their experience of physical discomfort. They often fear pain as they do death.

They have brittle nails that can easily be peeled away. They crave dairy products along with eggs, milk, ice cream, and cheese. They also love pasta, breads, heavy foods, cream sauces, refined foods, and salt. This is another major remedy for those who suffer hypoglycemia, and so Calcareas crave sugar. They do not enjoy raw or whole foods.

Calcareas are at their worst during the full moon, which drives them crazy. They cannot sleep at this time, and their feelings of worry and fear are at their height.

They are also worse if they experience any shortness of breath from any ailment or exertion. They are immediately sure they are dying if they have shortness of breath.

All in all, they are at their best in three circumstances: when they are in the fresh air, when they are crying at the movies, and when they are constipated.

Calcarea is a remedy that bears repetition quite well and may be repeated as needed. The potency level 30C is perhaps the most effective, certainly for chronic digestive problems. High potencies of Calcarea should be used as a single dose only. This is a slow, deep-acting remedy. One dose is effective for up to sixty days.

Poster Child: It's very hard to find a poster child for this remedy type because most of them would rather die than be in the public eye. But television has recently given us a great example in comic Drew Carey. His character on the *Drew Carey Show* perfectly displays the character type, both in terms of physical body type and in personality and career.

LYCOPODIUM
The Counterfeit

Remedy Source: The remedy Lycopodium is taken from the spores of club moss, a plant natural to central Europe and North America. The spores of the plant are shaped like a wolf's paw, which gives the remedy its name: *lyco* means "wolf" and *podo* means "foot." Although the plant is inert in nature, the spores have explosive power. They have even been used to create the special effect of stage lightning in theaters.

Moss is one of the oldest surviving plants. It is at least 350 million years old and, for the most part, has existed all this time without changing. This attribute of the plant is valuable in understanding those who need the remedy Lycopodium. Think of it as the barnacle of the plant world; it latches itself onto a rock and stays there, never moving, never changing.

Samuel Hahnemann created the remedy. The story is that he became intrigued by the white powder that was used to coat pills to make them easier to swallow. That powder was taken from the spores of club moss. He created the remedy from the powder as an experiment, just to see if this seemingly benign substance had any curative power as a homeopathic. The remedy he made became one of the most important in the homeopathic pharmacy.

Situations That Suggest Lycopodium: Male issues: impotence, premature ejaculation, prostate disease; digestive disorders of all sorts: irritable bowel syndrome, colitis, Crohn's disease; eating disorders, especially bulimia. Also diabetes; liver disease: hepatitis and cirrhosis; kidney and urinary disease: kidney stones, urinary tract infection, cystitis; headache and migraine; allergies: rhinitis, asthma; infections of all sorts: colds, flu, bronchitis, otitis media, sinusitis; chronic fatigue; sarcoidosis; lupus.

Remedy Overview: Impotence is the key to understanding this remedy. Lycopodium is a constitutional remedy needed overwhelmingly by men, specifically by men whose fathers gave them the message that they would never be rich enough, smart enough, successful enough, or just plain man enough to earn that father's love. As a result, the son grows into a man who, in many ways, is just a large child: emotionally immature and given to overcompensating his feelings of low self-esteem by behavior that is aggressive if not downright abusive.

Inside, Lycopodiums feel impotent, worthless, and fearful. But they feel that their success in life, indeed their very existence, hangs on their ability to hide these feelings and instead to project a persona that is filled with confidence and, above all else, intelligence.

As a result, this inner feeling of impotence manifests itself as physical impotence and in other health issues surrounding male sexuality. The life's work of the Lycopodium becomes plugging the leaks in his life raft as they appear. The method that is most often chosen by Lycopodiums is blaming the other. If they cannot get an erection, it is the woman's fault: "This has never happened before." If they fail at work, it is the underling who is blamed and fired for the failure. This strategy leads the Lycopodium on a downward spiral of abusive behavior and self-destruction.

Remedy Theme: Impotence and ambition.

Remedy Motivation: Lack of self-confidence.

Emotional Portrait: There is a way that you can spot the Lycopodium boy early in life: He is the one who, although he has absolutely no skill for a sport, keeps right on playing, no matter how muddy, bloody, or tired he gets, because this is the sport his father most admires. Right there you have two patterns that become the central themes in the life of a Lycopodium: the need for his father's love and the willingness to take whatever abuse is necessary to attain the goal he selected or his father selected for him.

Often the Lycopodium child is somewhat shy with his peers, although he is just as likely as the Lycopodium adult to hide his inner feelings of inferiority with a persona that projects pure ego. Some Lycopodium boys lack the ability for this projection and instead turn their will toward intellectual pursuits, believing that they can gain respect by outdistancing all others in terms of grades, awards, and accomplishments.

Typically the Lycopodium child has a large head with a small and rather underdeveloped body. He tends to be sickly, especially with allergies and respiratory infections. He can appear to be a tiny old person instead of a child. With his thin arms and legs and large head, he gives the impression of being much older than he is.

The inner troubles of the Lycopodium child often manifest themselves in nightmares. The child doesn't want to be alone at night anyway, as Lycopodium depends on the opinions of others in order to feel good about himself and tends to crumble a bit when there is no one to impress or argue with. He wakes screaming. His typical fears are also more adult than childish in nature, and he likely fears his own death at an early age. Lycopodium fears that he will not survive.

From childhood onward, the Lycopodium tends to polarize his personality into two facets: the public and the private. The private can become so private that it is unknown even to his wife and children. The Lycopodium, so fearful and so vulnerable, loses touch with the fact that our lives and our successes largely have more to do with our external behavior than with our interior motivations. The Lycopodium often sees himself as the victim of his life. He is a great rationalizer who always gives himself the benefit of the doubt for whatever he has done, whether lies that he has told or abuse that he has heaped on others.

This is an interesting aspect of the Lycopodium personality. He has a wonderful adaptive behavior in place when it comes to self-control. If you were his employer looking at the outer Lycopodium personality, it would seem as if no one is more self-controlled. To the teacher or the boss—or the father—he seems on top of everything, with all his tasks and assignments well in hand. On top of this, he seems the picture of appropriate behavior. He is well dressed and well behaved.

The internal Lycopodium is another story. Here we have a person who is driven and defined by a complete lack of self-discipline. He shows this in many ways. The simplest is probably his craving for sweets. The Lycopodium may go to the gym five days a week to keep in shape so that the public admires his build, but he cannot refuse himself any sweet thing. It is his reward to himself, not only for the work that he has done to earn the right to eat the sugar but also, and more important, because he has been so victimized by life, because he is so put-upon and misunderstood.

It is the same with drugs and sex. I wager that Lycopodium buys more cocaine than all the other remedy types combined. He loves the way it makes him feel powerful. This intoxication is something he cannot deny himself. Many white-collar abusers of drugs of all sorts, particularly cocaine, who look and act like successful and intelligent men at work, and who do their drugs on the side, reveling even in the fact that they are spending so much of the money that they worked so hard to get, are pure Lycopodium.

Sex works in the same way. The Lycopodium man sees a woman in a bar or at a desk in an office. He wants her in the same way that he wants the sugar or the cocaine, as a reward to himself for all the troubles he has to deal with in life. It usually is important to the Lycopodium that the woman be of a social status inferior to his own, or at least intellectually his inferior. The last thing a Lycopodium man wants in a sexual conquest is a woman who is his equal. That she could actually be his superior in some way is intolerable.

And so Lycopodium men are always on the lookout for a new sexual conquest, and, after they have rewarded themselves sexually, they immediately lose interest in the woman. After all, she was inferior, wasn't she?

This is the mating dance of the Lycopodium. For sex, he wants an inferior woman. As a wife, he must find an equal or a superior woman. Therefore, Lycopodium wants to marry the boss's daughter or a woman who is socially his superior. (He still doesn't like the idea of a woman who is intellectually his superior.) He especially wants a woman whose beauty speaks well of her husband's taste, wallet, and social position. He is looking for a trophy wife: a woman half his age, who stands a head taller than he does, and whose breasts threaten at any moment to explode.

The fact that the Lycopodium man may find himself unable to perform sexually with such a woman is another manifestation of the polarization of the remedy's personality. Just as long as she looks satisfied when they are out in public, he is likely to be fine. The relationship between the character played by Jack Nicholson and Ann-Margret in *Carnal Knowledge* is a perfect example of the Lycopodium courtship, marriage, and its aftermath.

Lycopodium lives most of his life in public. Thus, as long as his marriage looks good—as long as he is pretty sure that his friends envy his marriage—he is happy. In the same way, as long as it looks as if his children are well adjusted, well dressed, and loving to their old dad, he's happy. But let the mask slip, let the children misbehave in church or in a restaurant, and they are in for a very bad time when they get home. The Lycopodium type tends to love to sing in the church choir, or to be on the board of a homeless shelter, from whose lectern he can pontificate on family values and then go home and verbally or physically abuse his family for any and all embarrassment they caused him.

After behaving in this manner, Lycopodium usually starts out truly sorry, as he recognizes that he is treating his children exactly as his father treated him and that he is pushing his sons exactly as his father pushed him. But, over time, and with repeated bouts of abusive behavior, he convinces himself that, like sugar, he really can't deny himself the assertion of his personal power over his family and that they should work to understand him better, should see that he is really the victim here, the victim of their thankless behavior.

This concept of inferiority/superiority is both an internal and an external pattern. Certainly, no one feels as inferior, or as phony, as do Lycopodiums.

Interestingly, however, they do not feel that they are phony socially by acting hypocritically. Instead, they feel that they are fakes in that they are fooling others. They feel that they have fooled their superiors into thinking that they are competent. Internally, Lycopodiums feel that they haven't the slightest idea how to complete the task at hand, that they will never be able to bring it in on time or perform up to the expected standard. Because of this, they work harder than everyone else. You suspect that they have terrier blood in their veins—they take that task in their teeth and shake it until it is dead.

When the boss looks at the Lycopodium, he sees a wonderful employee. He seldom sees the results of the drug taking that goes on after hours; the Lycopodium sweats that out at the gym. What he does see is someone who is clear eyed and well dressed—usually very expensively dressed—and who gets to work early and works late. The boss may notice that the Lycopodium tends to drive his own assistants a little hard, but it usually is interpreted that he cares about his work and about his employer.

For the assistant, it is another story. While the Lycopodium is perhaps the best employee you can have (except for the fact that he is quietly trying to get your job), he is the worst boss in the world. The Lycopodium boss is a total tyrant.

This is the other aspect of the inferior/superior pattern. As long as the Lycopodium has, for whatever reason, judged you to be his superior in some way (and as long as you, as the superior, don't have something he wants), he yields to you like a whipped dog, eyes to the floor. But if the Lycopodium perceives you as an inferior, then you are like the girl in the bar, someone to be used and disposed of.

The Lycopodium boss requires his employees to work when and for how long he tells them to work. He certainly is not above taking credit for any of his employees' work as his own. And he certainly is not above sexual harassment of low-level female employees.

At work or at home, Lycopodium does not abide disagreement from any underling—and remember, for Lycopodium, the wife and children are underlings. The worst insult to a Lycopodium is to disagree with him publicly. If an employee at a conference disagrees with Lycopodium's plans for the company, especially if the CEO is present, that employee can expect to be politely asked to come into the Lycopodium's office later that day. Once the door is closed, the employee is likely to hear abusive language the likes of which he has never heard before. Compared to what the wife will hear that evening, he is lucky.

Of course not all wife beaters are Lycopodiums and not all Lycopodiums are wife beaters, but the pattern of a deep schism between public and private behavior is central to the Lycopodium type, as is the quest for success to overcompensate for inner feelings of inferiority. Add to this the Lycopodium's lifelong tendency to toady to those perceived as superiors, while abusing those perceived as inferiors, and you have the essence of those needing the remedy.

Lycopodium is well known for his fears, the most pronounced of which is claustrophobia. Many Lycopodium types are unable to get into an elevator without a full-fledged panic attack. They also can be afraid of ghosts.

Almost every Lycopodium man can be said to be afraid of commitment and of marriage. But Lycopodium is also often afraid of people. Lycopodium men are likely to be afraid of other men in general. But a more important fear is the fear of being alone.

Like Arsenicum (which Lycopodium can resemble), Lycopodium does not want to be alone. But unlike Arsenicum, he does not want to be with other people either. Lycopodium likes to have people near but not with him. Often he wants to be in his den alone but have the rest of the family in the family room. He is greatly comforted by hearing their voices and the sound of the television set, but he does not want actually to have them in the same room.

The Lycopodium also has a deep fear of public speaking, although, like his usual feelings of inferiority, he covers this fear and appears self-assured and calm when speaking to a large group, although such an event causes him much gastric distress after the fact.

Only one thing makes a Lycopodium cry. He can cause a great deal of pain to the people around him. And he can bear up under a great deal of discomfort, emotional and physical. But when a Lycopodium is thanked, when his effort is recognized, when someone at last realizes how difficult it has been for him to be a Lycopodium and still function well, then the tears begin to flow. When the Lycopodium is thanked from the heart, then his wound is opened full and raw. This is especially true if the Lycopodium is thanked by a person he respects or feels is his superior. At that moment he feels loved by this father figure, if not by his father himself, and the floodgates open. At that moment, the wounded child can be revealed, for a time, in the Italian-suited body of the man. At that moment, if the Lycopodium can allow these painful emotions to be a catalyst to change, a healing can begin.

Physical Portrait: Physically, Lycopodium has two areas of weakness: his sexual organs and his gastrointestinal tract. The liver also tends to fall prey to disease. Nash lists the remedy among the trio of flatulent remedies (along with Chinchona and Carbo Vegetabilis).

It is by his flatulence that you often identify a Lycopodium. He is far more likely to wander into a homeopath's office for treatment of a digestive condition than for any psychological or sexual complaint. The Lycopodium has excessive flatulence, as if his verbal outgassing were matched by his body. He has a constant sensation that his abdomen is filled, particularly the lower abdomen. He feels full and bloated after just a few bites of food. He feels a swelling in the lower abdomen and is aware of the formation of gas. Often he says that he feels like a brewery, in that the food he has eaten feels like it is fermenting in his system. The Lycopodium feels uncomfortable after eating and unhooks his belt to get comfortable.

When the Lycopodium is bloated, he is irritable. Kent tells us that the smallest things, the crackling of a piece of paper, the ringing of bells, the slamming of doors, goes through his head like a knife. The patient feels anger from such things; he also feels faint.

A feeling of fainting, of shortness of breath along with bloating is common in Lycopodium. Nash warns us that these and other gastric symptoms common to Lycopodium can be warning signs of deeper liver troubles.

There is pain in the area of the liver, and the gastric symptoms get worse after eating onions or drinking liquor, particularly wine. Lycopodium also feels worse when he comes in contact with tobacco in any form.

Lycopodium has symptoms more often on the right side of his body, or they appear on the right and move left. Even in acute situations needing Lycopodium this is true. The Lycopodium sore throat starts on or is worse on the right side.

Lycopodium's symptoms tend to be worse, like clockwork, at 4 P.M. The Lycopodium may have a headache each day at this time or may feel faint.

In general, Lycopodiums feel better when warm and when drinking warm things. They are better if they loosen their clothing, particularly after eating, and if they uncover their heads. It is important to note that Lycopodiums must eat on time. Their symptoms grow worse if they do not eat regularly, and they often get a headache.

Lycopodium tends to crave warm things, which soothe his generally chilly system. He also tends to crave oysters, which he cannot digest, and cheeses of all sorts, which are guaranteed to make him ill. Usually the Lycopodium dislikes both coffee and meat, neither of which sits well in his system.

Age is important in the Lycopodium system, both mentally and physically. The Lycopodium loves the idea of himself as a whiz kid or a child genius. He tends to set goals for himself involving a deadline for having made a certain amount of money or achieved a certain goal. If he does not achieve what he set out to do, illness begins to set in, illness that tends to become chronic over time and shadow the Lycopodium's future.

Physically, aging is very stressful for Lycopodiums. Although they tend to be somewhat sickly children, they tend to grow to be strong adults. Often they pride themselves on never getting ill. On top of this, they hate doctors and do anything to avoid a trip to the doctor's office. So, as middle age comes on and chronic conditions take hold, Lycopodiums wait and wait before seeking help.

On top of this, age is a problem for them in its own right. They find that they cannot detox their system of the poisons they put in as easily as they could a few years ago. Further, they see themselves going bald early in life. This is typical of Lycopodiums, as is prematurely graying hair, especially at the temples. They consider this baldness to be a challenge to their masculinity. This stresses their system more, as does every single new wrinkle and every pound gained.

So they awaken one day to find themselves, in their own eyes and usually nobody else's, old and a failure. No one else has a midlife crisis with the intensity that the Lycopodium does. And no other type, after this crisis, goes into such a decline, becoming old before their time. They look again, as they did when they were very small, like the wizened elder, with thin limbs and a large head.

Poster Children: Almost all lawyers and politicians, particularly Dan Quayle, Prince Charles, and Ross Perot.

NATRUM
The Caretaker

Remedy Source: There are more than a dozen remedies in the Natrum family, all based on the substance sodium. The remedies included are compounds of polycrest types, fusing the issues of Sulphur, Arsenicum, and Phosphorus, among others, with Natrum's own qualities.

For my purposes, I use the remedy Natrum Muriaticum, taken from sodium chloride or common table salt. This chemical compound is found in nature in rocklike formations, in ocean water, in the atmosphere, and in the cells of plants and animals.

Natrum Muriaticum is one of Samuel Hahnemann's own remedies, but it was re-proved as a remedy by the Austrian Society of Provers.

Situations That Suggest Natrum Muriaticum: Emotional distress: grief, suicidal states, depression. Also sexual dysfunction; allergies and chemical sensitivities: environmental illness, chronic fatigue, hay fever and rhinitis, asthma. Also herpes and aphthae; contagious diseases: cold and flu, sore throat, fever, whooping cough; digestive disorders: dyspepsia, gastritis, constipation, colitis, ulcer; hemorrhoids; obesity; edema; goiter and Graves' disease; Addison's disease; joint and muscle pain: low back pain, sciatica, painful conditions of the spine; skin conditions: eczema and psoriasis, rash, ringworm, warts; eye troubles: myopia, eyestrain; headaches and migraine; heart disorders: arrhythmia and hypertension; varicose veins; anemia.

Remedy Overview: Think of the characteristics of salt, especially of how salt affects nutrition. If you eat a lot of salt for a long period of time, you slowly begin to see permanent changes to your system. Salt leaches moisture from everything around it and retains that moisture. In the same way, salt in your system retains fluids that usually are flushed out. This retention results in edema and dropsy. Further, too much salt in the diet changes the blood, leading to anemia.

The general feeling of retention, along with an almost overwhelming feeling of weakness and debility, is a hallmark of the remedy type. The third part of the picture common to the Natrum Mur type is denial. Natrum Murs have a highly developed emotional defense system, one that depends largely on selective memory.

Remedy Theme: Retention and denial.

Remedy Motivation: Grief, abandonment.

Emotional Portrait: In that Natrum Mur is made up of salt, and salt is a part of every organ in our body and a major component of our environment, this remedy, along with Sulphur and Thuja, has a curative impact on nearly every person who takes it. Some homeopaths liken Natrum Mur to the ocean. Natrum Mur represents the unconscious mind, the mind that can be known to us only in our dreams.

Like the unconscious, Natrum Mur has a great deal to do with the riddle of our own perceptions, our own memories. It is a memory that clears away the denial and wishful thinking, allowing us to face the reality of ourselves uncolored by the overwhelming retention of old hurts and the denial of past injuries.

It is the riddle of the Natrum Mur that she cannot recall exactly what these hurts were and why she feels so sad. At the same time, she is unable to let these hurts go and move on in her life from the past that now traps her.

Again, let's consider the chemical action of salt as a method of better understanding this remedy. Just as salt absorbs and retains, it preserves. And this action of preserving is an important part of the overall constitution.

The Natrum Mur is most commonly female. She seeks to preserve the past literally. Often she lives almost entirely in the past. Since it is often called the widow's remedy, think about a widow when you think about Natrum Mur. Think about Queen Victoria in her later years, after the death of Prince Albert. Think about the quote that we most identify with her: "We are not amused."

The widow who has moved, in her grief and loss, into Natrum Mur has on a very vital level closed down. She identifies herself now by her loss as some chronically ill people identify themselves by their diseases, or as most of us identify ourselves by our careers. And, in a very real way, her grief becomes her career. She is seeking to retain and preserve the memory of her husband, as her younger counterpart Natrums seek to preserve the memory of their children's childhoods by keeping old bedrooms exactly as they were left, leaving the children to sleep in single beds and look at posters of defunct rock groups when they come home from college to visit.

In the same way, the Natrum preserves her husband's possessions and her memories of him. In that Natrum dance of retention and denial, she works over the memories in her unconscious mind, so that what begins to resurface in her active memory is only the happy side of the marriage. The Natrum who was married to a brutal man remembers only the joyous first year or a happy Christmas. The rest is forgotten. If a child tries to remind her of the truth, she changes the subject. Usually this is done by saying, "Let's not spoil your visit." Then she goes into the kitchen to get some cake. This is said with a combination of sorrow and wistfulness. And the child lets the subject go.

It is interesting to note that, for someone who lives so very much in the past and who all but ignores the future, the Natrum commonly talks in terms of the present. She says, "Can't we just have a nice Christmas?" if anyone is doing anything she sees as disruptive. But she sees the present as fodder for future memories of the past, and she seeks, in the moment, to make those memories as pleasant as possible by censoring anything that might disrupt her selected memory.

Family relationships are all-important to Natrum Mur, starting with her relationships with her parents. The very fact that the child has moved into the Natrum Mur constitution points to a disrupted relationship with one of her parents. Natrum Mur, as a grief remedy, carries with it strong feelings of abandonment, as well as feelings of rejection and of not being loved. The child who moves into a Natrum Mur constitution at a young age feels that she is not loved. This is common in children of divorce, and it is at a time of divorce that most children become Natrum Murs. The child who was once open and laughing suddenly becomes quiet, as she silently blames herself for her parents' divorce and begins to feel that she is not loved by the noncustodial parent.

It is important to note that, from the parents' point of view, nothing may seem to be wrong with this child. Her silence may easily be interpreted as the way she tries to stay out from under foot during a very difficult time. Or worse, the parents may notice nothing at all, as they are going through their own process of grief and anger at the moment.

Natrum Murs, young and old, typically have a terrible time trying to express what they are feeling. They seem to want others to read their minds or, more difficult, read their hearts. While Natrum Mur may internally be in agony, she does not shed a tear—this is the leading remedy for those who want to cry but can't—or speak a word of her needs. The only way anyone who knows homeopathy may become aware of the problem is that the child begins to show Natrum symptoms. Suddenly, at the time of divorce, she has headaches or allergies or becomes myopic.

Another time a child may move into Natrum Mur is when her mother goes back to work. The child who interprets this as abandonment, who moves into grief in this situation, is likely to move into a Natrum Mur constitution.

It is also common for the oldest child, particularly if that child is a girl, to become a Natrum Mur; it is through raising this child that the parents learn the job of parenting. If they put a good deal of responsibility on the child, and if she takes to the task of becoming a smaller version of her mother for the younger children, she may take on the Natrum Mur constitution.

But most people move into Natrum Mur at a later time in life. For many the constitution is set in place after the first experience of love. Natrum

Murs often see themselves as, and in fact often are, unlucky in love. They are arch romantics and firmly believe that they have a soul mate whom they have only to meet in order to be happy forever.

And yet they seem to do everything in their power to choose the worst possible person as that mate. Natrums, who tend to be somewhat conservative, solid students with career and educational goals, amaze their parents when they insist that they must, at age seventeen, marry a boy in a black leather jacket with earrings in both ears. The parents are unprepared for this event, unless they, like their Natrum, have been studying *Wuthering Heights* for insights into Heathcliff's character.

In relationships, as in everything else, Natrum tends to absorb whatever it touches. So when the girl touches the boy, she absorbs him, with every intention of retaining him for all time. When that boy says that he is too young to settle down and breaks up with her, the Natrum can respond only with quiet grief and a sense of betrayal.

It can be the plague of a lifetime, this pattern of relationships. The Natrum Mur tends to be almost stubborn in her refusal to learn about relationships. She chooses men who are beneath her, whom all her friends warn her about. But, with her mind busy selecting memories for future use, she refuses to listen. Later, she revisits her grief, as she withdraws further and further into herself and her memories.

As a person moves deeper into this type, she tends more and more not to want to be touched. It makes her ill at ease. Mothers can even reach the point that they do not really want their children near them. It begins to seem that they have an invisible wall around them. Those they love can see and hear them, but, on a profound level, they are unable to get very close.

Often it takes years for others to realize that they really know nothing about what is going on inside a Natrum Mur. They are so very good at changing the topic and at playing on everyone else's natural desire to talk about themselves that no one may notice that they never reveal anything about themselves and never ask for anything from anyone.

The last thing that any Natrum Mur wants is to be beholden to anyone, to take anything at all from anyone else. This is true on the emotional level as well as the physical. Natrum Mur is always worse if someone tries to comfort her. She becomes very angry and lashes out. (And, in that Natrum Mur stores up all the hurts of a lifetime, never letting any slight go, when someone invades her space, presumes to touch her, and then offers sympathy, implying that she can understand the emotional torment the Natrum is experiencing, well, it all becomes too much. That person experiences the full flow that has up to that moment been retained. Very quickly, the emotional outburst ends. And, at least for the Natrum, is forgotten.) The only way it is safe to console a Natrum Mur is to make her laugh. She loves to laugh. She loves to go to movies that make her laugh. And when she laughs, two things happen: She becomes a lighter, more rational person, and she begins to cry. It is as if in the moment of laughter her true nature comes forth. For the moment she does not have to bear the burden of the past. She can let it go and let it out. And, in that moment, the tears can flow. She says that they are tears of laughter, and, oh, how she loves shedding them.

The way Natrum Mur manages to deflect her own needs is to focus on the needs of others. As with love relationships, Natrums tend to form very loyal friendships very quickly. While they reveal next to nothing about themselves, they very skillfully find out every detail about the other's life and do everything in their power to support and nurture that person in every sort of need.

They are among the best constitutional types to have as a friend or for a parent. They almost overwhelm their loved one—friend, relative, or pet—with love. They show their love in tangible ways, with pies and cakes and cookies, with kind words and thoughtful gifts, but not often with physical touch. Even with those they love most, they would just as soon remain at a physical distance.

The anger comes out in the Natrum Mur when she feels that she is being taken advantage of, or when she begins to feel invisible. It takes only a little attention to make her happy. She would just as soon there be no fuss about her birthday or Christmas. But, if the other person actually takes her seriously when she says not to make that fuss, all hell breaks loose.

It is important for those with Natrums close to them to remember that they are not lying when they speak less than the truth. They are working out of a wound of abandonment and grief that has taught them that if you honestly tell people what you need or want, they will use this information to hurt you. Those close to Natrums must also remember that they are not purposely being oblique, it is just the only way they can express themselves. If you want to help them, just help them, without emotional outburst. If you want to give them money, then say, without passion, "Take this." Don't make a big deal out of it. If they can learn over time that it is safe to tell you what they want, they can begin to step out from behind that wall toward freedom.

Above all else, if you want to truly help them, make them laugh. Laughter, for all of us, but more for the Natrum Mur, is a powerful tool for healing.

Physical Portrait: Possibly the first thing you think of with a Natrum Mur is a headache. She tends toward headaches and takes them on with any emotional slight, especially if she feels embarrassed or senses that someone is getting too close. For the Natrum, the headache is a protective device, an excuse to go to the bedroom and lie down, quietly and alone.

In fact, it is a keynote of all the ailments of Natrum Mur that she improves when she just quietly lies down, when she gets to be alone. This remedy is often considered the constitutional equivalent of the acute remedy Ignatia, which shares the general improvement of all symptoms when left alone. Surely Greta Garbo was one or the other, in that her motto was "I want to be alone."

It is also a general symptom of the headache and all the various aches and pains of Natrum Mur that the symptoms come on when the patient awakens in the morning, before she even gets out of bed, and that the symptoms grow worse as the sun rises and begin to fade as the sun sets. She is always worse in the day, particularly in the direct sunshine, and better in the evening or in the shade.

In general, the Natrum Mur experiences a worsening of all her symptoms when she is near the ocean. This is unfortunate—there is no place the Natrum would rather be. She is drawn to the ocean, may even dream of the ocean, but is overwhelmed by it. Her physical symptoms, especially allergic symptoms, grow so bad at the ocean that she has to go home.

Putting these together, then, the worst place of all for the Natrum Mur is at the beach. Look for her to get a terrible headache at the beach, or a wild bout of hay fever. The hay fever of Natrum Mur is always worse in summer, always worse in high heat, always much worse when the sun is shining. The Natrum commonly feels great itching with her allergies, with the sensation of a worm crawling in a nostril being keynote. At these times, the Natrum can be made better only by closing herself in a cool dark room and lying down.

A Natrum Mur suddenly becomes myopic. In becoming nearsighted, the Natrum is again protecting herself. Her range of vision becomes smaller and smaller, allowing her to feel safe in this narrow range. Her vision typically blurs when she feels threatened or overly tired.

Exhaustion, too, plays an important part in the Natrum constitution. Both physically and mentally, she becomes exhausted, taking to her room once again as a method of recharging her energy.

In general, the Natrum Mur is warm-blooded and does not want to be in too warm or stuffy a place, although she tends to prefer to be indoors than out. She feels at her worst at about ten in the morning, as the sun begins truly to heat the day. She is given to vertigo, especially when she looks into the distance, when she faces the myopic blur. She has a tendency to fall when she experiences vertigo and to pitch toward the left.

Natrum Mur is an important remedy for colds and for allergies, both of which have the same symptom of mucus that is like raw egg white, with much sneezing. As this is an important remedy for those with cold sores, it is commonly the most helpful remedy for colds that are accompanied by sores. It is also common for the Natrum Mur to have a crack in the middle of her lower lip or in the corners of her mouth.

Natrums crave salt and sour flavors, they like lemon, they love chocolate. They either love or hate milk. In the same way, they either love or hate bread and other baked goods. Natrums are very thirsty people and tend to drink large quantities of cold water. They tend to be averse to slimy foods, especially egg white.

The Natrum Mur has pain in the lower back. The pain is usually chronic and psychosomatic in origin, coming on or growing worse when she is trapped in her grief. She also tends to have problems with her extremities: cracked nails, peeling of the fingertips, and skin conditions like eczema, psoriasis, and ringworm. She often has hangnails and as a habit chews her fingernails.

The wide range of physical symptoms covered in the Natrum Mur type speaks to the range and depth of the remedy. Natrum Muriaticum, as a grief remedy, springs forth as a type from one of the most basic emotions common to humanity. It is a deep remedy, slow acting and long acting in its curative power. It is a complex remedy, sometimes easily recognized in an individual, sometimes apparent only when one considers what one does not know about an individual and not what one does know.

A dose of Natrum Mur can be active for up to fifty days. It is, in various schools of homeopathy, used in potencies ranging from the very lowest to the very highest and is wonderfully effective in all of them. High potencies, however, work best in a single dose, while lower potencies may be repeated as needed.

Poster Children: Aunt Bee from *The Andy Griffith Show* is a perfect Natrum Muriaticum, always putting Andy and Opie's needs ahead of her own, and always feeling a little angry about it. Sue Ann Niven, from *The Mary Tyler Moore Show*, is another example, one that stresses the sexuality of the remedy and the verbally abusive barbs that can flow from the Natrum's mouth. One has to consider fictional characters in the selection of a Natrum example, in that they tend not to want to become famous. They want, instead, to be loved.

NUX
The Aggressor

Remedy Source: While there are two major remedies that begin with the word Nux, Nux Moschata and Nux Vomica, they are not, in reality, related remedies. The word *Nux* is Latin for "nut," so all these remedies really have in common is that they are both taken from the nut of a tree. Nux Moschata is made from nutmeg. The vastly more important remedy, and the one that we will use here as an essential constitutional remedy, is Nux Vomica, which means "poison nut."

The full name of the remedy gives away the type of poison: Strychnos Nux Vomica. It is taken from the gray seeds of a tree of the Loganiaceae order, and these seeds contain strychnine, or rat poison. The seeds are said to be incredibly bitter as well as highly toxic. The seeds are contained within an orange fruit that itself is benign and is eaten by birds.

The substance of the seeds is used medicinally in India, most often in cases of snakebite, but also in various fevers. The Strychnos Nux Vomica tree is related to the Saint-Ignatius's-bean, making Ignatia and Nux Vomica related remedies.

The remedy Nux Vomica was created by Samuel Hahnemann.

Situations That Suggest Nux Vomica: Constipation, especially chronic constipation; Crohn's disease; hemorrhoids; influenza. Also diarrhea, colitis, irritable bowel syndrome; heart disease: high blood pressure; liver disease; cerebral accidents; spasms and twitches of all sorts: epilepsy; kidney stones; endometriosis; fibrositis; sleep disorders: insomnia, nightmares; addictions: coffee, tea, drugs, alcohol, tobacco. Also coughs and cold, asthma, chronic fatigue, multiple sclerosis, environmental illness, neuralgic pains.

Remedy Overview: If you met my landlord, Ed, you would know everything you need to know about the remedy. Ed is a type A personality. There is never a moment when he is not too busy to listen to your problem. But when he wants to talk to you, he just appears at your door at any time that is convenient to him, day or night. He never calls first; it gives him a great advantage to take you by surprise.

Everything for Ed is a struggle, and it is a struggle he must always win. He tries to win first by simple intimidation. If that does not work, he lies. (He smiles then, and that's how you know that he's lying. It is the only time he smiles.) It never occurs to Ed that any problem could be solved by simple cooperation. He feels that it lessens his personal power to work with others; he must instead defeat them.

Ed has a certain bitterness to him. Being near him is like being near a thunderstorm. You never know when the lightning will strike. He acquired this attitude early in life as a defensive posture. He feels that if he is mean enough, people will pretty much let him do whatever he wants and will leave him alone.

Like most Nux types, the core reason that Ed pushes everyone around and away is that he has no idea how to communicate and is terrified of having to talk to people. Like most Nux types, Ed, at his core, is motivated not by anger but by fear.

Ed, as is typical of the type, is more cunning than he is smart. Most Nux people ultimately destroy themselves in any situation. They react in the moment without a thought to the ultimate price that they will have to pay for their cruel behavior. As a matter of fact, I cannot think of a more appropriate career choice for a Nux than a landlord, who can greatly enjoy withholding the heat in winter and the water pressure in summer, and still take people's money while abusing them.

Like most middle-aged Nux types, Ed is well on the way to his first heart attack. His red face and constant rage are testaments to his high blood pressure. Like most Nuxes, he will likely have that attack by age sixty, after which his body's aches and pains will force him to calm down.

Like many Nuxes, Ed is accident prone. When objects and tools defy their will by not doing what they are supposed to do, Nuxes incorporate those objects into their rage reaction, often injuring themselves in the process. Once, when a power saw failed to perform to his expectations, Ed nearly cut his own arm off during his tantrum. For the weeks in which he was on potent painkillers, Ed was a different person, almost pleasant. But as soon as he was well, we were once more off to the races.

Ed resembles the majority of Nuxes physically as well, with the aforementioned red face. He is a shortish man, but very solid and stocky in build. Like most Nuxes, he has lost most of his hair and wears a little wool cap from September to spring. Ed hates to be cold, which makes him even meaner.

Like most Nuxes, Ed is a medley of twitches—eye twitches, facial tics—which get worse when he gets mad, which is most of the time. He gives those with whom he must deal the Look. The Look says, Don't mess with me, I'll kill you. He also never smiles with his eyes. Like most Nuxy types, his eyes look cold and almost dead.

Remedy Theme: Struggle, aggressive behavior.

Remedy Motivation: Anger, covering deep fear.

Emotional Portrait: It was a Nux who came up with the idea of winning by intimidation. Nux types believe in two things: (1) that we are all here on this planet to compete, and (2) that they must win the contest by intimidating all the others.

This could seem a bit like Lycopodium, but there is a major difference in the two types (both by and large male remedies). The Lycopodium chooses battles with those he knows he can beat, who are physically weaker, or stupider, or, most often, poorer. Nux picks a fight at any time with anyone. He is the pit bull of humanity. And he is willing to go down swinging and unafraid. Think of Captain Kirk on *Star Trek*, a character who could be physically driven to his knees by evil aliens, but whose spirit would never bow. Think of him barking orders or shouting, "Don't tell me no, Mister!" and you get the idea of the type.

Nux types are perhaps the most sensitive people on Earth, always making sure that they haven't been insulted in some subtle way that they haven't quite understood. They are aware that, like dogs, they can sometimes be fooled by the tone of a human's voice and not catch the full meaning of the words, so they are on guard.

The Nux sensitivity runs through all levels of being. Just as he is hypersensitive to insult, he is hypersensitive to cold. He refuses to let you even crack open a car window. And it is almost impossible for the Nux to get warm again once he is cold. Classic homeopaths say that they had only to look at a patient with a Nux cold or flu to know that the patient needed this remedy, as no other remedy is so well covered and yet so cold.

Nuxes can't stand noise. You can spot the apartment buildings in which a Nux lives; all his neighbors are tiptoeing around trying not to set him off again.

And that's just what Nuxes count on and how they live their lives: betting that you will do anything not to set them off. They give themselves full and fully rationalized permission to do whatever they have to do to get their way. They are, in their way, even more self-centered than Sulphurs. Take the way they drive, for example. Nuxes usually own the blackest cars (they love black everything, it is their favorite color), and they love to drive fast. They cut you off and then swear at you for being in their way. All the way to work, they are changing lanes, speeding then braking then speeding again, all because driving, like everything else, is competition for them. If they can get to the exit ten full seconds ahead of you, then they have won.

Even the Nux child is competitive, and even he falls prey to the illness of stress, particularly to digestive disorders. This child is a terrible loser and would rather lie and cheat than lose. Somehow he never understands that winning by cheating is worse than losing. This child never admits that he has done anything wrong, or even that he has made a mistake. Again, he attempts to lie his way out of the situation.

Nux children are incredibly jealous of their brothers and sisters, especially if the siblings display any sort of talent or skill. The Nux actually feels better about himself if he is able to undermine the self-confidence of others. This is, unfortunately, a trait he never seems to outgrow.

The Nux type forms around the notion that they are not good enough, and they almost violently fight against this message. Nuxes have a violent anger against one or both parents and charge that parent with both neglect and abuse. And, truly, Nuxes are often children who have been abused and who have elected to take over the role of abuser in order to seize the power of the tyrant for themselves. At their core, they see themselves as pitiful persons who are just trying to protect themselves from the evil all around them. Like Lycopodiums, they feel misunderstood. Unlike Lycopodiums, Nuxes are often driven deep into despair. They suddenly and violently commit suicide.

A core motivation for Nux is general impatience. They feel that others are just lagging behind. As bosses, they feel that it is necessary to abuse employees in order to get them to behave and keep up. They are also demanding and difficult husbands and fathers who lack any ability to show love and compassion and are more concerned with the fact that dinner is not on the table on time than with the needs and wants of the family.

Nuxes tend to move into careers that allow them to have power. They love to carry weapons of all sorts, so look for them in the military and police force. They are also happy being night watchmen, when the weapons are real but the dangers are less. As they are pit bulls who throw themselves into the line of fire, they can be very good police or soldiers. Ironically, the people at whom they are hurling themselves are likely Nuxes as well, as those who are not motivated toward the good of society make for happy criminals, especially when they are able to take their rage out on a victim who is not getting his wallet out fast enough.

Enough cannot be said about the addictive nature of the Nux personality. They love uppers of all sorts, particularly coffee, which speeds them up and helps them to feel powerful. But they need downers. Nuxes, even at their best, have trouble sleeping. As they become involved with stimulants of any sort, they lose the power to sleep almost altogether.

Let me take you through the daily pattern of a Nux. Start just before dawn. After an evening of tossing and turning, or thinking about the day that has passed and about anything he should have done and didn't, should have said and didn't, the Nux finally falls into a deep, heavy sleep. An hour or two later, his alarm rings and he pulls himself out of bed.

His family knows better than to talk to the Nux when he comes downstairs. He is mean in the morning. And his wife knows to have the coffee ready. He needs the coffee both to wake up and to allow him to pass a stool. His family knows by the expression on his face that the coffee has just "kicked in," and no one gets in his way as he rushes toward the bathroom. His constipation is as chronic as his insomnia, and the family knows better than to interfere.

After breakfast, he rushes to his car and drives like a maniac to work. He gets to his office and gets more coffee. (Usually, Nuxes are heavy coffee drinkers, thinking nothing of drinking a dozen cups a day. Just as often they are addicted to cigarettes.) He needs to smoke when he drinks his coffee for the full buzz effect that the two together bring.

He barks his way through the day, doing his work. If he works in a corporation, he is likely in middle management, as his aggressive nature takes him part of the way up the corporate ladder, but his abrasive personality limits promotions. He is unlikely to get much exercise, and his sedentary lifestyle increases his constipation.

Throughout the day, the Nux's head buzzes more and more, a combination of caffeine, nicotine, and sleep deprivation. By the time the workday is done and he is racing home, he is hardly fit to drive safely. But this doesn't encourage him to slow down. No, he drives all the faster in his race to get home.

At home he demands a drink to relax. If he doesn't go home for this, he habitually attends happy hours at local bars. He usually feels that alcohol is the tool that best allows him to unwind after a hard day. He carries his martini to the dinner table with him or switches to red wine, which Nux types tend to love. For dinner he wants meat and potatoes—steak is usually his favorite—and eats a little salad if it has cheese on it. After dinner, having eaten too much too quickly and having had a good deal of alcohol, he falls asleep in his chair in front of the television.

His family has been trained to let a sleeping Nux lie, so they do not wake him. He awakens from his snoring after the eleven o'clock news and moves from his chair to his bed. There, sleep eludes him, and he tosses and turns again, a mixture of chemicals churning in his system, until the hour before dawn when he falls into deep and dreamless slumber.

It's not easy being a Nux. Because of their chronic exhaustion, they use rage to fuel their day. They ignore the fact that, although they feel good for a short time while angry, they feel much worse later after the anger has waned. It is especially common for the Nux type to get a headache after throwing a tantrum. At this time, also, when they have spent their rage, they are sensitive to light, to sounds, and to smells. Nux types, perhaps more than any other remedy, are sensitive to odors of all sorts, especially to perfumes, which literally cause them to feel faint.

The remedy Nux, therefore, is a valuable curative tool for those who have been chemically poisoned and those who are environmentally ill. It is also considered the homeopathic universal antidote, in that it undoes the effects of most remedies or medicines, homeopathic or allopathic.

Nux proves, perhaps better than any other remedy, the homeopathic belief that the stronger the poison, the stronger the cure.

Physical Portrait: I call them Chock Full o' Nux, and they are toxic people who, due to their diets and their lack of exercise, are largely responsible for the toxins in their system. But people who are bombarded with other, more environmental sorts of toxins, people who live under high-tension wires, for instance, may also take on a Nux constitution. A characteristic anger comes on with symptoms. A person who has the same sorts of symptoms but who shows no sign of irritability needs some other remedy. There is the characteristic oversensitivity to cold, light, noise, and smells, and the characteristic twitch or spasm or nervous habit, such as jingling coins in the pants pocket. Some part of the body, usually the colon, is likely to be in spasm as well, causing a chronic discomfort that helps to drive the anger.

These spasms, and, indeed, all these general symptoms, are made worse by eating. Nuxes are also worse when touched, and they dislike and distrust touch. They are also, although they never seem to understand this, worse when they are angry. They also tend to be worse if they do any physical labor, which they seek to avoid.

In general, they are also worse in dry weather. Nuxes like wet weather, as long as it does not make them cold. They are also worse when drinking and are given to powerful hangovers. Nux is, in fact, the best acute remedy for hangovers and is especially helpful if it is taken before drinking is begun and then repeated after the fact.

The Nux is plagued by headaches. The head pain is worse when there is noise and during any form of mental activity. It is particularly worse in bright light.

Their constipation, unlike that of Calcarea, drives Nuxes crazy. They try anything to get rid of the constipation. They tend to feel cramping and sharp pains in the abdomen after eating or after anger, but these pains never seem to bring on a relieving bowel movement. Nux also tends to have headaches that tie in with the constipation, being bilious in nature.

Nux, therefore, is also a useful acute remedy to consider for colic in children. Look for the child to seem angry and to arch the back angrily from the pain.

The Nux type tends to crave spicy foods that act as stimulants in the system. They also crave meat, especially red meat, fat, alcohol, coffee, and tobacco. They are given to developing peptic ulcers and gastritis, all brought on from a combination of their diet and lifestyle.

Nux also is a general remedy for allergies and colds when the usual symptoms of the remedy are in place. These conditions come on slowly, the cold taking days or weeks finally to take hold. The nose flows freely in the day, particularly in the early morning on waking, and is entirely stopped up at night. The patient sneezes in the morning but not at night.

Nux types are given to chronic coughs. These too are worse in the morning, especially when still in bed. The cough is shallow and dry, and may become their personal nervous habit as they cough relentlessly during the day.

Asthma is also common. Unlike the cough, the asthma is at night, especially at 3 A.M., and worse in cold weather.

High blood pressure is almost essential to the remedy type. The Nux feels chronic heart pain. This remedy probably has more vulnerability in the heart than in any other organ. Nuxes often lose their health to a circulatory ailment, leaving them in their final years rather impotent, angry husks. If the heart attack or stroke does not cripple them, or force them to change, it likely kills them on the spot. Nuxes have a habit of dropping dead, their heart having given out without warning. It is also common for Nuxes to mistake heartburn for a heart attack, or vice versa. They may also have panic attacks that they mistake for heart attacks.

Nux is perhaps most helpful in the 30C potency, which gets to the guts of the situation, although a higher potency may be needed for those who have given way totally to their anger.

It is used for a wide range of acute cases, as well as in constitutional treatments. Often Nux is the first remedy given in cases that involve a dependence on allopathic medicine or a coffee habit.

It is helpful to know that Nux works especially well if it is given for the first time just before bedtime, as it soothes the patient and helps him sleep.

Poster Child: To really get to know Nux Vomica, watch reruns of *All in the Family*. Archie Bunker is the Nux's Nux.

PHOSPHORUS
The Charmer

Remedy Source: This remedy is created from the element phosphorus. The element is known for its pale yellow color and its distinctive odor. Like sulfur, phosphorus is found in regions surrounding volcanoes. And, like many of the other remedy types that form the essential constitutions, phosphorus is found in all of our bodies, as a part of our bones.

Phosphorus was discovered by 1673, and soon after it was used therapeutically. Alchemists considered it to be an essential element, the "light bearer." The name *phosphorus* refers to its luminescence. Physicians and alchemists alike used the substance, in the form of "luminous pills," to cure everything from fevers to diarrhea to tuberculosis.

Samuel Hahnemann turned the element into the homeopathic remedy.

Situations That Suggest Phosphorus: Upper respiratory diseases: asthma, cold and flu, sore throat, bronchitis, pneumonia; respiratory infections of all sorts; chronic otitis, tinnitus; emphysema; tuberculosis. Also chronic laryngitis; preacher's throat; heart disease: congestive heart failure, valvular heart disease; hypertension; skin disorders: ichthyosis, skin ulcers, eczema, psoriasis; disorders of the blood: hemophilia. Also headache; vertigo; Ménière's disease; arthritis; rheumatism; neuralgia; seizure disorders: epilepsy and petit mal; senility; phobias; low blood sugar and diabetes; eye and vision troubles: amblyopia, detached retina, retinitis, optic neuritis, glaucoma, flashes of light in front of the eyes; nose bleeds; pyorrhea with easily bleeding gums, excessive bleeding from dental procedures; excessive bleeding after any operation.

Remedy Overview: We are told a good deal of nonsense about this constitutional type in our homeopathic literature. We are told that, as a group, these people are just not very bright. We are also told that they are perky and bubbly, and they are even compared to the bubbles that rise up in champagne.

But we have learned a good deal about human intelligence and about how it works. In the past, IQ ruled the roost, and the activities of the left brain were those that were both measured and praised. Recently, however, we have been introduced to the concept of EQ, or emotional quotient, and have learned a bit more both about the necessity of developing our right-brain activity and about how to measure it.

And while average Phosphorus types may not rate highly in terms of left-brain intelligence, they are off the charts in terms of their right brain. Phosphorus types usually gravitate to careers in the arts, in which creativity is prized over math skills, or to work that involves public speaking and motivation and sales, or careers in human services. They love to persuade people and to help others. Like President Bill Clinton, they feel your pain.

The other thing we are told is that Phosphorus types are natural psychics who have the power to read minds. This is not true. What is true is that Phosphorus types tend to live in their own bodies a little less than do other people. They tend to need physical pain to anchor themselves entirely in their body (which is why they so hate physical pain—they don't want to feel trapped in their bodies). Phosphorus types have problems with boundaries, and they see their own body as the biggest boundary of all, so they tend to float out of it whenever possible.

They are not psychics, but they are all naturally empathetic. They do not know or care what you are thinking, but they know what you are feeling. It is on this level of feelings that Phosphorus types live their lives. They communicate on an incredibly visceral level, manipulating others with emotions and not with words.

Remedy Theme: Manipulation through charm.

Remedy Motivation: The need for love.

Emotional Portrait: Perhaps more than any other constitutional type, Phosphorus is aware of the world around him. He can sense changes in that world, on both a physical and an emotional level, better than can any other type. The Phosphorus type is often referred to as being a "human barometer"; he can sense changes in the weather even days away. This is especially true of oncoming rain, especially storms, which can throw the Phosphorus system for a loop. He may get headaches before a storm, or panic attacks. When the storm arrives, something in the Phosphorus awakens, as it also awakens with physical pain. He becomes fully aware and fully incorporated with his own body in a way that he never can without the storm, or without such tools and crutches as sex, spicy foods, or drugs.

The Phosphorus child seems to be aware from birth. These children seem actually to be seeing you, almost from birth. They look you directly in the eye with their own piercing eyes and seem to be able to look right into your heart. They seem to be able to understand your every feeling and thought.

It is important to remember that, even as babies, the Phosphorus type is open. They are available emotionally. In the same way, they are truly trusting of human nature, often seeing, as Melanie Wilkes does in *Gone With the Wind*, only the essential goodness in human nature.

The Phosphorus child exhibits a strongly curious nature. And, as Calcarea learns by putting things in his mouth, the Phosphorus learns by seeing. It is as if from birth he wants to travel, to take flight, to see everything there is to see.

Phosphorus children are sympathetic and empathetic. They do not often cry, nor are they prone to tantrums. If they are held—Phosphorus types crave human touch—and told often enough that they are loved, they are the easiest children to raise.

However, Phosphorus children often exhibit deep fears. This is especially true if they do not feel that their home environment is a safe one or one in which they are truly loved. Look for them to fear ghosts. They have a deep fear of the dark as well and often want their parents to search the bedroom, especially checking the closet and under the bed, before turning off the light. Phosphorus children sleep with night-lights and their bedroom doors open. Even when they become adults, they usually cannot face the concept of a closed bedroom door without a good deal of fear. They are fearful of the future and convinced that something bad is about to happen. They should not be permitted to watch the news on television, especially just before bed. They absorb the negative news and turn it into pure fear, which is projected into their own near future. Phosphorus children also usually fear being alone. They want to sleep between their parents, or want their parents to sit by their bedside until they fall asleep.

Illness enhances and deepens Phosphorus fears. The Phosphorus child with an ear infection, for instance (ear infections are very, very common to the type), needs his mother's physical touch in order to allay his fears and soothe his pain and allow him to fall asleep.

Other common fears, in adults as well as children, include earthquakes, insects, and water. Many Phosphorus types never learn to swim because they deeply fear water. Some are unable to travel over bridges or even to fly over water without feeling panic. Some Phosphorus types fear insanity; their boundaries have so eroded that they can no longer block out the pain of others. This is the Phosphorus who can no longer bear to go to the mall because he feels the unhappiness of thousands of other people, all milling around him. This instability of boundaries also reveals itself in fear for other people. Phosphorus types can drive themselves to the edge of their own endurance with fear for those they love. The child becomes sure that his father has been killed when he is fifteen minutes late getting home from work. He reaches out for his father with all this vital force, seeking to protect his father no matter what cost to himself.

If there is one central lesson that every Phosphorus needs to learn it is pacing. Phosphoruses tend to let their energy flow as they think it needs to flow, with no thought to their own needs or their own future. Phosphorus children are hyperactive for a time and then fall exhausted to the floor. They never pace themselves and often forget to eat. You see them flying around the room like tornado funnels, only to find them twenty minutes later asleep under the dining room table. No other child falls asleep as deeply as does the Phosphorus child. He is carried upstairs, undressed, and put to bed without ever stirring.

In fact, if there is one thing that Phosphoruses love as much as they do other people, it is sleep. They can and often do sleep as much as ten hours a day. They have vivid, colorful dreams and awaken totally refreshed and recharged from their sleep. Yet, due to their ongoing emotional outpouring, they exhaust themselves again the next day and fall, exhausted, into bed again, ready for a revivifying sleep.

As Phosphorus children grow, they tend, through multiple hurts and betrayals, to begin to direct their emotional needs. They begin the search for the "other," the partner who will enable them to travel forth into the world, see what there is to see, do what there is to do, and then return home feeling safe and sound.

Having somewhere to go at the end of the day is of vital importance to the Phosphorus, as is having the other present when he gets there. For Phosphorus, the most stressful time of day is twilight. All physical and emotional symptoms grow worse then. If he does not have a home he can consider his own, he falls prey to panic and to fear.

Hollywood is home to many a Phosphorus. The entire drive of their life, from the earliest years until death, is the need to connect with others on a visceral level, the need to feel loved. In order to feel loved, the Phosphorus does and is anything the object of desire requires.

This need to connect can it itself become an addiction, or it can lead to a number of other addictions. Phosphorus types tend to become addicted to sex or applause.

They seek approval and love. If they cannot find the soul mate they so desire, they seek the approval of the crowd. Therefore, many Phosphorus types are in show business, sharing their heart with the crowd in exchange for approval.

If we study the lives of some classic Hollywood types, we uncover an understanding of the type. Hollywood icons Marilyn Monroe, Montgomery

Clift, and Judy Garland are all prime examples of the type. Each was totally open on an emotional level—or at least projected an illusionary openness—to the public. Each flew from relationship to relationship, giving each new partner the same total attention while the attempt was being made, then leaving each one just as totally when that relationship was, in his or her mind, over. Each turned to typical Phosphorus crutches for assistance when the vital force was overwhelmed. And each followed the typical Phosphorus pattern of collapse, followed by recharging and then by return.

In the first aspect, consider particularly Judy Garland, who was so adept at projecting her own emotions and at absorbing the emotions of her fans that it came to matter very little whether she could, on a given night, sing. Her fans wanted her, not her talent, with a desire that bordered on the religious. Only a Phosphorus can draw out and receive such affection from the crowd, and only a Phosphorus can be so in need of it.

The second aspect can become one of the most dangerous of all Phosphorus traits. They want to connect instantly and totally with another person, anyone who catches their eye. And so no one gives you so intense a relationship as does a Phosphorus. No one connects with you so quickly, or makes your heart pound as hard. Phosphorus types seem to know you, to see right through you. And they are loaded with charm. What they say doesn't matter, you just stare into their eyes, willing to believe most everything they tell you. Your love seems to be all that matters in the world. But if you give them your love, they suddenly move on, forgetting about you because there are literally billions of other people in the world for them to connect with and from whom they also need love.

This can make for a good time. Phosphorus types make you feel really, really good about yourself, as if you were the best-looking, wittiest person on Earth. Their attention is focused on you and only on you. It is as if some heavenly spotlight is illuminating you from within. They give you the ten most intense seconds of your life—then move on to their next target.

Phosphoruses, caught up in the hunt, often do not notice the broken hearts they leave in their wake. Nor do they notice that, over time, their ability to connect profoundly and intensely leads them down dangerous paths. Some Phosphorus types who move deeply into the remedy endanger themselves while looking for Mr. Goodbar; others open themselves up to dangerous sexual and chemical habits as they seek the universal union with the other.

The other danger of this pattern is that, over time, Phosphorus types become pathetic in their need for connection. They can grow into grotesque emotional leeches. They will always be "on," always in need of the next emotional stimulus. This will drive them in time to some sort of addiction that replaces the need to connect, or to a life in which they face the ongoing rejection of younger and younger people whom they try in vain to attract.

Julia Roberts, who is a total Phosphorus type, already shows this pattern. She has become engaged to many of her leading men. And she also displays strongly the next trait: that of breaking down and disappearing, only to come back reinvented, more spectacular than before.

This traces itself back to the little Phosphorus who fell asleep under the table. As an adult, that pattern turns into one of emotional bingeing and purging. For a time, the Phosphorus is everywhere, at the center of every activity and every party. The Phosphorus actor makes three movies a year and goes on every talk show to promote his work. Then he disappears. For a month, a year, two years, he is gone. Look under the dining room table, because that's where he is.

Some go to the hospital to recover and, often, to dry out. Others simply shut down and return to their sleep pattern in order to recharge. At this point there is no getting them to move. It is not even worth the attempt. They do not respond and, truly, do not even want to connect with others. They pull into themselves, into their food and into their books, as they begin to recover.

Then, one day, they are ready. They have a new outfit, a new hairdo. They have lost weight and look fantastic. Their eyes are brighter than they have been in years. They may suddenly change their home, their relationship, or their career. They may even change their name. They have reinvented themselves, and they are back.

As adults and as children, Phosphorus types need advice. They do quite well with psychotherapy, and the combination of therapy and homeopathy can do them a great deal of good. They need to learn to come more fully into their own bodies and into their own lives. They must learn that, if they are fully in their own body and fully aware, they will not be more cut off from others, but instead will be able to communicate in a simpler and more wholesome way.

They also need to learn pacing. They will not need to reinvent themselves if they do not destroy themselves in the first place. If they allow their day to have both activity and rest, they will not exhaust themselves.

And they need to learn that they do not need alcohol, drugs, or sex as a drug, just as they do not need spicy foods to awaken their digestion.

Phosphorus types who do not learn these lessons tend not to live very long lives. Like Jim Morrison, they live hard, die young, and leave a beautiful corpse.

Physical Portrait: Phosphorus types show weakness in their ears, throats, and chests. Phosphorus children particularly have almost constant earaches and infections. Every cold moves quickly into the chest. Most respiratory ailments start in the throat. Sore throats are very common and are improved by cold liquids—Phosphorous types want an entire tray of ice cubes emptied into their drink.

Phosphorus often reacts to stress with a sore throat—sore throat from exhaustion, from over use of the voice, with allergies. Allergies, especially plain old hay fever, are very common to the type.

Allergies manifest with the loss of the voice. Phosphorus types lose their voice entirely and usually painlessly. It is as if the voice had been stolen from them. They dehydrate quickly when they are speaking in public and need liquids to keep their voice. Often, their lips are very dry with dehydration.

Phosphorus types also typically have a cough. The cough may cause them a great deal of discomfort in their chest. It hurts deep down when they cough, and they cannot stop coughing.

As children Phosphorus types usually have very thin bodies, with the chests being particularly underdeveloped. Even as adults, they tend toward very thin chests, arms, and legs. If they gain weight, they tend to gain it all on the stomach or on the hips. The face, too, shows weight gain, while the chest stays very thin. The shoulders are typically narrow.

Phosphorus types are given to gastric troubles, such as ulcers and vomiting blood, which is, like the blood of the Phosphorus nosebleed, very red. Their gastric disorders are accompanied by nausea and vomiting. They desire cold drinks and are greatly improved by them, until those cold things are warmed in their stomach. Then their nausea increases, with the Phosphorus often throwing up the now-warm liquid.

They crave ice cream, chocolate, cold foods and drinks, salty and spicy foods. They like milk, although they cannot digest it. They like meat, fish, eggs, cheese, sweets. They don't want warm foods and drinks. They become ill after eating the spicy foods they so crave but cannot digest.

They are tremendously thirsty people, perhaps the most thirsty of all types. A normal thirst counterindicates the remedy type.

Phosphorus types are troubled by belching and indigestion. They are given to diarrhea that can be sudden, violent, and very painful. The pain in Phosphorus is similar to Arsenicum and Sulphur in that it is burning in nature. This is especially true of diarrhea.

The Phosphorus person is apt to have skin conditions as well—dry skin and red, itching patches of eczema or psoriasis.

In general, Phosphorus types run a little on the chilly side, although body temperature tends not to be an issue with them. They do, however, tend to be better when cold things are taken internally and when warm applications are placed on them externally. They are given to great aggravations from changes in the weather and do not do well living in places with weather extremes. They are very sensitive to their environment on an aesthetic level as well and never are happy or able to function very well in any place they do not consider beautiful. They want to be surrounded by beautiful sights, sounds, smells, and people.

They want to be touched and are improved in every way by touching or rubbing. They want a back rub every day and feel much better for it. Some Phosphorus types want a back rub more than they want sex or food.

They are worse when fasting and, like Lycopodium, need to eat regular meals. They tend to do better eating very simple, small meals several times a day than larger meals less often. They often do best eating only one food at a time, making one small meal out of fruit, another with just roasted chicken, which they love.

You can spot them by their sleep position. Phosphorus types cannot fall asleep on their left side. They do not like to shift onto the left even briefly. Typically, they have to be in a fetal position on their right side to fall asleep. As sleep is so very important to them, Phosphorus types have elaborate nighttime rituals, with several steps that bring them just a bit closer to their beloved sleep.

Perhaps the Phosphorus so loves sleep because it finally and totally frees him from the restriction of his body, allowing him to be anyone or to travel anywhere during those few precious nighttime hours. Perhaps it is because all boundaries are finally down and all laws of physics that the Phosphorous finds so restrictive erased that this type finds sleep so refreshing. It finally gives him his heart's desire.

Poster Child: President and allergic voice-loser Bill Clinton.

PULSATILLA
The Marshmallow

Remedy Source: Pulsatilla is created from the anemone, or windflower, which grows naturally in northern and central Europe and is particularly abundant in Great Britain. It grows best in regions with sandy soil, on hills and pastures that receive a great deal of sun. The plant is a perennial that blooms twice a year, in May and September.

This flowering plant is also called the pasqueflower because it blooms during the Easter season each year. The violet-purple flowers have been traditionally used in the creation of dye used to color Easter eggs.

Dioscorides in his materia medica lists the anemone as a remedy for headache and ophthamalia.

Pulsatilla is a remedy created by Hahnemann. About the remedy, he wrote, "This powerful plant produces many symptoms on the healthy human body which often correspond to the marks symptoms commonly met with, hence, also, they admit of frequent homeopathic employment and often do good." In other words, this is a homeopathic remedy of the first order. It covers a wide range of symptoms, making it both an important remedy in acute situations and for a wide range of constitutional effects.

Situations That Suggest Pulsatilla: Women's health issues: PMS, pregnancy, menopause, puberty, uterine prolapse, labor pains, dysmenorrhea, inflamed ovaries; allergies and respiratory complaints: hay fever, asthma, bronchitis, sinusitis, colds and flus in their later stage. Also mumps, measles, conjunctivitis, chicken pox; eye troubles: obstructed tear duct, cataract, styles. Also heart palpitations and vertigo; digestive troubles: heartburn, diarrhea; mental anguish: fear, depression, hysteria. Also pain.

Remedy Overview: The classical idea of this remedy is a woman who is soft and yielding. This is true, but we should look at this remedy a little more clearly. Our society has redefined not only our assigned gender roles but also our constitutional types. Just as women entering the job market have taken over the once male remedies of Nux Vomica and Lycopodium, and are having those remedies' traditional heart attacks and ulcers, men are now moving into the range of Pulsatilla.

This is most usually a woman's remedy, just as Nux is still usually a man's, but we can no longer slot this or any remedy completely. Our constitution is largely determined by our environment, our stresses, and how we react to those stresses, so when you place a woman in a cutthroat environment, expect her to take on more and more of the traditional male ailments along with the traditional male role.

The same is true for men. As men are freed to explore their natural roles, rather than feeling that they have to live their lives as society says they should, they are exploring some new constitutional types. And we are seeing more and more of a mix of genders in what once was a pretty clear constitutional game.

Whether female or male, Pulsatillas combine two traits: They are soft in their bodies and their spirits, and they are changeable. In body, mind, and spirit they can be counted on to change. Their symptoms change as quickly as their minds.

Pulsatillas lack a clear direction of self and, often, a clear direction in life. They look to their parents and to their mates in particular to give their lives shape. Shape is a very important part of this remedy as well. As Phosphorus lacks boundaries, Pulsatilla lacks shape. They are amorphous and yielding, like clay that is just sitting on the potter's wheel, waiting. The Pulsatilla lucky enough to happen upon a potter who is willing to put the time and energy into this structuring process develops into a loving and centered person, one who is naturally among the most nurturing persons on Earth.

But such Henry Higginses are rare, and most Pulsatillas instead seek out the strongest person in the room, the most alpha of the alpha males available in the gene pool, and thrill to his dominance. As a yielding and feminine type, the Pulsatilla—male or female—prizes nothing more than masculinity. This can become problematic.

Pulsatillas often project themselves into a victim role, believing that life itself is shaping them. This is particularly true for those who lacked solid parental direction. These Pulsatillas tend to say yes to everything, because they are unsure when to say no. Therefore, when some tattooed lug says that they should get married, the Pulsatilla, at once thrilled just looking at this guy and unsure of what she should do in this situation, marries him, even though he has already cheated on her and hasn't had a job in the two years since he got out of prison.

This gives the Pulsatilla a reputation for not being very intelligent. Sometimes, sorry to say, the reputation seems well deserved, as Pulsatilla tends to make mistakes like this one again and again.

Worse, once she has said yes to this guy, she blocks out her friends' warnings with a stubbornness that seems to belie her type. At all the wrong moments in life, Pulsatilla seems to develop a powerful personality.

After she is married to this man, she works to make him happy and accepts his abuse as if it were in her job description. As she basically sees herself as "fortune's fool," she takes to sighing and crying and eating as her defenses against her bad marriage and her life.

Pulsatillas never seem to give themselves a chance. They seem never to have any real ambitions and tend to get only the education their parents force them to get. Like their bodies, their minds lack shape. They never develop themselves past a basic, needy role, as if they were frozen in an infantile state.

Perhaps for this reason they are incredible in their skill with children; something in themselves recognizes the needs of this blank slate they are holding in their arms. No other type works so that her children have it better in every way than she did. No other type takes parenting so seriously or works so hard at it.

Remedy Theme: Softness, changeability.

Remedy Motivation: Avoidance, fear.

Emotional Portrait: Classically, this type is compared to the weather on an April day. Or as Will Rogers might have put it, if you don't like her present mood, wait a moment.

No other type changes moods as frequently as does Pulsatilla. Where Ignatia can rocket between laughing and crying, both with the same dramatic intensity, Pulsatilla has the full palette of emotions available to her at all times and for all occasions. Mostly she makes you, as Ignatia does, wonder what you did or said that upset her so. But unlike Ignatia, this wonderment is not tinged with the feeling that you are being emotionally blackmailed. Instead, you feel that this is a poor, sweet, innocent child who has somehow ended up sitting next to evil you. You want to take her in your arms and comfort her. And, in fact, no other type seems as open and available to comforting as Pulsatilla. And no other type takes comforting with such aplomb. Like a sort of emotional prostitute, the Pulsatilla will, if you are not educated in the ways of comforting the sad and the helpless, teach you the niceties of the practice: how to rock someone in your arms (Pulsatilla loves that rocking action), how to go out and buy flowers and gifts, and how to apologize even if you think you were right.

Pulsatilla is so good at this sort of thing, where Ignatia is more direct in her approach, that it takes you years to realize that you are still being emotionally blackmailed.

It is not that Pulsatilla is helpless; it is that she sees herself as helpless. In reality, Pulsatilla has a potent arsenal of weapons to get her own way. These are adaptive behaviors that are usually developed in turmoil, as Pulsatilla usually grows up in a family situation in which she feels unsafe. Pulsatilla women usually feel that men, while overwhelming and thrilling, are also unsafe. So they develop feminine wiles as a way of keeping themselves safe and the men in line. The Pulsatilla woman who to the outside world looks like Blanche DuBois trapped with that brute Stanley, is more often sister Stella, who is in firm control of everything that goes on in that household.

The first weapon, and in many ways the greatest, is tears. Pulsatilla cries more often and for more varied reasons than does any other constitutional type. Along with Sepia, Pulsatilla cries in the practitioner's office when she is talking about her own symptoms. She cries at sad movies and at comedies. She cries when she looks at her old yearbooks. She cries and cries and cries if her feelings are hurt.

These tears keep people both off balance and in line. The Pulsatilla has been wounded. The drill now is that everything must stop and she must be comforted. Unlike the Ignatia, who runs to her room to cry, making you go after her and tap on the door so that you can be locked out and forced to hear her cry, and unlike the Sepia, who cries with such an angry look on her face that you are too afraid to comfort her, the Pulsatilla stands or sits right where she is and turns to a puddle of tears right in front of your eyes, at once confrontational in her tears and oblivious of your presence, making you deal with it. And, indeed, there is nothing else to be done—you must deal with whatever you've done and work very hard to restore her to an even keel.

If you do not respond, or do not jump quickly enough to comfort, the Pulsatilla moves on to questions—"Don't you love me? Why don't you love me? What's wrong with me?" and variations of this theme—until she receives an answer. If the answer is a good one, and you move on to the comforting stage, the whole event is over quickly. But if the response is a bad one— "How could I love anyone who makes me feel like I am choking all the time?"—the Pulsatilla ups the ante and increases the emotional barrage. You are split in your reactions: Should you stay for more of this, or should you flee, knowing that the reckoning will be worse later?

Usually, you end up in a bar saying something like, "Women, can't live with them, can't live without them."

The Pulsatilla type usually is also quite shy. She never wants to speak in public or attract undue attention (that is, any attention that is not due her from her victim status). Yet few people are as skilled at a visceral connection with others as is the Pulsatilla. It is as if she can connect with the inner child that we didn't even know that we had. She can pull this child out of our gut and spend the afternoon rocking it in a rocking chair.

The Pulsatilla invites you into her kitchen and into her life. She feeds you and nurtures you, and by day's end she has drawn your whole life's story out of you. This having been done, she now loves you and offers her unconditional love—just as long as you are willing to join the roster of people who stand and scratch their heads, wondering what they did to make her cry, and then comfort her in her time of need.

This is what makes life so difficult not only for Pulsatillas but also for the people around them. What makes them seem so wonderful when they are young—their innocence, their openness, their emotional availability— becomes sheer torture when they get older. Then they start to act too young for their years.

A good deal of this is a mask. The Pulsatilla has, through living, gained a good deal of sophistication and something of a backbone, yet she falls back on this adaptation when threatened.

In fact, some Pulsatillas do not seem very Pulsatillaish at all. From time to time, you find those in whom the adaptation is placed on the physical level, around the concept of changeability.

As a counterpoint to the emotional changeability of the Pulsatilla, we have the constitution's characteristic dogmatism.

Pulsatillas are conservative by nature. They dress in a conservative manner and certainly do not want to put up with anything that is in any way unpleasant.

The same follows through in their environment, as the Laura Ashley Pulsatillas of yesteryear have yielded a new crop of Martha Stewart Pulsatillas. They respond to gentle colors and gentle sounds. They like pastels, and they are usually fond of the color yellow. They want a yellow kitchen.

They do not allow rude language or rough behavior, especially from strangers. Like Kathy Bates's role in Fried Green Tomatoes, the Pulsatilla who has been knocked aside by a rushing teen will burst into tears in wonderment that anyone can be so cruel.

Pulsatillas often are very religious, or very political. They are conservative in their outlook, so this weeping, yielding marshmallow of a person can become the most stubborn media watchdog, organizing protests and boycotts, if she feels that the action of the other threatens her convictions, or especially if she feels that the behavior threatens her children.

Again and again you find Pulsatillas in the center of any controversy that concerns children. They work hard against the right to abortion, they are very involved in their children's school, and they make sure that no suspected homosexuals get anywhere near their children.

As her children get older, an interesting thing happens. Pulsatilla, who communicates so easily with young children, doesn't know what to make of adolescents. She becomes confused and tearful when wondering what happened to her own children. And she loses interest in the children whose lives she so protected in the embryo stage once they are born and are likely candidates for public support.

The same woman who fought against abortion rights also fights against welfare and never questions the mental knot she has tied. Instead, she cries and sighs over her own plight or that of some newer, younger child.

Pulsatilla is a fear remedy and, especially, an avoidance remedy. A Pulsatilla goes out of her way to avoid confrontation and anger in others. She almost never gives herself permission to be angry; at best she is capable of being peeved. At odd moments, however, she displays a real anger, bursting into shouts and tears at the same time. As she is usually so mild, her anger has major impact on those around her.

Since she is vague, her fears are likely to be somewhat vague as well. Mostly she fears that a big man (usually of another race) is going to hit her over the head. She crosses the street to avoid what she fears. And, if she is deep in the remedy, she withdraws from the world more and more as time goes on, in order to avoid that which she fears. Pulsatillas feel that they are choking when they are in stuffy or small spaces, and they have a deep claustrophobia. They are also, usually, afraid of heights.

The sensation of disgust is very strong in Pulsatilla. This woman, who usually is so nice, suddenly becomes a barbed creature who shoves her plate away or slams closed a book or turns off the television and slams down the remote. When the Pulsatilla is upset by the content of a speech or of writing, especially when it violates her moral or religious code, her sense of disgust is total and intense. At that moment, her usually somewhat vague mind clears and she is direct in her words and in her action. Watch out. A disgusted Pulsatilla is not to be trifled with. Don't attempt to comfort her, just stay out of her way as she goes to the telephone or to get her perfumed stationery in order to communicate her disgust to the parties responsible.

Physical Portrait: Changeability is the whole story here. Everything in Pulsatilla's physical condition changes as much as her moods do. In cases of diarrhea, no two stools are alike. In cases involving pain, the pain refuses to be centralized and steady in its symptoms. Instead, the pain moves about the body without rhyme or reason.

In fact, the Pulsatilla case often totally lacks rhyme or reason—which is one way you know that it is a Pulsatilla case. Practitioners may use the remedy much in the same way as they do Sulphur, to open a case and uncover what is going on, when the case taken makes little or no sense.

Pulsatilla may be the required remedy for women who develop incontinence, particularly if they urinate when they cough. The desire to urinate comes on suddenly and uncontrollably, and the urine has a strong smell.

Pulsatilla is also the first remedy to consider if symptoms come on after eating fatty foods, or from becoming too warm in an enclosed space. It is the first remedy to consider in cases of phantom pregnancy.

General weakness in any or all of three areas of the body usually physically determines the Pulsatilla type: the respiratory system, the circulatory system, and the hormonal system.

Pulsatillas usually have trouble breathing. This may actually have a physical basis, as with allergies, or it can be an emotionally based situation, with many Pulsatillas reacting to stress by feeling that they cannot breathe. This can often be accompanied with heart palpitations and/or vertigo.

In the circulatory system, the Pulsatilla is flushed and pressured. Her skin is pink. She is seemingly overfilled with blood. These symptoms, as with most of Pulsatilla's, are improved by a cool environment, which lessens the flush.

But it is the hormones that cause the most trouble. Most women move into the Pulsatilla constitution at times of hormonal change: puberty, pregnancy, or menopause, times when the balance of the hormones changes and dictates change to the entire system. Women who move into the Pulsatilla type at any of these times begin to gain weight suddenly.

In general, the Pulsatilla type is plump, if not downright fat. She is very concerned about her weight and has a great deal of trouble shedding pounds. The skin of a Pulsatilla is specific to the type. Pulsatillas have exceedingly soft skin. If you poke your fingertip into their skin, the dent remains for a good long while.

Pulsatillas are warm-blooded people. They want to be outdoors if the air is fresh and it is not too hot. They do not like to go into the sun for very long, and sunshine aggravates their complaints. They feel much better in cool or cold weather. They love to apply the words *crisp* and *fresh* to weather and to food, and they love anything to which they can apply those adjectives. The Pulsatilla wants to keep the windows open in order to let in fresh air. They actually begin to feel faint if they must stay in a closed, stuffy room.

Like Phosphoruses, Pulsatillas are at their worst at twilight. It brings out all that is melancholic in their nature.

They crave butter, although they do not digest it well. They also love dairy products, especially whipped cream. They crave cheese, ice cream, and peanut butter. They usually hate fatty foods, especially pork.

Finally, Pulsatilla is well known for the color of her discharges. Traditionally everything that comes out of her body, from mucus to diarrhea, has a yellow-green hue and in texture resembles a cloud, or that whipped cream she loves. The discharges pour out painlessly and copiously. Sometimes, as in the case of a cold, all you have to see are those discharges and you know what remedy to give.

Pulsatilla is a wonderfully benign remedy that may be repeated as needed in acute cases. In constitutional care, however, it should be given in a single dose of high potency. One dose of the remedy works for between one and two months.

Poster Children: Pulsatillas seem to have gone out of style in recent years. But the works of British Victorian writers, especially Charles Dickens, are crowded with them. In American fiction, the prime example is probably Melanie Wilkes in *Gone With the Wind.* But I say that on television, we are given the best modern example of Pulsatilla in Poppin' Fresh, the Pillsbury Dough Boy.

RHUS
The Codependent

Remedy Source: The Rhus family of remedies comes from a group of plants that act as irritants on the skin. The most important of this group, and the remedy I consider here, is Rhus Toxicodendron, which is taken from poison ivy. The second most important is Rhus Venenata, made from poison elder. Other remedies in the group include Rhus Diversiloba (poison oak) and Rhus Glabra (poison sumac).

Rhus Toxicodendron is also known as snow rose. It grows in the shape of a shrub, with an erect stem, to a height of two to four feet. It is native to North America and was introduced from here to Great Britain. The leaves of the plant are used in the creation of the remedy. They must be gathered at sunset just before the flowering stage. This remedy was created by Hahnemann.

Situations That Suggest Rhus Tox: Joint and muscle pain: low back pain, connective tissue disease, torticolis, tendonitis, sciatica, housemaid's knee, lumbago, sprains and strains of all sorts; physical trauma; rheumatism and rheumatoid arthritis. Also herpes and shingles; poison ivy and poison oak; smallpox and chicken pox; measles; laryngitis and preacher's throat; skin conditions: rash, warts, wen, scarlatina, abscesses, acne rosacea; fevers of unknown origin; hemorrhages of all sorts.

Remedy Overview: A usual symptom of poison ivy gives us an important clue to the nature of this remedy: Those who are covered with poison ivy often say, along with the intense itching, that they feel as if their skin were shrinking all over their body. In the same way, the Rhus Tox type feels trapped in the skin, and it feels overly tight and confining.

Often this remedy is referred to as a "rusty hinge." By this we mean that the person needing this remedy, after a period of quiet or of rest, feels as if the joints have stiffened and, in becoming stiff, have become painful. The Rhus type seeks slow, steady movement as a method of avoiding stiffness and pain.

The same principle applies to the Rhus type on an emotional and mental level. When they move through a period of quiet and rest, they feel that they stiffen up, and this stiff sensation is painful, so they seek movement on the emotional and/or mental level in order to attain the fluidity that eludes them in their natural state.

It is important to understand that those belonging to this type nearly always must be discovered by their physical symptoms, and all but the most seriously ill may be nearly symptom free on the emotional and mental level, or their symptoms may be considered well within the range of normal human behavior. The Rhus type evolves a mask of cheerfulness that serves them at all times. It is by their own bodies that they are betrayed, in that the body, after a time, simply refuses to play along any longer.

Mentally, Rhus types tend to be clear and practical thinkers. They tend to approach problem solving practically and not too creatively. Throughout their lives, they tend to be future oriented and to stress the fact that the past is past and that we can't, no matter how much we may want to, change it. Although they may be holding on to a good many emotional hurts, they choose, while not denying these pains, to focus their attention on the future.

The Rhus motto is, "I've got to keep moving." This is their major mechanism to avoid pain on the mental as well as the physical plane.

Remedy Theme: Awkward, painful compliance, painful humor, sensation of being trapped.

Remedy Motivation: Lack of fluidity, loneliness.

Emotional Portrait: There is no way to overstate the importance of this remedy, or the difficulty of recognizing it on an emotional level. This is so true that I am tempted to begin the section with the physical traits.

They are not more important than the emotional, but they are a lot easier to recognize.

Rhus types are cheerful. They are dead set on being positive in their attitude, and it even seems that the more physical pain they are in, the more positive they become.

And yet you can sense the struggle it is for them to maintain this positive stance. There is a struggle behind the humor, a strain. Rhuses seem as strained on the emotional level as they are on the physical. In addition, they tend to be somewhat awkward.

Rhus types are never totally at ease with other people, especially with strangers or those they believe have power over them, teachers and doctors especially. Rhuses often willingly defer their personal power to another person. Further, they enjoy helping and serving in any way they can. (I can't help but conclude that the rheumatoid arthritis that many Rhus types develop is the way the body stops the mind from inhabiting this servile position. The hand literally curls up, preventing further passing of trays, for example.)

On first meeting a Rhus, you may confuse him with a Phosphorus. He seems so friendly and so willing to be a part of your life and help you in any way he can. But over time you see that this openness and willingness to help is not his natural state but one that requires a great deal of work for him.

Rhuses often feel tight, enclosed, and cut off. They have great emotional needs but don't have the slightest idea of how to communicate those needs to others. They are lonely, and this basic loneliness often motivates them in all their dealings with others. If this connection works, if they are able to buy affection with their actions, Rhuses settle into a lifetime of service.

But if they find that such behavior patterns are not a solution to their chronic loneliness, Rhuses move deeper and deeper into the constitutional pattern and become more and more serious. The person who at one time resembled a loving Phosphorus now resembles a Sepia or a Nux Vomica— work oriented, aggressive, and somewhat bitter.

Most Rhus types are exercise junkies. They fill our yoga and aerobics classes. When they loosen themselves up physically, they find that they also loosen themselves up emotionally. They count on the warmth and exhaustion that exercise spreads throughout their body to let them feel a warm glow of camaraderie with the people around them. Often the people they meet at exercise class are the favorite people in their lives; they equate these folks with these happy surroundings.

The Rhus who is not permitted to exercise, through illness, injury, or deadlines at work, undergoes an extreme personality change. The Rhus who was so mild-mannered and funny, with a joke for all occasions, becomes moody, angry, and increasingly rigid.

In the same way, Rhus types respond to emotional warmth with the same relaxation response that they have for physical warmth. Perhaps no other type so loves warmth, especially damp warmth. A hot shower is the balm for all their ills. And a warm person who showers them with attention and kindness brings a calm relaxation to Rhuses, who bloom under this influence to become healthy and balanced.

But, like Pulsatilla and Phosphorus, Rhus tends to become involved with those who withhold warmth. This situation brings out the whole range of codependent behaviors in the Rhus Tox. As he feels emotional cooling, he begins to tighten and to live life in a constant state of tension.

In this pattern, Rhus undertakes service to this person and comes to seem once again imprisoned in his own body or skin. Some Rhus types caught in an unhealthful emotional situation turn again to exercise. Others simply continue with the pattern of codependency, often blaming themselves for the behavior of others until the body puts a stop to the pattern.

It is important to understand that, for whatever reason, Rhus types are highly unlikely at any time to draw a line and to put an end to an abusive situation. It is only the body that can free them, moving them into a pain position in which they must take action.

When Rhuses love, they love with every fiber of their being. If you tell them as a friend that perhaps their marriage is not as well rounded as it could be, that perhaps they could be a little more selfish, they leap to their mate's defense with an intensity that suggests you made some sort of physical threat. Rhus, a remedy based in the physical, tends to take every sort of emotional strain and place it in the physical. Thus, a Rhus becomes physically restless when anxious.

If there should actually be some sort of physical threat against a loved one, Rhuses throw their bodies directly in the line of fire. They happily take a bullet for the sake of those they love.

This is all the more interesting because a Rhus's greatest fear in life is of physical pain. Because Rhus is such a pain remedy in general, it shows the full courage common to the type that he happily takes on pain for the sake of love. In the same way, he endures physical pain that a loved one causes. A black eye can be rationalized as his own fault, and he might feel he became too physically worked up by an argument. Should anyone even suggest that the husband or wife had no right to strike out, the Rhus will fly into a rage to "protect" his or her mate, telling everyone to mind his own business.

The Rhus almost never seeks treatment for an emotional or mental problem and finds excuses to cover the wounds that have been inflicted on him. The wise practitioner learns to identify him by his physical complaints, as the body reveals what the lips will never say.

Rhus types generally are very superstitious. Their minds are filled with fixed ideas of how things must be done. If these ideas are challenged, or if their rituals are ignored, they become very, very worried, anxious, and even angry.

The anger in Rhus Tox is a rare thing. It either plays off this need for rituals, or it is a part of the remedy's typical impatience.

Rhus Tox is listed by Nash as one of the restless trio of homeopathic remedies, along with Aconite and Arsenicum. It is easy to acknowledge this trait on the physical level: They need to keep moving in order to avoid pain and therefore always seem to be in motion, especially during changes in the weather.

Emotionally Rhuses are restless as well. There is a need for some passion to drive them. They are impatient with anything they feel is too calm or too quiet. They stir things up emotionally in many situations just in order to feel some sort of emotional movement. They pick a fight to feel something again, to feel more alive.

As they feel imprisoned in their own skin, lonely as they are, they come to feel imprisoned in a marriage if it does not contain enough passion. The Rhus who becomes imprisoned emotionally usually displays that emotion on a physical level. He takes on joint pains or arthritis as a method of showing that he feels he cannot escape his unhappiness.

A major fear of the type tells us much about their internal troubles. While other types fear death or ghosts, Rhus Tox types most often fear that they will lose control and kill someone. This takes the remedy's sensation of imprisonment and its loneliness to the deepest level. While Rhuses are too codependent to release themselves from a bad situation, in their hearts they recognize their environment's toxicity. They come to fear that some night they will just lose control and kill their spouse while he or she sleeps. The target of their fear can be any person in their life who makes them feel cold or tight, who enhances their deepest feeling that their life is not under their control.

Control issues are central to the troubles of Rhus Tox. With their need for ritual behavior, those deep in the type are likely to fall prey to compulsive behavior. At this level of illness, they can resemble a deep Arsenicum—fearful of cold, in need of warmth, restless, and compulsive in their need for order. Their thoughts become fixed, as tight and hard as their joints. They need new ideas, new philosophies, as much as they need that warm shower.

If there is one thing that all Rhus Tox types fear, it is a thunderstorm. This touches off their control issues. They fear the wildness of the storm and its intense power. Because they cannot control the storm, or even their overwhelming response to it, they tend to fall apart before and during the storm. Before the storm, the Rhus Tox has a headache, or rheumatic pains. During the storm, he cowers like a frightened animal.

They are like Phosphorus types in their ability to predict changes in the weather and sense the coming storm a day or two away. But unlike Phosphorus, their sensitivity ends with the storm. While they are wildly loyal and protective, they have no skill in sensing the wants and needs of others. They need to be told what you want, and may need to be told more than once. They are down-to-earth, practical people who, as they tend to overextend themselves mentally and physically, tend to have poor memories. Coupled with their poor communication skills, they can sometimes appear to be stubbornly refusing to do something when in truth they don't know how to tell you that they simply forgot.

It cannot be overstated that the weather has a major impact on the Rhus type, on the mind as well as the body. Rhuses cannot bear cold, especially damp cold. They are worse in any weather change from dry to wet. And they are especially worse if they become wet, such as getting caught in a cold November rain. Even overcast days can be difficult, with damp, foggy weather affecting them like a physical and emotional blow. If you expect a Rhus to think clearly on a foggy morning, you will be disappointed. Although Phosphorus is sensitive to the weather and to its changes, he is no more or less sensitive to the weather than to anything else. Rhus Tox, however, is almost part of the weather and never finds it possible to disconnect from the weather environment. Life in the wrong climate is difficult at best. They need to come to understand that as the weather changes, they too change. They had better make sure that they live where the weather works for them and not against them.

Physical Portrait: The rheumatic pains associated with this remedy type are almost without end: muscular rheumatism, TMJ, fibrosis, iritis, stiff neck, lower back pain that is worse when sitting still, sciatica, stiff knees, rheumatic inflammation of joints, and any or all rheumatic pains that are worse in cold and damp and better in warmth, and especially from rubbing or from continued gentle motion. This is a physical pain remedy, and the type and intensity of the pain largely define the person's quality of life.

There is often a history of rheumatic fever in this constitutional type. A history that includes intense bouts of chicken pox, measles, or mumps is also common.

Fevers, too, are covered in the type: typhoid fever, influenza with fever and body ache, measles, pneumonia, and scarlet fever. The fever contains the following symptoms: The patient must change position often in order to be comfortable; the patient has fever blisters around the mouth; the patient's tongue is dry and sore and red at the tip, is swollen, and has the patient's teeth marks along the sides; the patient becomes apprehensive with fever, especially at night; the patient is very thirsty with fever and drinks a great deal; and the patient's fever is worse in wet weather.

Rhus Tox is one of the remedies that many persons new to homeopathy discover early on as an acute remedy. It is of great use in situations that involve physical trauma, as long as patients follow the general Rhus symptoms. All ailments that are brought on by overlifting or overstretching, such as the back that is thrown into spasm when the patient attempts to lift a heavy box, and aches and pains that come on after the patient sits or lies on the damp ground, can be greatly helped by Rhus Tox.

The injured or affected parts of the body may feel paralyzed. The pain sensation often is accompanied by numbness. Pain travels from the point of the injury into the limbs, especially in cases of sciatica.

This is an especially good remedy for singers, whose voices become hoarse from overuse. The sore or hoarse throat that needs Rhus Tox is soothed by warm drinks and made worse by cold drinks. Typically, in keeping with Rhus's general symptoms, the singer who is unable to sing feels better when speaking quietly, as speaking is to the voice what gentle motion is to the body.

The improvement of pain by the application of warmth is a general symptom of Rhus, as is the need for gentle motion. Rhus pain is worse on first motion and grows less with sustained motion. But it must be noted that, if the Rhus does not stop moving in time, the pain suddenly returns as the injured part is reinjured by the ongoing motion.

Rhus Tox is an important remedy for parts of the body that have been repeatedly injured, particularly the ankle. Ankles are swollen when sprained, and the injury follows the general Rhus symptom portrait.

Rhus Tox is greatly helpful in situations that involve rashes of all sorts that mirror in some way the redness and itch of poison ivy. The rash is better with warmth and worse with cold. The rash usually is a patch of small red vesicles that are made much worse by scratching. The patient wants to take a hot shower in order to lessen the itch and feel that the skin is not too tight. He may even want to put scalding water on the rash to stop the itching. The rashes improved by Rhus Tox, especially eczema, are worse in winter, wet weather, and in a warm bed at night, which dramatically increases the itching.

Rhus Tox is an important remedy for those with arthritis. The arthritis pains are worse in the night and when the patient is in bed. They also are worse first thing in the morning. Patients have trouble sleeping and toss and turn a good deal as they try to get in a comfortable position. The pain of the arthritis is improved by bathing in hot water and is better in dry weather. The patient needs to keep moving in order to soothe the pain. The pain is common in the left shoulder.

Rhus Tox is a helpful remedy for bursitis, especially in the left shoulder, and tendonitis. Affected limbs become restless, and the patient has to keep moving the arm or leg in order to lower the level of pain. In general, Rhus types tend always to have restless limbs and may move their limbs, especially their legs, almost constantly in order to keep them from stiffening. Rhus Tox is also suggested by joints that crack when moved.

Rhus Tox is the major remedy for herpes, especially genital herpes. There are eruptions on the inner thighs and on the mouth, fever blisters on the lips, and cracks at the corner of the mouth. Rhus Tox often expresses itself with bright red skin eruptions on the tip of the nose.

Rhus Tox also often shows itself on the tongue. Characteristic to the type is a tongue with a bright red tip and a red triangular patch.

In general, Rhus Tox is a remedy given to left-sided symptoms, or to symptoms that begin on the left and travel right. Symptoms become aggravated in drafts. Autumn is the most stressful time of year, as the weather changes from warm to cold and dry to wet. The Rhus Tox patient is so sensitive to wet and cold weather that it may be said that he is literally allergic to the dampness in the way that Sulphur is to pollen.

The Rhus Tox type has ailments that return periodically, almost ritually. This can even be true of their physical traumas, their strains and sprains. They tend to injure themselves in the same way again and again.

The Rhus Tox type moves somewhat awkwardly, even when not in pain. They seem as if they cannot quite trust their body not to hurt and not to fail them.

In general, Rhus Tox is a thirsty remedy. They love to drink and want either cold water or cold milk. If they are having symptoms in their throat, however, they want only warm things. Like Arsenicum, they tend to want to sip their drinks, although they may be very thirsty. They tend to crave oysters and cheese and sweets.

In their dreams, Rhus Toxes often see themselves being poisoned. They often mirror this feeling when they have a fever or great pain, when again they insist they are being poisoned. They also dream of physical exertion, of rowing a boat or swimming.

Rhus Tox can be given in any potency as a constitutional, although the 30C and 200C potencies are most common. In acute cases of pain, strain, or sprain, high potencies may be required and in multiple doses.

Those who are highly susceptible to poison ivy may want to use Rhus Tox preventatively. If the remedy is taken at least a month before the poison ivy season, a single dose of 200C usually is effective. But if the patient already has the rash, do not give a high potency, as it causes the rash to express and cover the whole body. The remedy must be given in a very low potency like a 6X.

Poster Children: Batman. He is a classic do-gooder, rigid in his thinking and judgments. He is driven by loneliness and loss. Having been injured numerous times, he must keep moving to keep the pain in check.

Also actresses Rosalind Russell and Donna Reed. Modern actress Meg Ryan follows the type as well.

SEPIA
The Bitch

Remedy Source: The remedy Sepia is created from the ink of the cuttlefish. It is a brownish-black juice.

While the ancients had considered the cuttlefish to be a source of therapeutic substances, including the meat, bone, and eggs, it was Hahnemann who came upon the idea that the ink could be made into a powerful homeopathic remedy. It is ironic to note that this most powerful of the women's remedies was first created homeopathically as a constitutional treatment for a man.

Situations That Suggest Sepia: Women's health issues: endometriosis, PMS, menopause, pregnancy, miscarriage, uterine pain, vaginitis, incontinence in times of stress, hirsutism, female baldness. Also anemia and chronic fatigue syndrome; digestive disorders: dyspepsia, constipation, rectal pain, pruritis ani, peptic ulcer; sexual dysfunction: low libido, painful intercourse; liver ailments: toxic liver, liver spots, jaundice; mental disorders: depression, hysteria. Also nosebleed; anal bleeding; varicose veins; skin diseases: seborrhea, warts, ringworm, rash; cystitis; gonorrhea; herpes; toothache. Also whooping cough, cough, bronchitis. Also sciatica, low back pain.

Remedy Overview: Gravity weighs heavily upon Sepias. All their aches and pains push down on them; everything hurts in a downward direction. In the same way, Sepias feel an emotional gravity and feel that the effort it takes to function mentally and emotionally throughout the entire day also pushes down on them. They tend to feel that life is hard, involving a great deal of struggle.

Because of this, they tend to make life as hard as possible for those around them. Sepias are hard taskmasters. They require complete loyalty not only to them but to their every whim. It is characteristic of this type that, as employers, they go through many employees. They quickly fire any who does not jump high enough when required, and working for a Sepia requires a great deal of jumping, as well as late hours and low pay. Those they find acceptable often quit, feeling that pleasing this royal creature is just not worth it.

Sepias present themselves as princess or queen. They do not allow themselves to be questioned and, if they are, are likely to refuse to answer. They also insist that, as employer, they be allowed to set not only the direction and pace of the work but the emotional tone of the workplace as well. It is quite important to Sepias that those they employ be happy in their employment and that they continually express their gratitude for being allowed to continue on the job.

I jumped to the level of employer somewhat automatically when considering Sepia. It is hard indeed to imagine the Sepia who is a mere employee. Yet they often are, as they work their way up. They are behind the executive secretary's desk in the CEO's suite. They are tenured professors in colleges and universities. They then make themselves indispensable. As total professionals and perfectionists, they get the job done perfectly. They tend to have wonderful minds for business and excellent organizational skills.

Remedy Theme: Rude and aggressive behavior, perfectionism.

Remedy Motivation: Disappointment.

Emotional Portrait: The central issue facing the Sepia is disappointment. Something in her life has deeply wounded her and made her rigid and controlling. The classical homeopaths sometimes express it as the golden-haired bride who, years into the marriage, finds that her hair is brown with disappointment. These are bitter people, who often feel that their only mistake was in believing it when someone said, "I love you."

Typically, the Sepia, out of a feeling of disappointment specific to one relationship or common to all of her life, becomes cold to the very people she should love most. Mothers may feel nothing for their children. This may happen immediately after the birth of the child, when the mother, in postpartum depression, fails to bond with her child, or it may happen as a result of some behavior or failure on the part of the child. Sepias are noted for their conditional love. Their children often tell tales of emotional and verbal abuse. The Sepia mother can drive her children mercilessly to achieve, until she drives a permanent wedge into the relationship.

Sepias also behave coldly to their husbands. They may feel love, but they are unable to communicate that love. It is typical that women needing Sepia have a general aversion to men and that the men needing the remedy have a general aversion to women. Both men and women needing Sepia have an aversion to sexual intimacy, especially with their mates. Both have a low libido.

The emotional ailments of Sepia begin with the increasing sense of gravity. The Sepia typically moves into stasis to protect herself. Feeling that life is just too hard and that the struggle takes too much out of her, she stops trying to move forward and begins to freeze in place. This freezing process ultimately prevents her from joining in emotional involvement of any sort. The usual outlet for the Sepia's emotions is her work, which interests her more as her emotional relationships interest her less.

Many Sepias struggle with this concept of heavy gravity by exercise. The Sepia takes exercise class more seriously than does the Rhus, who tends to become warm, happy, and relaxed by exercise. The Sepia just gets more tired, but she knows that this is the only way she can keep gravity in check.

Sepias especially love swimming and dancing. During these activities they let down their guard. It is also these activities that can become totally and obsessively addictive.

An example of this love of dancing is Leona Helmsley, who is most certainly our Poster Child. As a Sepia, Leona is a tough cookie, one whose frozen face shows the world just how tough she thinks life is. And yet, when she met her beloved Harry, she met him while dancing, falling in love with the man before their first dance ended. This is typical of the type. Dancing moves them, and warms them as heavy exercise will for Rhus Tox.

Leona also loves swimming. At the time of her troubles with the IRS I remember reading that she swam every day in the pool at her Greenwich, Connecticut, estate. And that, as she swam her laps, she required a servant to stand on either side of the pool, holding a shrimp on a toothpick. She would swim a lap, lift her head out of the water and bite the shrimp off the toothpick. Any servant who held the shrimp too high or too low was fired. Whether the story is true or not, it so elaborates on all things Sepia that I include it here.

Leona also tells us another fact about Sepia. When I saw her on all the talk shows before she was put in prison, I noticed that as she told her story of government abuse, she would invariably burst into tears. Like Pulsatilla, Sepia cries when she tells you her troubles, but she does so while holding her face and body totally rigid. She cries because life is so hard and so unfair, but not because she wants to be comforted. Her face is stone, and her expression warns you to keep away.

Zelda Fitzgerald illustrates the compulsive nature of the type. As the young wife of F. Scott Fitzgerald, she was famous for her beauty and wit. But after a time, especially after the birth of her daughter, she withdrew from those she loved and began instead to display more and more anger. As is common of the type, she had great difficulty controlling her temper. Finally, she took her first ballet lesson. And, true to the type, she became obsessed with ballet. She took lessons every day and danced and danced the day away in her private studio in the attic. No one dared to enter her studio or to interrupt her dancing.

Zelda finally became famous for her erratic behavior, her emotional breakdowns, and her many stays in mental hospitals. She was among the first patients to be diagnosed with schizophrenia. Her illness, both physical and mental, paralleled the remedy Sepia.

Sepias love thunderstorms. A good loud thunderstorm awakens something that is dormant within them: passion. While the thunderstorm lasts, gravity is lessened.

A thunderstorm brings out in the Sepia type the person she was before gravity grew so heavy. She is filled with excitement, like a child on Christmas Eve. She has humor other than sarcasm. Her eyes glow.

The Sepia runs to the window when the storm comes. She wants to go out into the storm, even to feel as if she is part of the storm. Many Sepias dance while the storm rages outdoors.

———

Sepias refer to themselves as strong women. They are proud of their perfectionism. Unfortunately, most Sepias are very difficult. They are cruel and, like Lycopodiums, often feel that life is competition. In order for them to win, you must lose. They are jealous, both in terms of emotional relationships and career success. They feel better about themselves when others face failure.

At the same time, Sepias have a strong sense of fairness and of justice. For this reason, they sometimes hold their behavior in check or feel a great deal of guilt about the ways they treat others. Sepia is aware of what is going on inside of her, of all the changes that she is experiencing on the mental and physical levels. She just feels helpless to do anything about these changes. She fears them.

This often is the case when the Sepia constitution comes on, as it often does, during periods of hormonal change in the woman's body. When she becomes pregnant, or when she faces menopause, the Sepia is fearful of what is happening in her system, even if she is quite aware rationally that the changes are natural and normal. They still are quite fearful to her, and she doesn't know how to communicate that fact. Since the struggle was hard already, these hormonal changes often make the Sepia isolate herself, if not physically then certainly emotionally, bringing on that keynote emotional coldness to the ones she loves.

This Sepia is deeply worried. She projects to the future with the worst-case scenario. She often fears, in spite of her present success, that she will die in poverty. This makes her lie awake at night worrying about the future. This also motivates the Sepia to be one of the most miserly of the constitutional types. She seeks to control money, to dam it up. In her ongoing competition with others, the ability to turn every simple agreement into a business negotiation is hard to resist. She feels joy at being on the winning side financially.

The urge within every Sepia, which motivates a good deal of her behavior, is to go away. Whereas other types are very home oriented and look at the home as their place of comfort and rest, Sepias would like to flee, to go somewhere new, somewhere where they do not know anyone.

Sepia tends to enjoy being alone and even thrives in her moments of solitude. She is averse to company and certainly must be telephoned for permission before even her closest friend drops by for a visit. But Sepia is not good if she is alone too often or for too long. She does not like total solitude and becomes deeply fearful if she feels abandoned.

Surprisingly, Sepia is wonderful at a party. No matter what is going on inside of her, she rises to the occasion and is filled with wit and humor. She takes to the dance floor, whirling her way through the evening. Those who meet Sepia for the first time at a party are surprised the next time they see her. She is a totally different human being.

Most Sepias dress in a very conservative, almost sexless, manner. They are understated, even when they have money enough to buy whatever they want. They tend to have very good taste and stress the excellence of a piece of clothing or jewelry over its popular style: A good piece of jewelry blends right in with your body, it doesn't jump out at you. Further, they say that a good haircut is one that has others saying that the Sepia looks nice, not that she just got her hair cut. And it is a short, practical haircut.

Sepia can be a very difficult patient to treat, because she is often in despair of her recovery. She usually has been aware of physical or emotional problems for some time before she goes to see a practitioner of any sort. During that time she has convinced herself that she is incurable.

Over time and with much struggle, Sepia finally yields to gravity. She gives up. With no hope of a future, she begins to crumble inward. The positive outcome of this stance is that once most Sepias reach this level, they finally do get help. Homeopathy can be a powerful tool in allowing them to overcome gravity and in teaching them to fly.

Physical Portrait: The typical Sepia is a somewhat tall and thin woman with a narrow pelvis. She is a bit masculine in build and movement. Her skin tends to be somewhat mottled, often with yellow undertones and a yellow saddle across her nose.

Her most common ailments cluster around the events in a woman's life that involve hormonal changes: puberty, pregnancy, and, especially, menopause. Sepia is our leading remedy for women in menopause. In pregnancy, she is given to terrible bouts of morning sickness. She craves odd foods, usually involving pickles, which all Sepias enjoy.

In menopause, she experiences hot flashes, exhaustion, irritability, and the feeling of heavy gravity, the feeling that she is very heavy and being drawn earthward.

Sepia is a major "not well since" remedy—many people needing the remedy have not been well since childbirth or menopause. Allopathic medicine has increased this category: Many women find themselves not well since beginning estrogen replacement therapy or since they began taking birth control pills. Sepia is an important remedy in both these situations.

The Sepia feels a general weakness in the area of the pelvis. She experiences bearing down or pulling down sensations, during which she feels that she must cross her legs in order to keep her internal organs in place.

With the exception of times she is having hot flashes, Sepia generally is a chilly person and is very sensitive to cold air. If she is prone to any chronic condition, extreme chills accompany the other symptoms. Sepia is traditionally chilly even in a warm room.

Because of the feeling of heavy gravity, Sepia feels weak even after a short walk. She feels burning pains in various parts of her body, pains that are made much worse by walking.

When Sepia feels weak, it is usually sudden. She feels as if her legs were giving out under her. During these moments of fainting, she often feels a rush of blood throughout her system or heart palpitations.

Pains in the joints and in the interior organs are common to the type, and these pains have the unique characteristic of moving from below upward. Her pains are, in general, improved by warmth, especially the warmth of bed. She is also better if she crosses her limbs during pain or pulls her legs up under her when she is in bed.

Sepias frequently experience chronic pain in the area of the liver, which is relieved by lying on the right side. The pain is shooting, and is either brought on or made worse by riding in a moving vehicle. This pain too is relieved by lying down.

Her symptoms of chronic disease come on every twenty-eight days as part of her regular cycle. This cyclic flow of symptoms even appears in the men who need this remedy.

The Sepia is beset with headaches, often occurring in a cyclical pattern. The pain is shooting, tending to center over the left eye. Often it, too, travels from below upward and from the occiput (the base of the head) up over the head to the forehead. Her headaches are typically worse just before her period, and the Sepia often experiences nausea and vomiting during her headaches. It is a keynote symptom of her headache that, during the headache, a Sepia may experience a desire for sex.

The Sepia commonly complains of a salty or sour taste in her mouth, or that everything tastes salty.

She typically has either a huge appetite or no appetite at all. As is often the case with pregnant women, she may not be able to stand even the smell of cooking food. She tends to crave sour things: pickles, vinegar. She craves salt, bread, and chocolate and other sweet things. She eats quickly. She becomes suddenly hungry and just as suddenly finds herself full.

Many Sepias are allergic to milk. Yet some Sepias crave milk, while others hate it. Most also hate meat and any other fatty food.

The Sepia type is attracted to both alcohol and drugs. Her system may have been worn into chronic weakness by the abuse of either or both.

In most cases treated by Sepia, there is a general improvement of energy and a feeling that, although the symptoms are still in place, they are more bearable. The most important transition for the Sepia in terms of healing usually takes place when she begins to believe that she can be well once again. At that moment, you see the lifting of the heavy gravity off her back, her pelvis, and, most of all, her face.

Sepia is used in all potencies, but most often between 30C and 1M. This works best in the single dose and does not bear repetition well. Many constitutional cases involving Sepia have been ruined by giving the remedy too often.

One dose of Sepia works actively in the system for up to fifty days.

Poster Children: Certainly Leona Helmsley and Zelda Fitzgerald. In fact, most of the institutionalized wives of authors fit the type, especially T. S. Eliot's wife, Vivien. Barbra Streisand best typifies the constitutional type. No one is more of a perfectionist, and certainly no one has a more dominant personality.

SILICA
The Coward

Remedy Source: Silica is made from pure flint or quartz, one of the most common substances on Earth. Of all the remedies available in the homeopathic pharmacy, Silica is one of the few whose base substances are without therapeutic merit. I would be interested to discover what caused Hahnemann even to suspect that flint could be made into a homeopathic remedy. I can only imagine his surprise when it turned out to be among our most important remedies.

Both Earth's mantle and the sands of the sea are composed of silica. And many plants take in silica as well, making it part of their own support system. So when we think of the substance from which the remedy is made, we must first consider how common it is in our lives. We must also consider that its function is largely that of offering support and strength to anything of which it is part. These two considerations underlie the remedy as well:

It is one of the most needed remedies, speaking to issues common to us all, and it is a remedy that offers both strength and support to those who need it.

Situations That Suggest Silica: Failure to thrive; digestive disorders: constipation, food allergy, gastric headaches, distended abdomen, lost appetite; diabetes; rickets; weakness of bones and joints: tooth decay, TMJ, fractures, bursitis, hip-joint pain, coccyx pain; ingrown nails; whitlow. Also anemia, night sweats; chronic swollen glands; ear disorders: Ménière's disease, vertigo; rheumatism; immune dysfunction: keloids, wounds that won't heal; foreign bodies in skin. Also mania, homesickness.

Remedy Overview: Picture the rolling orb of Jell-O the Earth would be if all the Silica were to disappear from its mantle, and you get the idea of the remedy type.

Remedy Theme: Compulsive behavior, cowardly behavior.

Remedy Motivation: Lack of strength, low self-esteem.

Emotional Portrait: There is no other type as refined as the Silica. They have an innate sense of what is good and correct, and that sense can serve them very well. No other type, not even the Phosphorus with his innate appreciation of beauty, can be so aware of the detail that makes or breaks the successful environment. It must have been a Silica who first told us, "God is in the details."

The Silica is usually a weak youth, scrawny and somewhat underweight. He has no athletic skills, being very fearful of his body. This fear is usually well founded; the Silica is likely to have a poorly developed skeletal system. His body actually is likely to fail him in time of need. So the Silica reacts to a sport that involves body contact as he would a physical assault.

This tends to make young Silicas loners. And, as they feel that they were shortchanged when it comes to bone and muscle development, they often live almost entirely in their heads. They are slim and often somewhat small (even tall Silicas tend to have small skeletons) and present themselves first and foremost as aesthetes and intellectuals, so they often are confused with Arsenicums. This confusion can become enhanced in that, like Arsenicum, the Silica type is very tight, very organized, and very controlling.

But there are striking differences between the types. Control issues for Silicas extend only to their own lives. While you may feel a little worried about going to their house, that you will sit in the wrong chair or use the wrong fork, you need not hesitate to invite them to your house. They are perfect guests, relaxed, humorous, and generous. And they know when to leave.

In fact, they know every rule of decorum required in society. Picture the Noel Coward character, wearing an ascot and sipping champagne, and you have the perfect Silica type. Picture that character's butler, and you picture an even truer Silica.

The Silica child can be somewhat coy and manipulative of his parents. He learns early that chronic ill health and a predisposition to communicable diseases of all sorts can translate into personal power. He learns that helplessness can be very powerful.

In the practitioner's office, the Silica child often whispers his answers to the questions the practitioner asks into the parent's ear, for the parent to relay to the practitioner. This predicts the type's inability to communicate and his adult method of control—saying one thing and doing another.

The word *proper* is central to the understanding of Silica. Arsenicum has neither his cool sense of right and wrong nor his stiff upper lip.

Silicas, because of their feeling of a lack of strength and support from within, often become pillars of society. They love to create things where nothing has been before. They love to build, to make foundations. Silicas are drawn to architecture, where they can experience both the solid joy of construction and the aesthetic joy of creating beauty. Some of the world's finest architects, including Philip Johnson, were and are Silica types.

Those who do not design or create buildings often care for them. They are excellent butlers or servants, as I said, and also are wonderful caretakers who treat a building as if it were their own. The other great career for a Silica is decoration. And again, some of the best and most famous were Silica types.

Within his realm of expertise, the Silica is solid in his confidence. But outside that realm, and especially in the realm of human emotions, he feels helpless. It's like taking the butler out of the great hall of a British home and putting him in a cowboy bar. No other type gets out of its element so completely as does a Silica.

And no type has such a poor self-image. Although Silica often presents to the world a person who is a bit tight, a bit stiff, and certainly clear and direct in his thinking, the internal Silica is often a product of the childhood full of vulnerability and loneliness. They often complain as patients that they can never think clearly: a poor memory, an ongoing sense of confusion, and a fear of being overwhelmed.

When they move deeper into this type, Silicas want to build not only physical walls for others to enjoy but also emotional walls around themselves. They withdraw into themselves and into their role in society. They are less and less willing to speak up and give an opinion. They fear deeply what others are thinking about them and what they will think if they give an opinion about something. Many Silicas complain that they actually have a good many deeply held convictions, but they feel it is not safe to give them. Others will think ill of them for speaking up or, worse, will ridicule them in public if they speak their mind.

But because the Silica does have deep convictions, and because he does know what he wants even if he doesn't tell anyone what that is, he tends to take on a more passive-aggressive behavior pattern as he moves more deeply into the type. He appears to be quite yielding, agreeing to anything anyone wants of him, and then he does what he likes and what he intended on doing from the beginning, even though he refused to let anyone in on that secret. Thus the people around the Silica become wary of working or living with him. Mostly he just seems a bit asleep, a bit vague. But some Silicas after a time become the most stubborn people on Earth, and some of the most infuriating. They never reveal what they think, but they never do anything they do not want to do.

Sleep is the great refuge for the Silica, as it is for the Phosphorus. The Silica, especially one who feels stressed, returns to the bedroom as if he were returning to the womb. And, as a simple type, the Silica is as greatly refreshed by sleep as he is by eating.

Silicas typically have problems with food. Like Arsenicums, they are highly aware of the trouble and have a memorized list of what they can and cannot eat. Silicas have trouble assimilating many different foods and are better off keeping to a very simple diet. They are also better if they eat several small meals in a day instead of two or three big ones.

The Silica is naturally slim and it may be difficult for him to gain weight. In fact, the type is often underweight. But the Silica who gains weight invariably does so in the area of the stomach. Silicas can have great distended abdomens, but they will keep the thin necks that are common to the type.

Silica is a remedy type that has many fears, and most have to deal with performance anxiety. The Silica deeply fears speaking in public and would choose death as the easier alternative. The Silica also fears deadlines and tests. This is the best acute remedy for those who feel anxious before a test.

The type is given to chronic low-grade anxiety that while never keeping them from functioning keeps them always a little on guard and prevents them from ever feeling truly relaxed. The only place that they tend to relax is at home. And home—those four walls—is of extreme importance to Silicas. They cannot be happy in an ugly home or one that is in disarray. This does not reflect the Arsenicum nature, with the need for things to be spotless. Silicas aren't overly clean, although they do prize cleanliness as being next to Godliness. Instead, the space must be aesthetically pure. The Silica with Victorian taste may have a very cluttered home, but it will purely reflect his taste and his own personal style. That home is his boundary from the world, a place where he can relax.

Homesickness is very common to this type. They do not want to go away from home. Instead, they want to create their dream surroundings within their home and then stay there. Silicas are very happy if they can work from their home, and they are happy to have others in their home, but only those with the good taste to recognize the home for its many wonderful qualities and the good manners to treat the Silica's home as if it were their own.

Silica has a natural gift for details, but this gift becomes more and more of a burden as the Silica moves deeper into the type. Then the details can become his entire focus. He loses the ability to see the big picture, seeing only an endless number of details. And, as each detail equals a decision that has to be made, the Silica becomes bogged down in these details and overwhelmed with the project. Classical homeopaths express it as, "He will think only of pins." Silica types can, when they enter a deep stage of illness, become totally compulsive in their behavior. At this stage, they have to follow a prescribed path each and every day, tending to every detail, and those near them must do so as well.

The Silica who has entered this level of illness in time comes to resemble a statue. He holds himself rigidly, and his face seems flat and devoid of emotions.

It is typical for the Silica constitution to be formed around feelings of abandonment. The Silica child may actually have been physically abandoned by a parent—usually the father—or he may have lost that parent due to a divorce. If the parent is still a physical part of the household, he may have a career that takes him away for extended periods of time, or he may just be emotionally distant. In any case, the Silica child interprets the circumstances in terms of abandonment and uses these feelings to form a self-image.

Everything else about the Silica type comes out of their self-image. They feel that they are not as good as others. They put a good deal of energy into trying to please those from whom they want love and approval. Their fear of speaking (which can manifest itself in children who learn to talk late, or who refuse to speak) can be directly traced back to this lack of self-esteem, as can their rigid body (poised at all times to receive verbal or physical blows) and their passive-aggressive nature (they cannot speak up for themselves, though they know their own minds).

Silica is perhaps the most sensitive type of all. Like Phosphoruses, Silicas can be natural psychics and literally feel the pains that others experience. They often manifest this sensitivity with clairvoyance, having dreams or seeing visions of events that have yet to occur. They are also sensitive to weather and feel ongoing changes in the weather as they do changes in upcoming events. And they have a great sensitivity to the moon. Silicas experience intense emotions, positive or negative, when the moon is full and increased feelings of abandonment during the phase of the new moon.

Physical Portrait: Almost from the first, this remedy type exhibits a lack of endurance. Silicas are slow in their development and milestones: slow to walk, talk, toilet train. Each new milestone represents a huge leap for the Silica child, for whom mere existence can be almost overwhelming.

Silica infants may have failure to thrive. They are not able to digest even the simplest foods. Further, they are angry children, always crying and very stubborn. They cling to the toy they want as if their life depends on it. And that is how they see things, in terms of survival. Silica's sense of survival is easily upset, and he cannot discern what is truly threatening from what is merely against his wishes.

Somewhere in those early years, usually by age five, Silicas are on the way to fulfilling the traditional portrait. As they learn what is and is not truly threatening, they become placid and cerebral children. They often seem mentally advanced, as they are serious and reasonable. If you explain what you want to a Silica child, and why you want it, you are likely to get it.

Failure to thrive continues in Silica children. Like Phosphorus children, they exhibit weakness to every illness that comes into the schoolroom. They get every ear infection and every cold, missing many days of school. They typically are underweight and have circles either under or around their eyes.

This general lack of stamina is characteristic of the type throughout life. They will grow to be slim people, with narrow shoulders, thin necks, and huge heads. It is as if all the calcium in their system rushed up to protect the brain, as it is the most important thing in the world to them, leaving very little left for the rest of the body.

They may have frail health: weakness in their upper respiratory tract and three or more colds every year. In addition, the type is given to chronic low-grade fevers and infections of all sorts, because the immune system is naturally weak. They lack the ability ever to throw off an illness completely, so they have chronically swollen lymph glands that are sensitive to the touch. Night sweats are also common.

But it is the metabolism of the Silica that is the weakest feature. Because they cannot seem to assimilate nutrients properly, they have weak bones, teeth, fingernails, and toenails. Their skin has many abscesses and wounds that do not heal. They are also given to chronic infections of the gums, and their gums bleed any time they are touched.

The Silica's skin is unhealthy. It doesn't heal and may have keloids or scars of all sorts. There also may be chronic acne that does not clear after adolescence. The skin is full of pus, as every sort of wound the Silica receives seems to become infected instantly, and the infection lingers.

The Silica type is known for his sweat. The whole body can be very sweaty, and that sweat typically has a sour smell. Since the Silica is such a refined person, he will most likely be more embarrassed by the sweat than by any other physical complaint. He may well go into the practitioner's office for the first time due to the crisis that the sweating creates.

The Silica's feet are particularly sweaty. The sweat is offensive to everyone nearby. The Silica often makes the mistake of trying to suppress his sweat, especially this foot sweat, but he becomes much worse in general, much more given to weakness and to disease, if he suppresses his sweat. Silicas also become ill if their feet get wet. They are very protective of their feet and feel vulnerable when their feet are uncovered.

Silica types are known for their low vital force. In treatment, they must begin with a low potency and slowly build. The healing process for Silicas is one of slow growth. They are not so much returning to health as creating health as a new concept in their system. As they are slow in all milestones, they are slow to heal and must not be made to feel hurried in the process in any way.

Silicas also have low vital heat. They are chilly and much aggravated by cold weather, feeling the need at all times to be bundled up. They love nothing more than an open fire on a cold day and sit right next to the fire, staring into it. Under no circumstances do they yield their position near the fire.

And yet, Silicas are also aggravated by a warm room and from being in too stuffy a place. They most love that fireplace in a large, cold room (giving rise again to images of the great house of England). They also love to be bundled up in big, thick sweaters while walking about in cool rooms.

They do, however, hate drafts. Silicas, more than any other type, are likely to take ill from drafts. They also need to keep their heads covered on cold days to protect them from colds, sore throats, and earaches.

The illnesses that come on in Silica do so slowly and are chronic in nature. The illnesses also usually come on in childhood, as Silica as a type usually sets in as a childhood constitution. Some outgrow the type, moving on to another constitution, and they look back on their childhood asthma as a phase they went through.

For others, however, their entire lives are greatly defined by their constitution. More than any other type, the Silica's life becomes a list of things he must not do or cannot do as dictated by his constitution. The Silica who does not receive treatment becomes a prisoner of his type.

Although Silica is usually not considered a very helpful acute remedy, there is one acute use that is of vital importance: combating the ill effects of vaccination.

As vaccinations are created for a general populace and not for specific individuals, they can be very damaging to some individual systems. The Silica constitution can literally be created, artificially put into place, by a vaccine.

The child who is in need of Silica after a vaccination quickly exhibits the symptoms characteristic of the remedy type. His vital force and vital heat begin to fail. He may begin to have low-grade infections and fevers. He has night sweats the general sour sweat of the whole body, especially the feet, chronic swollen glands, and glands that are sensitive to the touch.

The child who has had Silica grafted on him begins to become more and more fearful. Like a Silica infant, he may begin to cry a good deal and become very difficult and very serious, as if everything were a life or death matter.

This particular situation requires only an acute treatment to clear away. But if left untreated, it can set in place a lifetime of illness. And although an acute treatment, it is a very serious treatment, one that should never be taken on by the layperson or parent but should remain the sole domain of the professional, who knows the appropriate potency and dosage. This treatment merits careful study; it is important to watch for signs of change in this child's basic constitution.

In general, Silica is a most benign remedy, which may be given freely and without fear in many situations. But the Silica types, due to their lack of vital force, tend to do better with lower potencies at first, building to higher potencies over a period of time. The patient first improves on the level of vital heat. He feels less chilly and, therefore, more at peace within himself and the environment.

Many practitioners report that Silica in very very low potencies, 6X or 9X, is most effective for the chronically ill.

One dose of the remedy remains effective for up to six weeks.

Poster Child: Marcel Proust, who wrote *Remembrance of Things Past* inside his cork-lined room.

THUJA
The Stranger

Remedy Source: Thuja remedy is taken from the *Thuja occidentalis*, also known as the arbor vitae, the white cedar, and the tree of life. The tree is a conifer native to North America and is found most commonly in the Laurel Highlands of Pennsylvania. The tree can grow up to fifty feet tall, with a diameter of up to twenty feet. It is a common garden tree that was introduced into Europe—France, specifically—from Canada. The French came to prize the tree, giving it an honored place in some of their most famous gardens.

Throughout history, the plant has been honored, if not thought of as a therapeutic. In the temples of ancient Greece, the branches of the arbor vitae were dried and burned as incense.

Samuel Hahnemann, knowledgeable as he was of the plant itself and its history, felt that it could make an excellent homeopathic remedy, but even he, upon proving the remedy, did not predict how important it would become in the modern world.

Situations That Suggest Thuja: The ill-effects of vaccination, gonorrhea, and the effects of suppressed gonorrhea; condylomata; syphilis; tumors: fibroids, uterine polyps and fibroids, uterine cysts, polyps of the ears, tumors of the eyes with inflammation; warts and growths of all sort; cancer; rheumatism and rheumatic pain: stiff neck, cracking joints, joint pain; epilepsy and seizures; digestive disorders: distended abdomen, food allergy, constipation, irritable bowel syndrome, anal fissure, rectal pain, hemorrhoids. Also hernia. Also chronic sinusitis; mental illness: depression and manic depression; behavior disorders; violent behavior; toothache and tooth decay.

Remedy Overview: Hahnemann first used Thuja in a case of warts, because the leaves of the tree historically had been used to rid the skin of warts. The remedy worked well against the condition and became a part of the homeopathic pharmacy, but it was not until the historic work of Burnett that we came to understand the full power of the remedy.

Burnett coined the term *vaccinosis* to describe those persons who had never been well since they received a vaccine. In his practice, he saw some children who changed on a basic and profound level when they were given a vaccination. They literally seemed to become other people.

Because of Burnett's research, we know more about the etiology of this constitutional type than we do of many others. It is generally believed that a person may move into the constitution identified as Thuja by any of three methods:

1. Through the ill effects of vaccines. Burnett believed that the vaccine would weld to the person an artificial miasm, a general weakness or tendency toward disease. He considered that these children belonged in the category of "never well since," as their entire vital force and all that shaped them as individuals became warped when the vaccine invaded their system. This is a deeper and more powerful response to vaccination than is the Silica response. Here, the child literally seems to change, becoming angrier and more destructive. High fevers are also quite common. Another vaccination response is the Antimonium, where the child seems to be drowning, has trouble breathing, and seems to be on the verge of death.

This artificial miasm, once within the child's system, proves to be as difficult to treat as any natural miasm.

2. The suppression of gonorrhea. The suppression of gonorrhea creates a miasm within the human system. These people develop rheumatic pains and the mental and physical characteristics of Thuja.

Perhaps more important, these characteristics can be inherited as a general weakness in the children of the person so treated. This is a true miasm, a true genetic weakness of an inherited sort.

In cases like this, the traits are shared among members of a family, or each member of the family demonstrates his own take on the miasm. These family histories are filled with drug and alcohol abuse, family violence, and sexual abuse. The family is an abusive place where the children feel that they have to learn to hide on every level in order to be safe.

3. Children of war. Children who are brought into an unsafe world, in wartime, do not have the security necessary to develop in a healthy manner. They do not have the necessary hygiene or even food to grow healthy. These children feel a deep level of survival crisis: They feel that if they survive they will have to learn to hide, to lie, and to steal—all basic skills of the Thuja type.

Children who are raised in environments that are similar to war zones take on the type as well. These children learn to think that their own survival is paramount, and the pain or even death of others is of little or no concern.

Remedy Theme: Violent behavior, invisibility, lies.

Remedy Motivation: Survival, alienation.

Emotional Portrait: A century ago, there was little need to understand the Thuja type. It was, by and large, considered an acute remedy, so there was no need to learn to deal with it on a constitutional level. But the world is now filled with Thujas, and more are being created every day, so it is vital that we consider the type one of our essential twelve.

Thuja is perhaps the major remedy that speaks to the miasm known as Sycosis, the miasm that is related to gonorrhea. As this is the dominant miasm in our age, we have to learn not only how to deal with and understand those affected by the miasm but also how to help these people heal, both for their sakes and our own. The future of society is threatened by this miasm and by the Thuja type. The average American lives in fear of violent crime and identifies violent crime as the premiere challenge of our day. As the majority of these crimes belong to the miasm Sycosis and the remedy Thuja, we had better give them our full attention.

Thuja, like Silica, often forms in early childhood, or can even be present as an inherited miasm at birth. Like Silica, this remedy type often is a child who exhibits a failure to thrive. It is as if he is not sure he even wants to survive.

This is true whether the constitution has been put in place by a vaccination or is an inherited miasm. The typical Thuja child is sweaty and feverish, but the sweat has an unusual sweet scent of honey and garlic.

Thuja children may cry a good deal, act out, even strike out. But they more often are quiet, seeking only to survive and to be left alone.

From the earliest time in life, a Thuja does not connect with other people. He may be highly dependent on his mother, but there is likely to be little emotional contact other than the child's ongoing need to be protected. He feels that he is in great need of protection every minute of his life.

A Thuja child trusts no one and nothing. He feels threatened at every turn. But unlike the Silica child, who feels threatened in much the same way, the Thuja child does not move into his head as a method of survival. His survival mechanism is to hide. His goal in life is to be invisible.

This is particularly true of Thuja children who live in abusive households. They learn to be invisible. Like tai chi masters, they learn to be where the punch is not. Even their teachers do not often call on them, or do not come to know them very well, because they have a gift for blending in, for blanking out their face so that the human eye passes them over.

This skill lasts them a lifetime, and again and again the Thuja passes us unnoticed. Even their neighbors and friends, if asked, will admit that they never knew them.

The second skill the Thuja learns is lying. There are no better liars on Earth. They look you in the eye with a blank stare and tell you a boldfaced lie. They can even convince themselves in the moment that the lie is true so that it can carry the full power of their personal conviction.

As they grow older, Thujas get better and better at lying, and lying becomes more and more central to their existence. Thujas lie about more and bigger things. They may even take on new identities, a whole new name and life history, in order to survive.

The concept of the Lie is central to Thuja. This is the lie that gave birth to all the others, and most often has a sexual nature. Children who are repeatedly sexually abused often move into a Thuja type, especially if their behavior adapts around that abuse, and they decide to abuse others as they were abused.

Every Thuja has the Lie. They feel that they must protect this lie at all costs. It may be something as simple as homosexuality, but for the Thuja it is a deep and shameful thing. Whatever the Lie is, he feels that it will destroy him if it is ever known. Thus, the homosexuality of Thuja usually involves underage children or violence. But the Lie, this sexual secret, can be anything, as long as keeping this secret a secret is the central focus of the Thuja's energy.

As Thuja most often combines violence with the Lie, this type can turn to rape and sexual assault as a way to force onto others the pain they have experienced.

The Thuja man who as a little child felt so helpless when he was abused now has absolutely no concern for the pain he causes others. He is immune to the pain of others and may even rejoice in it, because it makes the child in him feel big and strong.

As much of what Thuja is about is sexual, all hell breaks loose when that child hits puberty. This is the usual time that Thuja moves from being passive, just trying to be invisible and to survive, to being active—and violent. He uses his talents for invisibility and for lying to hunt other humans as animals stalk each other.

He learns to steal. One day it occurs to him that there is no reason why he should be trapped on a mere survival level when so many others have so much more. So he takes it. He burgles and robs. Many Thujas prefer to mug their victims directly, so they can blend violence with the simple act of robbery.

At this point, too, Thujas often turn to alcohol and drugs, especially if they were raised in homes in which both were used. They especially love marijuana, because it increases their highly sexual nature. They also like cold drinks, such as beer and margaritas.

The Thuja by nature is more cunning than intelligent. He has a visceral understanding of all the things that he may be required to do in order to survive, and he is willing to do any of them. Although some Thujas are good students and attain higher degrees of education, most stop their education early on, and most work with their hands. Most Thujas have jobs, as opposed to careers, and many change their jobs and their residences frequently to prevent being known.

The Thuja personality is highly addictive: drugs and alcohol, sweets of all sorts, chocolate.

Almost every one of them is addicted to pornography and to sex itself. Thujas are highly sexual people, with a powerful sex drive. Many masturbate frequently, until it also becomes a form of addiction.

On the emotional level, Thujas early on usually come to think of themselves as being different from other people. They may think of themselves as literally not being human. And yet, especially in their childhood, they yearn to fit in. They frantically try to identify with others and to have others accept them. Yet somehow they never fit in.

Thujas usually come into their sexuality very early, and because of this they seem to be living on a whole other level of existence from other children. They touch others in a way that other children don't. They have expressions on their faces that other children don't. It is as if, on an experiential level, they are far older than their years.

Also, because Thujas are often concerned with survival, an issue that other children don't even consider, and because they tend to come from violent homes, Thuja children have little basis for relationships with children of other types. They go to a friend's home and see a happy place. Yet they dare not bring their friend into their own home, because they never know from one day to the next what to expect from their home environment. It isn't safe, isn't a place you could take a friend.

We are creating these people ourselves—through vaccination, through our own drug use and the use of antibiotics in the treatment of venereal disease, a treatment that so drives the disease into our system that it is suppressed into invisibility, only to show itself in the next generation.

We are experiencing an increase in crime, and we are seeing violent crime at the hands of younger and younger children. We are seeing a generation that no longer considers the rights of others or the feelings of others as they react to the world around them with increased violence.

These children, as well as the adults of this type, represent the cost to our society of our repression, our suppression, and our denial. The longer it takes us to change the circumstances of these people's lives, the greater will be the cost—to the individuals unlucky enough somehow to threaten the Thuja's survival issues and to our society as a whole.

Physical Portrait: The physical aspects of the type become apparent in childhood. Many mothers notice that, although their child was born very healthy, he suddenly develops allergies after receiving vaccinations. Or the child suddenly loses weight or takes on low-grade fevers. The child who, until that time, was happy and calm, now cries at every noise and seems challenged on every level.

When Thuja children learn to talk, they mumble, or they start out speaking in a normal tone of voice but fade into a whisper by the end of every sentence. The children have deep fears, especially the fear that others don't like them. They violently and willfully do not want to go to school because they feel they have no friends there.

They also fear losing control. This can be on either a physical or emotional level. They feel that they are using all their power and all their will just to appear normal. Any more stress, they fear, will make usual functioning impossible.

Thujas have the sensation that there is something alive in them. This is especially common in situations involving digestive disorders. They feel that there is an animal alive in their abdomen. Sometimes they are sure that it is crying out to them. Sometimes they feel it in terms of internal motion and discomfort. The abdomen protrudes, further convincing them that something is in there. As part of their digestive disorders, early morning diarrhea may drive the Thuja out of bed and into the bathroom. The stool is expelled with a great deal of noise, gas, and discomfort. The stool is very liquid and gushes into the toilet.

In fevers, Thujas first feel a chill in the area of their thighs. They sweat with fever, but only on uncovered parts of the body. The sweat is sweetish, especially the sweat on the genitals.

Thujas have terrible headaches that feel as if a nail were being driven into the head. The headaches are worse on the left side of the forehead. The skin, particularly the skin on the forehead, is greasy. Some Thujas never look completely clean, as their hair and skin are always greasy.

Their skin is covered with sores: severe acne, fever blisters on the lips, warts and tumors on the face, and sties in the eyes. Warts are common all over their body, especially on the hands and fingers. Fibroids and skin tags are also common and likely appear on the sweaty areas of the body. Eczema and psoriasis are also very common.

The Thuja is one of the most rheumatic types of constitution. They have terrible rheumatic pain and cannot bear the damp. Everything is worse for them during damp weather. Headaches come on in damp weather.

The typical Thuja sleeps only on his left side. The Thuja type has a daily aggravation at 3 P.M., although some Thujas experience this aggravation at 3 A.M. and awaken at that time. Thuja types have terrible nightmares and dreams that cause them to wake up suddenly, terrified.

Thujas are worse in cold, damp air but also worse in the warmth of bed. Like Sulphurs, they may have to stick their feet out from under the covers in order to be able to sleep. They cannot bear coffee or tea, although some crave tea. They are allergic to tobacco and to onions and usually are not fond of meat.

The mother tincture may be applied directly to warts and skin tags. The remedy is useful in all potencies but is usually not used below 12C. The remedy is usually started at the lowest possible potency because the remedy typically causes wild aggravations that can last for weeks before improvement begins. The remedy can be given frequently in low potencies but should be used very infrequently in high potency. One dose in high potency usually does the trick.

Since most of us have been vaccinated, it is felt that Thuja, like Sulphur and Natrum Mur, is a remedy that can help a large part of the population. Up to 90 percent of those of us who were vaccinated might benefit from the remedy. And although Thuja can be of help to both men and women, it is the men in need of Thuja who are far more likely to act out with sexual violence.

Although clearing vaccinosis is an acute use of Thuja, it should never be undertaken by the layperson, as the remedy may uncover a deep and deeply suppressed pathology.

Thuja is effective against the ill effects of vaccination no matter how many years have passed since the vaccination. Like all other remedies, the action of Thuja is to express what has been suppressed. It is therefore the action of Thuja, in cases of suppressed gonorrhea, to reinstate the gonorrheal flow before cure can be completed.

Poster Children: Jeffrey Dahmer, as well as many other serial killers and rapists, including Ted Bundy and Richard Speck.

9

CONSIDERING
TRANSFORMATION:
MIASMIC
TREATMENTS

Transformational healing takes the concept of homeopathy to its deepest level. Acute treatments seek only to keep the general health on an even keel, and constitutional treatments work to bring about a general improvement of overall health, but only homeopathic treatments that work on the level of the miasm, the inborn genetic weaknesses common to everyone, can be truly transformational in their impact. Only they can truly set the patient free.

Acute treatments match the patient to his pain, using the principle of similars in the treatment of disease. Constitutional treatments match the patient to the persona of the remedy as well as with the totality of the symptoms. Transformation requires something more: Miasmic treatments require that we put the patient into the context of his family, his genetic pool. We have to look at the issues facing the patient—mental, emotional, and physical—in the context of the other issues and other symptoms present in the family. In other words, we can't just look at the picture, we also have to look at the frame.

In this process, we once more have to wrestle with the concept of science versus faith. Some people insist that, when we talk about miasms, we are talking about genetics, about inborn weaknesses and strengths. Others believe just as strongly that we are talking about karma, about the issues we have brought into this lifetime from other lifetimes. I believe that we are eternal beings and that we have many lives. We chose specific illnesses, specific weaknesses in this life such that by approaching our illness with faith and hope, we grow not just as bodies but as spirits as well.

I see the two approaches, the scientific and the mystical, as just another example of the three blind men trying to decide what an elephant looks like. One touches the trunk and thinks that it looks like a snake. One touches the flank and thinks that it must look like a wall. The third touches the tail and insists that it looks like a rope. But they are all touching the same animal, the elephant.

In the same way, the scientist looks at the inherited traits and sees genes, the guru looks at the same thing and sees karma. Either way, we do come into this life with a good deal of baggage. Many children are born with immune systems that are already so compromised that it takes very little for them to get ill. Add to this the suppressive treatments that they receive from birth onward, the vaccinations that they are required to receive by law, whether they want them or not, and the toxins that are present in our environment, our food, and our water, and you have circumstances that often lead to disaster. It is no wonder that we are leading lives that are more and more defined by multiple chronic conditions.

In that our present circumstances have been generations in the making, it is also no wonder that, as early as 1816, Samuel Hahnemann was predicting our current events.

ON BEING TAINTED

I am always amazed at the work Hahnemann did in his last twelve years of life. After all that struggle, after being hounded by the medical establishment and literally driven out of town multiple times, in his last years, after he had become respected at last for the work he had done, after he had finally made money enough to retire and relax, he set about to do his greatest work. And in doing so he risked everything that he had managed to build up.

At a time in his life when most of the others of his profession would be very happy to take their rest, Hahnemann, instead of focusing on the 80 percent of his patients who found excellent results with his methods, looked at the 20 percent who, although perhaps they were improved to some extent, did not achieve that state of freedom that can be considered totally healthy. In his final major work, *Chronic Diseases*, and in the final edition of *The Organon*, Hahnemann shows himself to be unlike so many others of his ilk. Often men and women who, through their own will, their own work, and their own unique insights, have developed some new system of thinking and doing refuse to critique or take a new look at the model they created. Yet Hahnemann was quite prepared to say that he was wrong in developing this new thing he called homeopathy. He had never, you see, moved from being a healer to being a guru, as so many others do. He desired instead to put his principles to the test yet again, in the hopes of finding what he called "the deeper disease."

The term that Hahnemann gave to these "deeper diseases" was *miasm*. The word itself means "taint" or "contamination." And it describes exactly what Hahnemann was seeing.

By this time in his career, Hahnemann had already made the move from curer to healer. He already was quite comfortable in discussing all disease as being conceptual in nature. And he already was working with healing in terms of the vital force. He saw the vital force as the conduit between our spirit and our body. And, in that he believed that spirit was perfect and could never become ill, Hahnemann felt that all illness was a block of some sort between the spirit and the body. In some way, we were being cut off from our own spirits, our own perfect selves. If you clear the block, then healing is restored.

The taint that Hahnemann named the miasm, however, was something more profound. It was an actual part of the vital force. Instead of a simple block, the vital force itself was contaminated. Therefore, unless that force itself underwent a healing process, the circumstances of illness inherent in the taint were in place for a lifetime—or for multiple lifetimes. These same traits, or others linked to them in the case of related illnesses, could and would be inherited by generation after generation.

As homeopath Y. R. Agrawal puts it, after twelve years of "experiments and critical observations," Hahnemann found that "certain diseases were easily cured with simple remedies or had a natural and spontaneous cure, but he was disappointed to see that many other patients returned with old complaints and/or with new symptoms. He studied all such cases carefully and deeply and the latent inherent defect or obstacle to cure was inferred to have been caused by some miasms which he named Psora, Syphilis, and Sycosis."

HAHNEMANN'S MIASMS

Although all three of the miasms that Hahnemann identified are created by the suppression of specific diseases during their infectious stages, it is incorrect to equate the miasm with the disease. The fact that a child inherited the Sycotic miasm from a parent does not mean that he has inherited gonorrhea. Instead it means that he has inherited a taint, a weakness in his own vital force that predisposes him not to the disease gonorrhea itself but to a panoply of disorders that are common to the miasm. Like a constitutional remedy, each miasm has a theme, and each carries with it the tendency toward illness.

Psora

Samuel Hahnemann tells us that Psora is the first miasm. It predates history. Miasm can also be translated to mean "stain" or "sin," and so Kent likens the miasm to original sin. In his *Lectures on Homeopathic Philosophy*, he writes, "Psora is the underlying cause, and is the primitive or primary disorder of the human race. It is a disordered state of the internal economy of the human race. This state expresses itself in the forms of varying chronic diseases, or chronic manifestations. If the human race had remained in a state of perfect order, Psora could not have existed. The susceptibility to Psora opens out a question altogether too broad to study among the sciences in a medical college. It is altogether too extensive, for it goes to the very primitive wrong of the human race, the very first sickness of the human race, that is the spiritual sickness, from which first state the race progressed into what may be called true susceptibility to Psora, which in turn laid the foundation for other diseases."

Psora, then, represents the issue of susceptibility in the human system. If we had nothing blocking us from our own pure spirit, we would never be ill. Psora, however, whether it is thought of as original sin, or as selfishness, or as self-defeat—all variations on the same theme—is this block. It is the ego and the will that insist that we can never be happy if everyone else is happy, in that their happiness, their success, their possessions devalue our own. Psora, this susceptibility to our own wounded ego, allows us to be susceptible to any of a number of diseases.

Kent continues by telling us that the concept of this miasm extends beyond our understanding of the disease from which it stems:

If we regard Psora as itch, we fail to understand, and fail to express thereby, anything like the original intention of Hahnemann. An itch is commonly supposed to be a limited thing, something superficial, caused by a little tiny bit of a mite that is supposed to have life, and when the little itch mite is destroyed, the cause of the itch is said to have been removed. What a folly!

From a small beginning with wonderful progress, Psora spreads out into the underlying states and manifests itself in the large portion of the chronic disease upon the human race. It embraces epilepsy, insanity, the malignant diseases, tumors, ulcers, catarrhs, and a great proportion of the eruptions. It progresses from simple states to the very highest degree of complexity, not always alone and by itself, but often by the villainous aid of drugging during generation after generation; for the physician has endeavored with all his power to drive it from the surface, and has thereby caused it to root itself deeper, to become more dense and invisible until the human race is almost threatened with extinction.

Kent wrote these words generations ago. They show that homeopaths have seen a bleak future and that's where we now appear to be.

As Psora is the least violent of the miasms, it is often thought to be somehow less threatening. But when we think of this miasm not as a rash but as the way we become susceptible to worse conditions, then we really know what we are working with. It's like the marijuana that our parents told us would lead to harder drugs.

The theme of this miasm can be expressed in a number of ways. It is the miasm of defect, and it involves all sorts of conditions, physical and mental. These conditions involve the dysfunction of a particular system or systems within the being rather than a specific pathology. Psora is also termed the miasm of self-defeat, in that through the aforementioned dysfunction the mind and body of the patient himself, rather than any outside or invading force, keep the patient from any desired goal.

Psoric folks just start to become some sort of success in life, are nearing the completion of work that they have spent so much time and energy on, and then somehow manage to mess it all up. They suddenly get sick with a mysterious disorder, or they simply turn and walk away. They are great abandoners; they feel that anything that losers like themselves would want to work on isn't worth the effort of working on anyway. Like the Sulphur, which as a remedy type belongs within this miasm, Psoric patients have such a poor self-image, wrapped as it is in such a large ego, that they never seem to live up to their early promise. Think of Orson Welles, of the tragedy that was his later life given his early promise, and you are thinking of the effects of Psora. Think also of the character played by Marcello Mastroianni in Fellini's 8½, who as a newly famous film director builds a huge launching pad in the middle of nowhere, telling everyone that it is the central scenery for his new film epic, only to stay awake at night wondering what the hell to do with it now that all the money is spent, and you are thinking of the heart of Psora. Give them a success and they'll build an empty launching pad with it every time.

The diseases of Psorics are the diseases of their own dysfunction and of their own wounded ego. They have illnesses for which there is no concrete cause. Suddenly they are environmentally ill. Suddenly they have severe allergies. Suddenly digestive disorders. Suddenly eczema and other skin conditions. Their illnesses are largely affected by, if not entirely controlled by, their mind and emotions. They are the schizophrenics who are much better when their spouses just put them in a hospital and leave them alone. In other words, if we can identify the original, specific wound out of which the Psoric patient is acting, if we can get to the root cause of his condition, then we can almost always greatly help that condition.

The functional disorders of Psora are reversible, even if the diseases that come out of this sphere of dysfunction often are not. Therefore, the patient who undergoes a correctly planned treatment of Psora may seem to become miraculously well.

Hyperfunction and hyperexcitation of all bodily processes are a trademark of this miasm. Take allergies, for example. An allergy to pollen does not represent the underactivity of the immune system. Quite the opposite, it represents the hyperactivity of the immune system, which treats more and more things as threats. It considers this benign little pollen a threat and makes the whole body go to war against the pollen. If the immune system were not so quick to react, and treated pollen as pollen, you would not have the symptoms we call allergy.

That's how it goes for the Psoric. It is as if their entire being were on alert at all times. Over time, it is as if their system recognizes everything they come into contact with as more and more of a threat. Therefore the allergy tendency, the tendency to see more and more benign things as a threat—which is a symbol of the whole miasm—takes hold on every level of being until it cripples the entire system. All the vital force is being used to survive against things that are not even threatening the system, not to grow or develop.

Psoric patients are the most "stuck" patients. The more deeply entrenched the miasm, the more they feel helpless, not just against the miasm and the specific diseases it brings but also against life itself. They inevitably seek some adaptive behavior, eating a pizza or getting drunk, that makes them feel better in the moment and totally ignore the cost of that behavior to their system in the long run. The Psorics rush to do destructive things. From alcohol to bad relationships to buying things that they cannot afford, they crave what does them most harm.

Besides allergies, the Psoric miasm includes all sorts of skin conditions, from dry skin to acne to psoriasis; as well as weak nails and hair. Also prematurely graying hair or early baldness.

Smells play a large part in the lives of Psorics. They have a great sense of smell or none at all. But they all are sensitive to smells, especially to chemical odors.

In that "stuck" state, Psorics often just want to physically stay still, especially when they feel ill. The urge to rest battles the urge to exercise, as the urge for chocolate cake battles the urge for celery. They love, especially when ill, to be entertained and want to be made happy by their favorite foods and television shows.

The Psorics are the ones doctors tell that if they are to get well they have to want to get well. Often, it seems that they in no way want to get well. They tell you that they know just what to do in order to feel better, but somehow they never get around to doing it. They are too worried about Stephanie on *The Bold and the Beautiful* to look after themselves.

Two areas of the Psoric body tend to have the greatest weakness: the circulatory and the digestive systems. The heart disease belonging to this miasm is functional. Patients have the sensation of a rush of blood to their chest. A feeling of fullness surrounds the heart, bringing on terror. They fear that they will die of a heart attack, although there is no real disease present. Their heart condition is greatly affected by their emotions. They often mistake panic attacks for heart attacks. Actual heart attack, and sudden death due to heart failure, is largely the domain of the Sycotic and Syphilitic miasms. The heart conditions of Psora bring discomfort and imprisonment due to fear, but not death.

The digestive disorders are numerous. The patients are born with, or develop, many food allergies and sensitivities. Their diet usually consists largely of the very same food, and so they have many pain symptoms associated with eating—gas, bloat, cramping, irritable bowel syndrome, colitis, the feeling that food is fermenting in their stomach, rumbling and gurgling of the digestive tract.

Their pains of all sorts are relieved by heat. Some pains improve with light pressure while others demand the loosening of clothing.

Patients treated homeopathically while they are only under the control of Psora have an excellent chance of total recovery, as this miasm, tricky as it is, still has not moved beyond the functional level. But few of us today, thanks to our genetic heritage and our ongoing suppressive treatments, have only Psora to deal with. Many of us have the Sycotic and the Syphilitic weight upon us as well, intertwined with the susceptibility to greater illness that Psora brings.

Sycosis

Homeopath J. H. Allen tells us, "Sycosis is a profoundly acting miasm. It acts upon every cell of the human organism, even to the very depth of the physical being." Because this miasm may lie latent in the human system for a number of years, only to burst forth at last with a violence that all but destroys the system, it is called "the sleeping volcano."

The term *Syscosis* comes from the Greek word for "fig." It was named for the fig warts, or skin tags, and the warts and growths of all sorts that are the usual first sign of the miasm's presence.

As it is the miasm of vaccinosis, it is, next to Psora, the most common miasm of our age. And, as it is the miasm of violence, it presents our largest single health threat.

Sycosis is created from the suppression of gonorrhea in its infectious stages. Given that this disease is rampant in our culture, it should come as no surprise that the miasm is active in literally millions of humans, deeply compromising their vital force and deeply affecting their bodies and their minds.

In the patient in whose system the miasm has been placed by the actual suppression of the gonorrheal infection, the miasm moves as follows: first the appearance of warts, skin tags, fibroids on the skin; next chronic rheumatic pains and chronic conditions including neuritis and neuralgia. Chronic digestive disorders such as Crohn's disease are also common. Patients who have the miasm artificially grafted onto their system often follow this same pattern of illness.

The diseases common to Sycosis are more violent in nature than are the diseases of Psora. The central pain is rheumatic. The patient is physically sensitive to his environment in the same way that he is psychically sensitive to his emotional environment. A central issue of the miasm is that the person feels threatened. This is not the hypersensitivity of Psora, but more fundamental: The Sycotic feels that someone or something is out to destroy him. Most often, he feels that his childhood home is toxic or unsafe. And the Sycotic, instead of becoming self-absorbed himself as the Psoric does, strikes back in order to survive.

Sycotics are largely reactive people who strike back out of fear and who always strike back with more force than is required. Because they feel so very unsafe, they kill in order to survive.

Sycotics place the responsibility for their actions on the shoulders of the other person: "Look what you made me do." They rationalize their actions, no matter how cruel and unnecessary they are, as the only thing they can do. Often they place the responsibility of their actions on some supernatural being: "The devil made me do it." But one thing is certain: It is never their fault.

Sycotics come to see their own pain and their own fear as somehow more important than those of anyone else. They tend to dehumanize their enemy and to ignore the pain they cause in others, as if the others are not as vitally human as they themselves are.

Sycosis is also considered to be the miasm of obsession. Sycotic types feel the need to assert themselves. They tend to feel invisible and powerless. This, coupled with that feeling that the world is not safe, moves the Sycotic to act out.

Sycotics misinterpret the concept of love. They are given to obsessive love. They tend to feel that if they love someone, then it goes without saying that their love is returned. And they become intent on having that object of their love. They do not let the fact that the other person does not want their love stand in their way. Thus in the Sycotic type we have stalkers of all sorts, obsessives of all sorts.

We also have rapists, as Sycotics may combine their obsessive and their violent natures, confusing love and power, or, in the end, settling for the ability to control the object of their warped love, willingly sacrificing any return of affection.

Of course not every Sycotic is an obsessive or violent person. But excess is the hallmark of the miasm. Different individuals in the miasm certainly differ in the manner in which they express this tendency, but all exhibit it to some degree, often with drugs and alcohol, or with pornography, and almost always with sex. All have a powerful sex drive.

Sycotics approach many things, particularly sex and drugs and rock and roll, with a roller-coaster approach. Sycotics tend to be cyclical in their approach to what they consider pleasure. The man who seems quiet and mild mannered in his suit every business day goes wild every weekend. He drinks, takes drugs, and finds a new sexual partner every Saturday if possible. Others use St. Patrick's Day or any other holiday as their excuse to indulge in excess. Others binge on drugs and sex of all sorts, until they feel the release of some inner tension that drives them.

Sycotics also tend to flee. Where Psorics abandon a project, usually just before it is done, Sycotics disappear. The clichéd husband who goes out for cigarettes and never returns home is influenced by the Sycotic miasm. Sycotics cannot bear responsibility. When under pressure, especially when expected to be responsible for the results of their excesses, they flee as if the devil were at their heels.

Sycotics have a general weakness in the upper respiratory system. They tend to catch colds easily. They tend to have chronic coughs and chronic sinusitis. They cannot breathe through their noses. These symptoms, as all others, are greatly exaggerated by damp or cold weather, or by a change in the weather from dry to wet.

Sycotics also tend to have a general weakness of metabolism. A part of their body may be emaciated. They may be anemic or have lymphatic disorders or diseases of the endocrine system. Diseases influenced by the Sycotic miasm affect the muscles and the soft tissue, not the bone.

Many of these pains manifest in the extremities. Joint pains of all sorts and pains that are better with gentle motions and gentle rubbing are typical. So is arthritis in all its forms or locations, especially rheumatoid arthritis.

Also, those in this miasm have all kinds of cysts and fibroids and tumors. In men, there are prostate ailments of all sorts. In women, diseases of the uterus and the reproductive system, especially ovarian cysts and uterine fibroids, are common.

Chicken pox and smallpox also belong to this miasm, as do herpes, all forms of ringworm and psoriasis, and moles. The Sycotic type tends to be covered in moles. Like warts, moles are the early dead giveaway of the presence of the miasm.

Syphilis

J. H. Allen waxes melodramatic on the subject of Syphilis, but it's still a great quote: "The wages of sin is death and the wages of sex sin is syphilis." The action of the miasm of Syphilis is deeper and more violent than that of either of Hahnemann's other miasms. It affects specific organs with violent pathology. And it weakens the skeletal system with a number of malformations and disease conditions. The miasm is also often referred to as the Leutic.

Classical homeopaths say that Syphilitic patients are easy to spot. They have large heads with soft sutures and fontanels that remain open in children long after they should normally be closed. The scalp is damp in both children and adults; there is a good deal of perspiration of the scalp. Look also for eye troubles, for astigmatism, deformed lenses, ulcerations of the cornea, and inability to tolerate light. Syphilitics tend to have dry lips, with cracks and fissures in and around the lips. They tend to have a dull or gray undertone to their skin, especially on their face.

Syphilis is the miasm of destruction. It creates irreversible conditions that tend to become infected. Every wound, every injury becomes infected. Syphilitic patients are slow to heal. Their immune systems tend to be sluggish and nonresponsive.

In the mental sphere, those affected by this miasm tend toward deep depression, especially clinical depression. Patients often experience feelings of jealousy, revenge, hatred, guilt, and suicide. This is the miasm of the planned suicide; the patient plots and plans all the details and leaves a note behind.

The miasm of Syphilis largely follows the flow of the disease Syphilis that has been suppressed into the system. In terms of the infectious disease, the viral condition creates chancre sores a week or two after sexual contact with an infected person. The chancre first appears as a pustule, which changes in character into a painful ulcer with a raised border. If this chancre is not properly treated, it moves deeper into the system through three stages of infection. The first stage is the chancre itself. At this level, the disease is easily treated. The second stage involves skin rashes and lesions on the mucous membranes, as well as pains in the bones and joints. The lymph nodes enlarge and are painful. The third stage of the disease moves it deeper into the mind, with insanity resulting.

Like the Psoric and Sycotic miasms, the Syphilitic miasm usually first shows itself on the skin as copper-colored, crescent-shaped eruptions around the joints. They are not sore and do not itch. Scaly patches appear on the skin, along with crusting and patches of thick and inflexible skin.

But the major attack of the Syphilitic miasm is on the skeletal system. Just as the second stage of the infection includes pains in joints and bones, the deeper miasm strikes the bones as well. The long bones of the upper and lower body are especially susceptible to the miasm. The bones develop poorly in the case of small children, or become weakened. Syphilitics may have soft bones or bones that curve. They may develop rickets and deformities of all sorts, especially of the feet. The teeth become weakened, soft, and decayed.

At the same time, those in this miasm have chronic swelling of the lymph glands, which are very sensitive to touch. They are given to long-term low-grade infections of all sorts. They are unable to heal completely or to completely throw off infections. They have fevers and night sweats.

The mental symptoms of the miasm, representing the third stage of the infection, are the most pronounced. Syphilitics tend toward depression and manic depression. They feel a mental oppression, as if they were fighting for their own mind. The anxiety and oppression are both worse at night.

Syphilitics become manic in the repetition of tasks. They wash their hands again and again. They develop systems by which tasks have to be completed, fearing any variation of this system.

They can become very forgetful. They don't remember why they entered a room or how to end the sentence they began. In a deep Syphilitic state, the patient's mind seems to shut down, with a "lizard brain"—the part of our human nature dedicated to the survival of the system at all costs— taking its place. They function on a basic animal level, with all conscious thought appearing to have shut down.

Syphilitics are human thermometers. They easily become too hot or too cold and have to control their environment and keep it in their comfort range. Food and drink as well can be taken into the body only at the proper temperature.

This is the miasm of violence. It leads to violent disease and violent behavior. Unlike the explosive nature of Sycotic violence, the Syphilitic plans his violence. This is the miasm of the cold-blooded murderer.

THE FOURTH AND FIFTH MIASMS

After Hahnemann's death a great controversy arose around his concept of miasms. Some homeopaths denounced the concept, along with everything else that Hahnemann accomplished in his last years. Others not only grasped Hahnemann's discoveries but completed the work that he left un-finished.

Since then, two other miasms, both reflecting newer disease conditions, have been added to Hahnemann's original three. Both carry the weight and the destructive power of Hahnemann's miasms. And both require careful and wise treatment to move away and clear.

Tuberculosis

The Tubercular miasm was identified through the work of Henry C. Allen and Antoine Nebel. For years, it was called Pseudo-Psora because it closely mirrors the destructive pattern of the Psoric miasm. Today, most practitioners consider the Tubercular miasm not to be a single miasm at all, but rather a condition in which the Psoric and the Syphilitic miasms have combined.

This being the case, Tuberculosis is a miasm of exhaustion. The failure to thrive that is so common to the Syphilitic miasm combines with the Psoric sense of depletion and lack of proper function. There are night sweats, fever, and rapid weight loss.

This miasm usually shows itself in early life and almost always is highly noticeable in its impact by a patient's twentieth birthday. The children of this miasm are thin. They have very narrow chests, as if the lungs were underdeveloped. They have a general weakness in the upper respiratory system and in the eyes, ears, nose, and throat.

Children with this miasm have beautiful eyes. Their eyes connect with the world around them from a very early age. There are all sorts of weaknesses of the visual system, especially amblyopia and strabismus. Their eyes tend always to look liquid. They have a gloss, a shine to them, and dilated pupils.

Children with this miasm seem always to have colds. They catch colds very easily, and the colds last a long time. The colds move into the chest and go deeper and deeper into the system. Every cold may move into bronchitis, or the cold goes into the ears. Pain in the ears, and ear infections of all sorts, is common to this type. It seems that every time they get sick they also get an ear infection. The ears are the first to signal illness coming on. In all upper respiratory troubles, when the child is getting ill, the child's ears turn bright red and feel burning hot to the touch. The same is true for the cheeks. A Tubercular child who is becoming ill often has bright red hot patches across his cheeks.

It is important to note that, no matter how painful and troublesome these ear infections are, by taking on the infection they protect the whole system and keep the infection from moving deeper. In keeping the infection at a surface level, the ears actually protect the lungs, a far more vulnerable organ in a Tubercular child, from becoming infected.

The nose and the throat also play a part in the Tubercular childhood health drama. Tubercular children typically have nosebleeds. They come on suddenly and can be quite difficult to stop. The blood is bright red.

Some Tubercular children have infections of the throat instead of the ears. The throat becomes very red with burning pains. The child wants cold drinks to soothe his throat. In this type of Tubercular child, upper respiratory infections move immediately into the chest and into a deeper illness.

———

As the Tubercular child grows, his symptom portrait shifts. The child displays an allergy to milk and milk products. Still some tubercular children love milk and ice cream and literally scream with rage if they are refused either. Others hate all milk products. Diarrhea is quite common after eating dairy products. This diarrhea grows worse after the appearance of the child's first teeth. In some children, there is a personality change as well—anger or even rage when the child consumes dairy. In some Tubercular types, it affects them as sugar activates others.

The other great vulnerability of Tubercular children is cold. They are sick all winter. Their whole system lacks vitality and needs heat and sunshine to build strength. They tend to have thin necks and hands, and sweaty palms. They tend to have trouble breathing. Their narrow chest is of no help here, as their lung capacity is reduced. They tire easily.

In later life, the Tubercular adult still has troubles with breathing; asthma is common. So are various types of chronic pain, including sciatica and neuralgia.

Tuberculosis is the miasm of heightened emotionalism and emotional perfectionism. The persons of this type tend to be right-brain dominant. They are creative thinkers and nonlogical and nonlinear. They are usually considered high-strung, what used to be called neurasthenic.

They are restless people. They want to keep moving, keep trying new things. They are future directed and tend to have few ties to their past, even to their family. Once they have moved on beyond a relationship or a situation, in their mind, it is gone. They keep their eyes on what is coming next. Tubercular people want to change jobs frequently. They reach middle age without a set career in mind. They tend to happen upon jobs and fall into relationships, seemingly without desire or will.

Like the sixties generation—which was perhaps the peak Tubercular time in United States history—they want to explore everything, go everywhere, and experience bliss. And, like the youth of the sixties, they feel that they can change the world. They feel that one person who dedicates himself to change can indeed make a difference. Further, they believe in true love and the idea of a soul mate. In other words, in all things, due to their heightened sense of emotionalism and romanticism, they are setting themselves up for disappointment.

Ailments come on from disappointment, especially after disappointment in love. If the illness is great enough, the Tubercular type becomes bitter, the angry drifter.

Camille, the prostitute who finds true love and then dies coughing up bright red blood, with her eyes flashing in candlelight, is the icon of the Tubercular type. Her fate represents the miasm completing its task.

Cancer

As the Tubercular miasm is a combination of Psora and Syphilis, Cancerism is the combination of Psora and Sycosis. The most recent miasm to be identified, its discovery was the product of research conducted by Leon Vannier.

Many consider Cancerism to be the most destructive miasm. Vannier thought Cancerism, which he called the Oncotic miasm, to be the miasm of adaptive failure. Others call it the "miasm of denial," keying in on the type's tendency toward selective memory and unusual strengths and weakness in family ties.

This is a miasm that, left untreated, changes the entire body. There are changes in body odor and in the body's discharges. And, usually most noticeable at first, there are changes in the conditions of the skin, moles and warts in particular. The skin takes on a mottled appearance, with deep freckling of various parts of the body.

In this miasm we have a true breakdown of immunity. The patient loses the ability to heal. Wounds and diseases of the skin are especially difficult to heal.

The patient has sudden weight loss and is in pain. The pains appear and disappear without pattern. They tend to be rather vague, both in location and in description. This miasm combines the chronic fatigue of the Psoric with the rheumatic pain of the Sycotic. So the weather affects the pains.

There is a certain coolness to the people of this miasm. They tend to stand back from the world. The issue of denial for the type often leads them to put physical distance between themselves and the thing that is being denied. They often cut themselves off from the world.

Their relationship with family either seems too close or too distant. They may still be living at home in middle age and taking care of an aging parent night and day, or they leave home at fifteen and never return. The adults of this type often have patches of memory missing from their childhoods. Their talent for denial becomes so strong that they literally lose the memory of entire parts of their life.

This is a miasm of insomnia. The insomnia of Tuberculosis stems from a mind that is too active to settle down and sleep. The insomnia of Cancers is deeper and more chronic. They can never sleep. They don't know why they can't sleep, and though they are exhausted, they walk the floor night after night after night.

They tend to worry about their health. Fears about pain and death are worse at night when they cannot sleep. They worry about deadly disease. They especially fear cancer.

The persons of this type are not easily comforted. They withdraw from those who offer them physical or emotional comfort. They do not trust others and tend to use their own emotional coolness as their defense in all situations in which they feel threatened.

As they age, they tend to wither and shrink away, as if their body, in keeping with their emotions, was simply withdrawing from life.

THE WEIGHT

Acute treatments are so easy. They are just a little jump start for the vital force. While the patient who is in a good deal of pain, or who even is in a life-threatening situation, may see it differently, your work is simple. Just look at the patient last week, or yesterday, just before the illness set in or the physical blow was received, and see how he has changed, see the totality of the symptoms both before and after the event, compare and contrast, and give the remedy that seems most similar to the situation at hand.

Often you don't even have to do this much work. You can just deal with the moment and give the remedy whose portrait is most similar to the patient. You can trust the remedy and trust the principles of homeopathy to pull the patient through.

In acute treatments, patients don't really have to do anything. They don't even have to think that you are sane or that there is any merit at all in homeopathy. It still works. Their vital force, their immune system, if you prefer, gets the tiny push that it needs to rebound into the healing response required. And the event ends and the patient returns to the level of health that he previously enjoyed, usually with a new appreciation for homeopathy.

In constitutional treatments, we work for something deeper. We try to unravel the Gordian knot that most of us have tied over our lifetime of suppression and rationalization. And, in doing so, we need, at some point, the patient's full attention. At some point he has to want to change.

Transformational healing, the process in which patients actually throw off the weight of the miasm or miasms that have been pulling them down since birth, though, requires that everyone—the patient, the practitioner, and often the patient's family—work together. All join in the activity with the goal of not just getting better but actually changing on a fundamental level. In removing the miasm that has imprisoned him, the patient finds that he not only gets rid of his headaches, but that at the end of the treatment, he seems like another person, one who has discovered the blessing in every illness and who sees that the negative motivations of hatred and of fear, far from being the justified responses to past hurt, are actually poisons that hurt everyone whose lives are touched by them.

This is hard work, sometimes long, hard work. This process is far more difficult and profound than any simple action, particularly the simple action of swallowing a pill. At this level of work, the patient must come to understand that the remedy is only a catalyst, an energy flow that can and will assist his own vital force in transformation. Energy that heals flows into the body from the spirit. Many people, even those who have survived cancer or who have battled their way back from a heart attack, may feel that it is unnecessary even to consider this concept of spirit. But it is possible to undergo the process of cure and never ever deal with the path of healing. Survival is not the goal—transformation is.

Whether the religious among us are right or wrong, whether our spirits live on after we die, we are here for a period of seventy or eighty years. And we arrived without a textbook.

The concept of education seems as inborn as is the search for healing. In Western culture we dedicate the first seventeen years of life to education. There are few processes to which we give so much time and energy. And yet, like healing, like religion, which we would really like to keep bottled up on the shelf, just to let out on Sunday, many trap education within the walls of the school building, when it should be a lifelong function.

We can do whatever we want to in the time we have. But three things seem to come up again and again: healing, education, and the search for understanding creation, whether by science, philosophy, or both. These are the instinctive functions of our lives. These three great themes arise in each of us. Even the greatest couch potato, contented with his bag of chips and football game, has a moment in which his heart stops and he realizes that he will die. And in that moment, he wonders, What the hell is going on here?

Transformational healing is so important in our lives because it intertwines these three great themes. It is impossible for any of us to be truly healed, to throw off the weight of our own illness and our own sin, without undergoing an educational process in addition to the process of healing. And, if we are to be free, we must all come to terms with our universe and the way it functions, most especially as concerns our own death.

So the treatment of miasms, the releasing of the weight that was placed upon us even before our birth, is so much more than taking homeopathic remedies. It is the process of learning and forgiving and truly letting go.

For those who have become truly well, the term *expression* takes on a new meaning. They are, at last, free to express their true selves and to live their lives truly as themselves, without the need for the multiple masks or crutches that most of us employ just to get us through the day. But reaching this state requires a process that takes more and more of our attention, until for a time it takes our full attention. It is a commitment. And it is the only way to throw off the weight.

In approaching the miasm in the individual, we must see that individual not just as a whole and unique being but also as a part of his lineage, and, ultimately, as part of humanity. Instead of further separating the patient out of the pack, making him more isolated in the illness, the transformational treatment in working with the miasm brings the patient closer to his family and allows him to be a more active and vital part of their society. As part of the educational process that is transformational healing, the patient must come to understand the motivations of others and the actions of his own diseases. And once he understands, he must forgive and let go. As freedom transforms the individual, it transforms the environment as well. Thus the successful miasmic treatment transforms not just the patient but also the family and the society.

TRANSFORMATIONAL TREATMENTS

In approaching the treatment of miasms, it is of vital importance that both the practitioner and patient agree that the presence of any or all miasms is never an excuse to further weld the victim role onto the patient. Like a disease, a miasm is not a curse or something to be fought against. It is a legacy and, in its way, a blessing.

Perhaps our single greatest weapon against all circumstances that appear negative is our faith. Faith tells us that there is a creative force behind all the events that take place in the universe, and that, because of this, we know that all things work together to the good.

The second greatest tool is our own sense of ourselves and our sense of humor. The person who takes any condition, from merely uncomfortable to life-threatening, and lets that condition define his life is well on the way to becoming professionally ill. Now or later, he tends to let others know of his ongoing struggle, instead of making the hard work look easy.

We must work to reduce the circumstances of pain in our own lives first by picturing the pain not as a giant but as a dwarf, and second by working to express this dwarf from our system through the use of homeopathics, or other modalities of treatment that have the same reactive impact upon that system.

The practitioner who works with the patient in transformational healing must be well versed in the miasms and in the materia medica of appropriate treatments. Further, he must follow the principles of homeopathic treatment, strictly adhering to the Three Laws of Cure, if complete transformation is to take place.

The Treatment of the Miasm: Psora

The first thing to remember in treating Psora is that you must always start with today, from the present moment, and work backward in time, uncovering and expressing what remains within. Give the remedy, most usually a polycrest or nosode, that is most similar in action to the patient's symptoms. As the remedy acts, expressing all that has been suppressed and increasing the vital force, old symptoms recur. As with constitutional treatment, this is the normal pattern of cure: Old aches and pains that have been suppressed come back again in successive order. If conditions of any sort come out on the skin, they should not be treated in any way—and patients should be aware of this before beginning treatment, so that they don't panic when the rashes start to appear and run to the dermatologist. Patients should be comforted by the fact that, as issues return to the skin, the system in general should feel stronger and more symptom free.

In some cases, the movement is forward and the expression of suppressed conditions is ongoing. Expect chronic sinus disorders of all sorts to get a good deal worse just before the ailments move out onto the skin. In simple cases like these, if the skin condition is left alone to run its course (the ongoing homeopathic treatment is, of course, going to be continued since it is not specific to the skin symptoms, but rather is setting up the expressive situation that is manifesting out on the skin), the miasm finally is totally removed from the system, interior and exterior. The patient is free from illness.

Some cases are far more complicated. There may have been organic changes within the body. Here, the patient takes the medicine and it works well for a while, then stops working. The cure comes to a sudden standstill. Here it is important to encourage the patient to continue treatment and not be too quick to move on to another medicine. Often in cases of Psora, various blocks and blind alleys occur in treatment. Often, if the treatment can continue—and this can take a good deal of patience on the part of the patient and the practitioner—healing once again begins. A nosode, a remedy made from tissue that is diseased in a manner similar to the disease from which the patient suffers, may be needed to break through the blind alleys. But remember, the patient must show the symptoms of the specific nosode remedy in order for it to be of help in the healing process. Simply because a person falls within the Psoric miasm does not mean that he needs Psorinum, the nosode taken from diseased pus. Another nosode may be called for. Match the remedy to the person, the person to the remedy. The practitioner who lacks knowledge of materia medica may rush for Psorinum in all Psoric cases, and then wonders why it doesn't work.

Most complicated cases of Psora involve hereditary ailments. In these cases, the itch does not respond immediately to any remedy. It is too central to the case. But if the miasm can be brought out onto the skin, or into some sort of mucus flow, then the interior illness is well on its way to being brought forth.

Sulphur, of course, is the most common and most helpful first treatment of any miasmic disease involving Psora. Often this remedy alone gets the disease in some form out onto the skin, or into a catarrhal flow, greatly helping the overall system. In this way, Sulphur should be thought of as not the constitutional remedy but as the "fuse to the bomb," the catalyst that begins the healing. Sulphur helps to show what is happening in the case and probably is not totally curative. The practitioner must watch to see what happens after two, three, or four doses of the medicine. Then he must watch for what may be needed next in terms of an anti-Psoric medicine. A common movement toward cure involves the use of a triad of remedies: Sulphur—Calcarea Carbonica—Lycopodium.

Remember that although Psora is thought to be the most benign miasm, speaking more often to susceptibility to disease than to disease conditions themselves, it is still a difficult miasm to overcome. This is especially true in cases of deep, inherited Psora, which seldom are cured with just one, or even two remedies.

Also, the Psoric patient must use every sort of backup to homeopathic treatment. Changes in diet and exercise are especially important. The Psoric patient must get up and move. Every part of the body that has fallen into dysfunction is improved by movement. Sedentary persons must begin to walk in the fresh air and exercise every day. Alcohol, coffee, and tea are to be avoided, as are sugar and chocolate.

The bad news, in general, for treating Psora: The process can be long and slow with many stops and starts. The good news: More than any other miasmic condition, Psora can be totally and completely reversed.

The Treatment of the Miasm: Sycosis

Sycosis is considered the disease of fig warts. These can appear on any part of the body but are most common on areas that sweat or that rub against clothing or on the genitals. Remember, we are talking about the miasm of Sycosis, not the disease of gonorrhea. These fig warts are a sign of the miasm, as are skin tags. To have either of these surgically removed is to have only the outward sign removed. The inner miasm remains.

The most common remedy used in the treatment of Sycosis is Thuja, which should be given in doses spaced well apart, potencies of below 30C weekly, potencies 30C and above farther apart. Thuja is a remedy of slow, deep action and wild aggravations. You do not want to give it in too high a potency unless that is specifically needed. Wait after giving the dose for a good long time.

From here, the case must be completely individualized to the patient. As Thuja opens the case (just as Sulphur did for Psora), the constitution of the patient becomes more apparent.

Again, the return of old symptoms means the beginning of recovery. Often, treatment of the Sycotic miasm involves aggravations, the temporary worsening of disease symptoms. It is because of these aggravations that wise practitioners give Sycotic remedies, Thuja especially, in low potencies. The aggravation, most especially the aggravation that comes on toward the end of treatment, while uncomfortable, is temporary and a sign of cure.

In Sycosis, as in Psora, when the flow begins, and the miasm manifests in mucus, the patient begins to feel much better overall. The headaches, neuralgias, and rheumatic conditions are lessened or cease altogether.

In treating Sycosis, it is important to stress a vegetarian diet. The only alcohol allowed is beer, which the Sycotic digests more easily than any other alcohol. The patient must drink a great deal of water.

The Treatment of the Miasm: Syphilis

Whether the miasm is latent or active, only constitutional treatment can remove the suppressed conditions of the Syphilitic miasm. Unlike Psora, it is not necessary in Syphilis that the original chancre appear again on the skin. The patient instead may have an ulcerated sore throat as the first real sign that the remedy is working. When the sore throat begins, the deeper problems subside. Also very common is iritis, which may appear instead of the sore throat.

It is very important with the Syphilitic miasm that you be sure of what you are targeting. Sulphur can be used against this miasm if only simple infections are present. If there is a deeper or more chronic infection, the most common homeopathic remedy is Mercurius, created from the metal mercury. Just as mercury was once used in the treatment of Syphilis, Mercurius is a powerful remedy used in the treatment of the miasm Syphilis.

Although dietary restrictions are not as vital in the treatment of Syphilis as they are with the Sycotic miasm, the patient should again be encouraged to drink large amounts of water and avoid foods that are difficult to digest. The diet should include plenty of fruits and vegetables and very little meat. Discourage sugar and salt and all alcohol.

The Treatment of Mixed Miasms

In the blending of the miasms, we find deeply individualized cases. Where one patient may blend Psora and Syphilis and create within himself the Tubercular miasm, another may never blend the two, although he may have Psora latent in his system and Syphilis active and dominant. Therefore, the treatments themselves must be highly individualized and reflect the core homeopathic philosophy of uniquity and wholeness.

But Hahnemann gives us a clue to treatment when he lists three things to look for in each case of mixed miasm:

1. We need to know when the infection took place, if possible. We want to find out whether this condition is inherited, or brought on through vaccination or through suppressive treatments.

2. We must try to uncover the period in which the miasms first made their presence known. When and how did the specific symptoms of the miasms each first appear?

3. We have to learn to recognize the external manifestations of the internal miasms. This tells us the specific manifestations of the miasms upon this individual system.

While I could easily have written hundreds of pages on the miasms and their symptoms, I've given only an overview. But we have to learn what the miasms each look like and how they may be totally individualized within a family unit. Further, we have to learn to look at ourselves, without sacrificing for a moment our unique and whole stance, as part of our own gene pool and as a part of the human system. The New Testament tells us that all Christians are part of the body of Christ. In the same way, we are all part of the body of humanity, with gifts and blessings to share as well as burdens to carry. Only by at last placing ourselves within the context of humanity and making ourselves no more or less worthy and miraculous than everyone else can we bring about a healing of the human body.

The price that we are now paying for the wounding of this human body by our suppressive responses to any pain we experience in our bodies, our minds, or our spirits, is that more and more of us have not just two or three miasms at work. Now there are children in whom all the miasms are present, and one day these children will become parents, parents who will further contribute to the general weight that sits upon their children from birth.

These patients with mixed miasms are, of course, the most difficult to treat. Look for, as the classical homeopaths say, "the weakness of the psoric, the destructiveness of the syphilitic, and the stubbornness of the sycotic" to all be combined in one person's body.

In treating such cases, start with today and try to recognize which miasm is dominant today. A first remedy must be selected on the basis of three or four outstanding symptoms that seem central to the case. Ignore all other symptoms. To uncover what is really going on here, this first remedy is used as Sulphur would be used in a case of simple Psora. If you try from the first to treat the whole case, the sheer number of symptoms at hand will likely keep you from ever coming up with just one remedy to use. That's why you choose to work with the dominant symptoms, as they reflect the dominant miasm. Once this first remedy has caused a healing action within the system, all those other symptoms, the ones that were once ignored, should be taken into consideration and the second remedy selected. This second remedy will be constitutional in nature in that it speaks to the patient's total symptom portrait.

Once you select the constitutional remedy, begin it at the lowest potency that will be effective. Once begun, the potency may be increased as needed. The strictly antimiasmal remedies, however, the nosodes that are used in direct similarity to specific miasms, should not be considered constitutional remedies. They should not be given regularly or ever in low potencies. They should be given only in a single dose and in a high potency to remove the blocks to healing.

———

Kent gives us the best advice concerning the treatment of miasms: "A great deal depends upon a physician's ability to perceive what constitutes a miasm. If he is dull of perception, he will intermingle symptoms that do not belong together."

None of us can work alone for transformation on such a deep level as a miasm. We must find the practitioner who is our perfect partner in transformation, one in whom we trust all the education, skill, and prayer that comes with his practice. The trust that we build in this healing relationship will grow and allow us to experience this trust in every aspect of our lives, where, up to now, we have experienced only anger and fear. The process of transformational healing, after all, allows us to turn our backs on our old lives and to begin walking a path of freedom, of hope, and of love.

CONCLUSION

The homeopath has already dispensed with much of
what is unnecessary and unimportant in orthodox
medicine, but he has yet further to go. I know that you
wish to look forward, for neither the knowledge of the
past nor the present is sufficient for
the seeker after the truth.

—*Edward Bach*

We are on the verge of a homeopathic revival, as we seem more willing than ever before really to stop and take a look at our health system and at our ongoing struggle against disease. That this second look is largely the product of a health care system on the verge of bankruptcy, and of a society that is seeing an increase instead of the promised eradication of infectious disease, makes for a certain urgency in our exploration of "alternative" health systems. And this is certainly a time of great challenge in our global culture. But this challenge, no matter how uncomfortable it makes the present moment and how uncertain it makes our future seem, will be, I believe, our salvation.

There are so many systems already in place: political systems, health systems, religious systems. We have to look finally to the heart of these systems and truly ask ourselves if they serve us as they were intended to, or if we have come to serve them. We have to throw off the condescending notion that the average person is incapable of making real decisions for himself and that what we humans want, in our hearts, is leadership from without. It seems to me that what we truly want, in our heart of hearts, is the ability to be in touch with the leadership within ourselves, the ability to hear that "still, small voice" and the strength to follow its dictates. Because it is the only game in town, we have learned to settle for the exterior leadership.

But now that the old systems seem to be breaking down under their own weight, we have to look for something new, for new ways to solve our same old problems. And part of this search will lead to a homeopathic revival—a revival that has already begun.

This revival will not be without cost. It will involve education: education of laypersons as to the true nature of their selves and reeducation of the professional as to the nature of disease and the treatment of persons with disease. If you think of the money that is already at stake in the health care system and in the maintaining of the status quo in that system, then it is obvious that this change won't come easily. Just as the last barrel of oil will be worth more money than all the other barrels that came before it, so too will the last injection of antibiotic be worth the prices of nations. This, however, will be true only if that barrel of oil and that shot of antibiotic have not already been replaced by some other tool. Those who make their money by the old process will put all the power that their money buys behind the continuing of the status quo, even if in doing so they lead us all down a path toward destruction.

The average person, the one who stands to profit by change and not from the status quo, is charged with taking on the leadership role here. When the old ways begin to break down, the old leaders can be counted on only to lead us in the old direction no matter how ultimately incorrect that direction is. As homeopathy once survived in this country only in the hands of laypersons, the laypersons once again will have to bring it into the forefront; their dollars and how they choose to spend them will largely define the future of medicine. They, unlike the practitioners, have no license to risk and nothing to lose by speaking up. But there are other costs that this change will exact, costs to our quality of life. Think of our desire, in any given moment, to be anesthetized to all pain. We can be healed only if we stop trying to cure things and work with the processes by which the universe is governed. This means that we must also choose to live our lives in ways that make our planet healthy, even if we must give up some of our comforts in order to do so. We simply have to stop seeing ourselves as the center of the universe (how little things have changed from the time we saw the sun revolving around Earth) and start seeing ourselves as one race on a planet with many types of life and as one speck of life in a living universe.

We must dedicate ourselves to this concept of change. We must learn to take responsibility for ourselves as individuals, as societies, and as a race. It's time to grow up.

The study of homeopathy is a lifelong activity. We can never say that we have truly mastered all the aspects of healing and transformation offered through this wonderful method of holistic medicine. In studying homeopathy, we must work equally in two arenas: philosophy and remedies. To be able to use these wonder remedies correctly, always homeopathically, never allopathically, we must be well versed in homeopathic philosophy. And to bring forth the philosophy in an active and dynamic way, we must know our homeopathic pharmacy in order always to be able to choose the needed remedy.

In order to best understand the workings of homeopathy, you should:

- Study *The Organon*. Only by reading Hahnemann's own work can we truly say that we understand the ways homeopathic healings can take place, or indeed what homeopathy truly is. It doesn't matter which translation or edition you use. It matters that you begin your study. If the language of the original translation is too awkward, study a modern translation.
- Study materia medica. Again, it doesn't matter which one. There are many in print, and each reveals the remedies as used by a specific homeopath. Many are in modern language and easy to understand. Pick one and start reading.

It is most important that you come to see the remedies not as groups of symptoms but as representative of individual people. Remedies speak to many physical symptoms, but more, they speak to emotional needs and quirks. These reveal the face of the remedy, the heart of the remedy when studied correctly. Always stress in your study the whole and full portrait of the remedy.

- Learn to use a repertory. Once more, it doesn't matter which one. But even when you are not looking up specific symptoms for a case, open the book. Look at how it is organized. Look what symptoms are included and where and how. As with materia medica, each repertory is the work of one homeopath. Symptoms are grouped as they made sense to that homeopath. So repertories are different from one another. Find the one created by the homeopath whose thinking is closest to how you yourself think. That repertory will be easiest for you to use.
- Find a support group. It becomes doubly difficult to learn homeopathy if you are trying to learn it alone. It is important to have a group—even a group of two or three—to turn to, to use as a sounding board in diagnosis and as a source of insight and argument when studying philosophy.

Twelve years ago, when I began my own study of homeopathy, I knew no one I could turn to for help and support. If my own practitioner had not formed a group of patients, I might never have truly entered into a study of homeopathy. Luckily, the years have brought a greater interest on the part of the general public in homeopathy. There are so many more books in print now then there were twelve years ago, so many more tapes available and lectures to attend. And there are study groups forming throughout the country. If there is one near you, join it. If not, form one. If you don't think that you know enough to start a study group, don't worry about it, just start it. At first, I stayed a page ahead of everyone else in my teaching. Your knowledge will grow through a study group, as well as your wisdom.

Study groups can approach homeopathy from any angle, from the study of *The Organon*, a study of remedies, a mixture of both, or from any other aspect of homeopathy that suits the members.

Most important, study groups offer a support system in which members can call each other for advice and wise council. They are, at their best, healing circles.

■ Experience homeopathic healing in your own life. Even if it is as simple as finding out firsthand that Apis is tremendously curative for a bee sting, each of us needs to experience firsthand the power of homeopathic healing.

For most of us, this means finding a homeopathic practitioner who can work with us as a partner in that healing process. Be sure to find one who understands the principles by which homeopathic cure comes about and who is experienced with the remedies themselves. I find that those who have already experienced homeopathic healings themselves are by far the most sensitive in applying both the principles and the remedies. Find the practitioner who suits your heart and your mind, who honors your words and your innate ability to heal.

Healing, like illness, is a process. Sometimes it is a long and difficult road. But the primary difficulty often seems to be not the symptoms themselves, not the physical pain experienced, but rather responding to the call to change. I have seen many people who decided that homeopathy was not for them. And not one of them, in my experience, turned away from homeopathy because the homeopathic process did not work for him. Rather, they turned away because homeopathy *does* work, because the remedies create change. And that change is very challenging to many people for whom medicine has always offered stasis, a freezing of chronic symptoms under the label of "controlling the progress of disease."

Many of us are professionally ill. Our symptoms, their ebb and flow, are what we do with our lives. Our jobs are how we make money. But our disease represents what we truly do with our lives.

Homeopathy offers a healing from this position of stasis. But it demands change. It demands a willingness to have our symptoms flow through us and past us. It demands that we be willing to stand there, strong and tall, and get on with our lives after our disease has deserted us. For many who define themselves in terms of their disease, this is a difficult notion—that they should have to define themselves by self rather than by symptoms of self.

This is the beauty of homeopathy. It allows us to strip away the layers, to scrape off the old paint and barnacles, and to discover that beneath all that is a strong, healthy, and happy core. It is because of our belief in these three things—strength, health, and happiness—that we study homeopathy.

In the years that I have studied homeopathy, one central idea has pressed itself ever more onto center stage: No matter how much one studies homeopathics, the remedies and their uses, if one does not study homeopathic theory—the philosophy that governs the practice—then one cannot practice homeopathy. You can use these wonderful remedies, and even use them well, but at best you are only practicing allopathy with homeopathic remedies. Your "cures" will be Band-Aids at best, suppressions at worst.

Homeopathy is a science. It is also an art. But above all, it is a philosophy, a way of thinking. Allopathy, for all of its techniques, all of its "medical miracles" and diagnostic tools, lacks a core philosophy, leaving it hollow at its center. The allopathic physician may take a Hippocratic oath, may promise to do no harm, but he promises nothing more, and as he trains himself to view disease dispassionately, he thrusts down his emotions and his spirit in order to practice his craft. Therefore, allopathy may be said to be the science of suppression, both in terms of its actions on the patient's being and on the practitioner's as well. Allopathy not only denies the need for a central philosophy, it ridicules it. The training of a medical doctor denies the very humanity of the future doctor, with inhuman hours and the stressing of the need to remain nonemotional, noninvolved.

Homeopathy offers something unique. It is a medical science whose efficacy has been established, but one that also recognizes the humanity of both the practitioner and the patient. Homeopathic healing demands a true and honest bond between patient and practitioner. In order for the patient to be healed, he must be educated and cared for. The patient must feel comfortable exploring the conundrum of who he is with his homeopathic practitioner. If the homeopath is truly able to identify who this person is *beneath* the surface layers, this person may be healed. In her *Earth Sea Trilogy*, Ursula K. Le Guin offers the theory that each of us is a magician and that we may order each piece of existence, from animal, mineral, and vegetable to man and woman, to do our wishes. They will oblige on one condition: that we call them by their true name. Not the name their parents gave them or they were given by friends in high school—their true name, the one that is written on their heart. This theme in these works of fiction comes close to a definition of the process of homeopathic healing for me: a search for the true name. Some know theirs but are afraid to say it aloud. Some do not say it because anger or hurt has blocked their willingness, and they must be tricked into speech. Some truly do not know their name, and they must search until they find it.

If all this sounds a bit too mystical, then understand why I have hidden this part at the end. It is mystical, I guess, but I also believe that it is the truth. No other healing process can be said to follow the laws of karma as well as does homeopathy. It recognizes through the miasms the baggage that we carry around with us. But more, it recognizes our need to express our true selves while ridding ourselves of this baggage.

If there's one thing I have learned by studying homeopathy, it is this: We have misplaced the center pole that holds up the entire structure. I have written and studied and even taught that the Law of Similars is the core part of homeopathic philosophy. And I was wrong. The core issue here is the need to *express*. Period. Very simple in thought, very hard to bring into reality.

Many of us whose lives seem rutted in the mundane may yearn to express ourselves in painting or poetry. And many have finally become wise enough in our psychotherapy to realize that we must not live in denial and cannot shove down our anger, our fear, our righteous indignation without ultimately creating emotional illness. So, too, we must finally realize that we cannot physically suppress our pain, our symptoms, without creating greater illness. Everything about our natures wishes to express itself, no matter what our life experience has been. If we experience love, we can breathe out wonderful music and laughter and dance. If we breathe in bad air of abuse and anger and fear, we breathe out loud noise and the poetry that comes from wrestling with angels. It is when we do not breathe out, when we hold our breath, that illness begins, that destruction begins. This is denial, suppression. This need to help each and every one of us to learn to express, to breathe out the good *and* the bad, is the heart of homeopathy.

I believe that the most perfect book on homeopathy would be one that never mentions the remedies. Not the Bach flowers or the classical Hahnemannian or the nosodes, sarcodes, or isodes. We need a book on the way we should think in order to get well and to help others get well. Because as long as our thinking is wrong—as long as we continue to search for the perfect homeopathic headache remedy—we cannot practice homeopathy.

Again, back to karma. If you can for a moment accept the philosophy of reincarnation, picture yourself not as a tabula rasa new baby but as an old soul with a new form, perhaps a new gender or skin color—but with old issues, issues to be worked out and a job to get done. This job is one of expression. By this I do not simply mean saying what needs to be said, although this is a part of the process. No, think of this as the physical weights that held down Scrooge's old partner, Jacob Marley, after his death. We are born into new bodies with old weights, and it is the function of our lives to remove those weights by facing them, by forgiving those we can, and asking for forgiveness where we must. By expressing, giving off, breathing out.

Our natural physical response to panic is to hold our breath. Many of us have held our breath for our entire life, as if we have been in a panic since birth. When we are truly honest with ourselves, how many of us are motivated daily by fear or by guilt?

How many of us who immediately answered, "Not me," are also the ones who ask, "Why can't we just have a nice Christmas?" after it has become apparent that there is serious anger or serious communication problems among the members of the family? These are the ones who would rather deny the anger and forestall the communication yet again in the vain hope that a quiet holiday means a loving family. This is denial, this is suppression, this is holding your breath.

I can remember all three of these—fear, guilt, and denial—as the three fates that so long governed my life. And I can remember years of having my life controlled and defined by disease. My illness told me what I could and could not do, as my own limitations limited the lives of those around me. I sought help. Honestly, I was the allopath's greatest fan. I went from one to another, happy for the moment of attention that each gave me, happy for each new medicine. But I didn't get any better. It wasn't until I got sick enough of being sick that I tried something that seemed ridiculous, something that I had made fun of, and something that ultimately worked.

What I see clearly now is that allopathy could not work for me because it involved suppression, not just of my physical symptoms but of my entire being—body, mind, and spirit. It was this very denial of being that was making me sick to begin with. I also see now that, while the homeopathic remedies I have been given over the years—and, believe me, I have been given them all at one time or another, in both wise and stupid prescriptions from wise and foolish practitioners—have been helpful in my healing process, it was truly the increasing expression of my being that brought about healing and continues to bring me healing daily. In other words, I attribute my own healing much more to homeopathic philosophy than I do to homeopathic remedies.

We need to live in a homeopathic way. We need to be true to ourselves and to others. We need to stop fearing ourselves and our emotions. We need to stop trying to avoid every bit of our pain and just let ourselves experience it. (To this day, people look at me shocked—both allopathic and homeopathic people—when I have a migraine and they ask me what I've taken for it and I say I don't take anything for it.) If our entire culture is built on anything at all, it's built on denial. We are a culture not only of painkillers that are made to look like candy, but also one that numbs the fears at the end of the day with a goodly dose of television. I'm not saying that these things don't have a place, but that place should not be on the altar of our lives.

Enough. Study homeopathy. Learn all the wacky words and terms and latinizations. It's fun, and it makes you feel as if you belong to a club, a secret society of sorts. Get involved in the politics. Learn to yell and scream and demand your rights as a free and intelligent being to control the health of your body, your mind, and your spirit. Become a partner in your own health. Learn the remedies. Not just as representatives of clumps of symptoms, but as representative of people. There are always those who can immediately tell you which remedy to think of when you see a red, swollen, hot bump. They're screaming "Apis" right now. But if we cannot see the human who needs the substance Apis to balance his being, then we cannot practice homeopathy. These remedies and their actions represent two things:

1. Human beings who themselves have a particular set of symptoms and a particular central issue of need.

2. The vital force of all things natural, from water to trees to rocks to the Earth itself. An energy that is truly alive.

The curative power of the remedies themselves is nothing but their aspect of vital force. That's how they can affect our vital force.

So study the remedies, and get to know them as people, not facts or lists of symptoms. But most important of all, study the theory of homeopathy. Learn the consequences of suppression.

Think about that for a moment: the consequences of suppression. If we as a culture could wrestle with that for a bit, think of the changes that could come about. And not just in terms of creating new careers in homeopathy.

Learn to express. Learn the philosophy of homeopathy. It is an insidious course of study. It begins by transforming medicine as you practice it. Then it worms its way into your diet and exercise program. Then it interferes with your TV and movie viewing, as you sit there thinking, "She's such an Arsenicum." And then it gets into your dreams.

Finally, and this is the really good part, it becomes part of your breathing.

A REDEFINITION OF
TERMS

I n beginning a study of homeopathy, we must first agree on the meaning of certain words, some of which, in slightly different ways, are used daily, others of which are peculiar to homeopathy.

TERMS RELATING TO HOMEOPATHIC PHILOSOPHY

Healing Versus Curing

In the second paragraph of *The Organon*, Hahnemann defines **curing:** "The highest ideal of cure is rapid, gentle and permanent restoration of the health or removal and annihilation of the disease in the whole extent, in the shortest, most reliable and most harmless way."

Modern homeopath George Vithoulkas refers to **healing** as "the restoration of happiness." Also simply as "freedom." He would have us see that healing involves the spiritual as well as the physical plane. Whereas Hahnemann, while acknowledging the spirit as the home of all illness, places

293

the physician's role (in the first paragraph of *The Organon*) in the physical realm: "The physician's high and only mission is to restore the sick to health, to cure, as it is termed."

Homeopathy Versus Allopathy

Homeopathy is derived from two Greek words, *homios*, meaning "similar" and *pathos* meaning "suffering." The term, as coined by Samuel Hahnemann, means "similar suffering." It refers to the first law of homeopathic cure, the Law of Similars: "Like cures like."

Allopathy is another medical term coined by Samuel Hahnemann and in popular use today. It also is derived from two Greek words: *allos*, meaning "different," and *pathos*.

Uniquity and Wholeness

Together, these two concepts reach the heart of homeopathy. While we often strive to heal ourselves with homeopathic remedies, we forget that the best-prepared homeopathic remedy *ceases to be homeopathic if it is used with allopathic methods*. By understanding both the concepts of uniquity and wholeness, we better prepare ourselves to adhere to the methods of homeopathic health.

The homeopath always treats the patient and not the sickness. The key to the treatment is in all that makes such a patient **unique**. When entering a homeopath's office, be prepared to answer questions that may seem a bit odd at first—matters of thirst, cravings and aversions, sleep positions, etc.

These questions help the homeopath learn as much about you as he can, to identify all the things about you that make you unique. Because, to a homeopath, we are all unique beings. The ways you remain healthy or become ill may or may not have anything to do with the ways I do the same. The ways you express an illness—the symptoms—may be very different from the ways I express the same illness.

Along this same line of thinking, we have the concept of **wholeness**. Allopathic thinking has, over the last fifty years or so, managed to divide us into many parts, many organs or systems of organs. To the homeopath, you are one whole being, and *no two symptoms can ever be unconnected in a whole being*. Therefore, when you are treated by a homeopath, your symptoms must all be considered. If your head hurts on the right side at 4 P.M.

and your legs twitch in bed at night, both of these symptoms are considered as equal parts of the whole being's condition.

That's why we never see homeopathic specialists, homeopathic heart specialists, or homeopathic allergists. Homeopathy rejects the concept of specialists and demands that the homeopath always look at the whole person.

When you are treated by a homeopath, you are treated as a unique and whole being, almost a universe unto yourself, a universe that runs by its own laws of harmony. The homeopath envisions the proper running of this unique being and brings the energy of that being back into balance.

Symptoms

In allopathy, symptoms represent the domination of illness over our bodies. In homeopathy, **symptoms** are considered to be good things. In the first place, they are the sign that our immune systems have kicked in to combat the disease. But more, they help to identify, through the specific symptoms displayed, the uniqueness of our nature. The manifestation of specific symptoms points the homeopath to the specific remedy needed to bring about the cure.

Further, for the homeopath, not all symptoms need to be painful. General hunger or thirst is an important symptom, as is body temperature or sleep position. None of these things has any direct connection to disease, yet all are important symptoms and may well lead the homeopath to the correct remedy.

A symptom or set of symptoms may be most clearly defined as the way or ways the body is expressing its unique and whole state. As long as we are alive, whether we are well or sick, we always are expressing symptoms.

Vital Force

There is in each of us an invisible force that allows our bodies to sustain life. Many cultures and healing systems include this concept—the dynamism of the ancient Greeks, the *chi* of Chinese medicine. Hahnemann referred to this as **vital force:** "In the healthy condition of man, the spiritual vital force, the dynamism that animates the material body, rules with unbounded sway, and retains all the parts of the organism in admirable, harmonious, vital operation as regards both sensations and functions, so that our indwelling, reason-gifted mind can freely employ this living, healthy instrument for higher purposes of our existence."

TERMS RELATING TO CASE TAKING

Case Taking

For the homeopath, the skills of **case taking** and repertorization are vital to the ability to select the correct remedy. The skill particular to case taking is that of being able truly to connect with your patient, the ability to completely listen to what the patient is telling you, as well as being able to use your own senses—vision, smell, hearing, and, often, touch—to take in all that comprises the "being" of the patient.

In taking the case, the homeopath learns what state is considered to be healthy by this particular patient and how the present circumstances differ from this norm.

Two books are essential after the case has been taken, the repertory and the materia medica. Both come in many forms and from many authors. This lack of standardization in these texts, far from weakening the homeopath's ability to cure, actually strengthens it. For homeopaths, like patients, are unique beings, and the many choices available to them in the form of homeopathic texts allow each to select the unique volume that can best be his tool for cure.

The **materia medica** is an alphabetical listing of remedy portraits. Each remedy is listed by Latin name and common name. Following is an overview of the actions that this particular remedy has been seen to have on humans.

The **repertory** lists symptoms. Following each symptom is a list of all remedies that have been shown effective for that symptom.

When the homeopath takes the information that he has gathered by matching the picture of symptoms (as found in the repertory) that are being experienced by the patient to the remedy portrait found in the materia medica, he can determine the remedy that will be helpful to the patient.

Modalities

Modalities are an important part of any case taking. Modalities can be part of our personal environment that affects us for better or worse. For the homeopath, there are two types of modality.

In our day-to-day lives, **modalities of being** are what make us feel better and what make us feel worse. Some persons are better when being touched; they want their neck rubbed when they feel stressed. Other people do not want to be touched and are worse when another person comes close. There are many types of modalities of being, the chief among them time of day (high and low energy), weather (changes of weather pattern, change of seasons), hunger, thirst, and sleep.

Modalities of symptoms speak specifically to the cluster of disease symptoms being experienced at the present moment. Therefore, the homeopath may ask what makes the sore throat feel better, hot or cold liquids. He may ask the patient if he feels warm, cool, or cold during the fever state. In acute treatments, modalities of symptoms are most helpful in determining treatment. In constitutional care, however, both modalities of symptoms and of being need to be discussed and considered.

Types of Disease

Kent says that "the first prescription is easy." By this he means that, with a modicum of ability in the arena of case taking, almost anyone should be able to find the first remedy to open a case. But, as the layers unfold, it is important to have the knowledge of chronic cases and miasmic medicine in order to treat effectively. For the homeopath, the knowledge of what constitutes an acute or chronic case is key.

Acute disease is a short story. The disease overwhelms the vital force in such a way as to have a beginning, a middle, and an end. This does not, however, mean that acute diseases are by nature mild. The ending of an acute condition may well be death.

Chronic disease is a soap opera. The disease condition here, once established, is not relieved by anything other than the death of the patient or proper homeopathic care.

Types of Treatment

Acute remedies speak to acute ailments. The usual functioning of the being has been changed by the rising of the vital force to offset disease. The symptoms, representing a new, unnatural "being" imposed on the natural person of the patient, are treated by a substance similar to their own actions, bringing about cure.

Constitutional remedies speak to the long-term being of the patient, the symptoms that have been in place for months or years. The remedies are so named in that one well-selected remedy speaks to the entire being—or constitution—of the patient.

Constitutional remedies may well shift throughout the lifetime of a person. Illness, trauma, accidents, and the like may create a new constitutional being. The constitutional types can layer one over another, decade after decade, like the layers of an onion. Through wise homeopathic treatment, a patient can move back through layers of illness to a core of health.

Because constitutional remedies do transform one into another throughout life, there may be said to be a third kind of remedy, the **birth remedy**. This is the remedy that speaks to the genetics specific to the child at birth, before life experiences transform the patient's being into other remedy pictures. It is important to have an idea of the birth remedy of a patient in a chronic case, because this is the target for the patient once he is cured. When the case is cleared, the patient arrives once again at the remedy of birth, this time in balance and health.

The homeopath must know the difference between acute and constitutional prescribing. A series of what may seem to be acute situations—ear infections, colds, specific pains, etc.—may instead be the signs of a deeper, chronic condition.

Miasms

For our purposes, consider **miasms** to be genetic weakness, inherited predisposition to specific diseases.

Miasms represent family illness, traits that are found exactly or similarly within many members of the same family. Therefore, if all members of a family have allergies, in treating a member of that family you may have to select a remedy that speaks to the family as well as to that one member of the family.

Miasmic cures are deep cures that reach down to the true cause of disease rather than deal with only the symptoms of that disorder. They are treatments that attempt to undo generations of suppressive treatments and suppressed diseases.

Most miasms relate to suppressed venereal diseases, syphilis and gonorrhea, and to the toll that the suppression of these diseases causes to future generations. (Remember, the miasm is an inborn weakness and not the disease itself; therefore, the person with the gonorrheal miasm may never have or have had gonorrhea.) Other miasms relate to specific diseases, tuberculosis and cancer. Hahnemann's first-discovered miasm, called Psora, relates to suppressed skin conditions and to the earliest diseases and allopathic treatments known to man.

Therefore, there may be said to be three levels of homeopathic treatment: acute, constitutional, and miasmic. The miasmic level of treatment is the deepest and most profound, with the greatest possibility of being truly transformational.

TERMS RELATING TO CARETAKING

The Laws of Cure

Homeopathy is practiced in many different ways by many different types of practitioners, but Hahnemann has laid down three laws by which homeopathy is properly practiced.

The Law of Similars states that like cures like. The *disease picture* of a case, the totality of the symptoms, is matched against the *remedy picture*, or full range of symptoms that a specific remedy treats. When these two match, cure takes place. Cure is the total removal of disease symptoms, the rapid, gentle, and permanent restoration of health.

The Law of Simplex states that the wise homeopath gives one remedy at a time. That well-chosen remedy speaks to the full range of symptoms that the patient is experiencing.

The Law of Minimum states that the properly selected remedy should be given in the lowest potency possible to effect cure and in the least number of doses possible to effect cure.

In general, the rule is that when a properly selected remedy has been given, the patient should stop taking the remedy just as soon as improvement has taken place. Therefore, homeopathics are always given "as needed." The remedy is repeated when symptoms begin once again to come forth. It is an allopathic concept that you should take your remedy twice a day for thirty days. This practice should always be questioned, if not refused.

As we have all seen, many health food stores sell homeopathic medicines that are made from several different remedies all gathered together around a common ailment, like allergy or insomnia. These medicines, by their very nature, break the Law of Simplex and can be considered sloppy homeopathy at best. While these medicines are helpful in acute emergency situations, if taken for a brief period of time, in the long term they not only stop being of any help at all but can actually complicate the case, making it far more difficult to resolve.

Potencies are chosen with five criteria in mind:

- Strength of vital force
- Physical nature of the disease
- Spiritual nature of the disease
- Chronic versus acute nature of the disease
- Kentian octave

Kentian octave: Homeopath James T. Kent noted a traditional progression of potency in the cure of chronic disease. He used the same remedy in eight increasing stages of potency: 6C, 9C, 12C, 30C, 200C, 1M, 10M, LM, CM. Cure often came about when, after CM potency had been reached, the patient once more took the 9C dosage.

Hering's Law

Named for Constantine Hering, a German-born homeopath and contemporary of Hahnemann's who moved his practice to Philadelphia, **Hering's law** states that cure takes place in the following ways:

- From the top of the head down to the bottom of the feet
- From the inside out—from the most important organs to the least important, the skin
- From the most recent symptoms to the most long term

Arndt-Schultz Law

The **Arndt-Schultz law** refers to biological activity and provides justification for the use of minute doses. The law states that small doses of drugs encourage life activity. Large material doses of drugs impede life activity, and very large doses destroy life activity. To put it simply, the size of the dose of the drug is inversely proportional to the positive effect of the drug.

SCHOOLS OF HOMEOPATHIC PRACTICE

Homeopathy today is made up of many types of practice, some of which would no doubt make Samuel Hahnemann regret ever having had any of these notions to begin with. Much of what is called homeopathy today would have been considered allopathic by the practitioners of Hahnemann's day. Certainly those who treat with combination remedies, or mix homeopathic remedies with herbal preparations, or who prescribe remedies based on simple pathology or deficiency, would have been considered allopaths by Hahnemann.

The **unicist school** of homeopathic practice advises the prescription of one remedy at a time, in keeping with Hahnemann's own Laws of Cure. This group is considered "classical" in its approach. The irony here is that the unicists consider themselves to be the only homeopaths and consider the pluralist school to be practicing a bastardized form of homeopathy at best, and pure allopathy at worst. The unicist school itself is divided into two groups.

The **pure Hahnemannian school** holds to the full doctrine of inductive practice and is science based. In practice, the homeopath gives only one remedy at a time, either in a single or repeated dose.

The **Kentian school** follows the practice of James Tyler Kent, perhaps America's greatest contributor to homeopathy, who blended his study of homeopathy with the philosophy of Swedenborg, adding a mystical layer to Hahnemann's doctrine of practice. Kentians tend to practice by giving one high-potency dose of the suggested remedy.

The **pluralist school** is the other major school of homeopathic philosophy. It looks more to the disease and the treatment of disease than to the person who is experiencing the disorder in health. In this manner and in their practice of medicine, the pluralists are far more similar to modern allopaths than to classical homeopaths. In practice, pluralists give more than one remedy at a time and may blend the use of homeopathics with that of herbal, energetic, or even allopathic medicines.

DRUGS, MEDICINES, AND REMEDIES

The terms *drug, medicine,* and *remedy* are all used freely in homeopathy, but they are not used interchangeably.

A **drug** is an unpolished substance. It is the herb itself, in the case of such drugs as feverfew or valerian.

Medicine is the polished drug, which has been potentized into the form of a homeopathic medicine. Drugs are "polished" in a two-step process.

In *dilution,* the drug is dissolved in water or alcohol, whichever is most successful as a medium, and then diluted with water. For remedies of the X scale of potency, the drug is diluted with 1 part substance to 9 parts water. For the C scale potencies, dilution is 1 part substance to 99 parts water. For potencies of the M scale, dilution is 1 part substance to 999 parts water.

Succussion is the process in which the diluted substance releases its healing energy. Succussion is basically shaking the diluted preparation. Hahnemann set down specific methods by which succussion would take place, methods that are still in use today. Hahnemann succussed his remedies with a quick turn of the wrist, followed by slamming the solution down on a leatherbound Bible.

The process of dilution and succussion together releases the curative effects of the remedy, while leaving the toxic nature of the drug itself behind. Research has shown us that, by the 12C level of potency, none of the original substance remains in the remedy. What remains, instead, is the energy pattern, the healing energy.

I confess that I haven't the vaguest idea how such a process could work. I also don't know how my CD player works. But, like my CD player, I know that this process *does* work, however it happens. I have seen the remedies work time and again, on animals as well as on humans, on believers as well as on those who think that homeopathy is one step below voodoo.

A **remedy** is an indicated medicine. When the homeopathic medicine appropriate to your specific case is identified and taken from the homeopathic pharmacy, that medicine is referred to as a remedy.

A *similar* is any one of a group of remedies, all of which may speak to a majority of a patient's symptoms, and any of which may move the patient closer to health.

The *simillimum* is the exact, correct remedy, given in the exact, correct potency and the exact, correct number of doses to effect a total cure.

The Remedies: Preparations and Potencies

The homeopathic medicines are prepared in specific potencies on three basic scales.

Mother tincture is raw substance diluted in water or alcohol or ground into powder with milk sugar. This is the 0 potency from which all other potencies are made through dilution and succussion.

The **decimal scale** is a system of dilution in which the ratio of substance to water (or alcohol) is 1:9. At each level, one part of the diluted substance is diluted again at the same ratio. The decimal scale is referred to with an X.

On the **centesimal scale**, the ratio of dilution is 1:99, 1 part substance to 99 parts water. The levels of dilution are the same as above, only the ratio of dilution changes. The centesimal scale is referred to with a C.

The **millennial scale** is a continuation of the C scale. The step in dilution after 999C, instead of being called 1,000C is called 1M, standing for the Roman numeral for 1,000. The scale then continues to 10M, LM (50,000 dilutions), and CM (100,000 dilutions). This scale is referred to with an M.

A central mystery of homeopathic healing is that the more diluted the substance becomes, the more potent the homeopathic remedy. Therefore, the M-scale remedies are vastly more powerful than the X-scale remedies. And so, too, is the M scale's power of aggravation in the curing of a case. This scale, therefore, is to be used sparingly and wisely.

All homeopathic remedies taken orally are placed in their liquid form onto beads of milk sugar. When dried, these pellets are placed on or under the patient's tongue. Hahnemann chose milk sugar because his experiments identified it as the least medicinal substance he could find. Colored pellets are never used; Hahnemann felt that the coloring process itself created a medicinal effect.

Homeopathic remedies should never be touched by the hands of either the patient or the practitioner. Instead, the number of pellets desired, usually two or three, should be tipped from the remedy bottle into that bottle's cap and then dropped onto the patient's tongue. Not touching the pellets ensures that no chemical of any sort, perfume or otherwise, damages the remedy's potency before the dose is injested.

Provings

The methods by which homeopathic remedies are tested on healthy human subjects are called **provings**. Hahnemann was the pioneer in the concept of testing medicines on healthy humans. Subjects in a double-blind study are given a remedy on a regular basis (usually for twelve weeks). They keep a strict diary of how that remedy alters their usual symptom structure, how their energy, cravings, etc., are changed. The diaries are compiled to see the dominant actions of the remedy.

Proving may also come about by the unwise use of a homeopathic remedy in treatment of illness. If the remedy is taken too often, or repeated after the illness has been removed, symptoms reappear, just as they did for those who originally tested the remedy. These provings are temporary, however, and disappear as soon as the patient stops taking the remedy.

Aggravations

When a proper homeopathic remedy is employed, the patient may at first experience a temporary worsening of his symptoms. This flare-up of symptoms is called an **aggravation**. Many modern homeopaths use these aggravations as a guidepost to having selected the correct remedy, but classical homeopaths sought to avoid aggravations because they felt that any pain led to a weakening of the overall system.

Aggravations, by their very nature, are a sign that the correct remedy has been given but in too high a potency. They should never last more than two or three days at most, except in cases of the remedies called nosodes, in which aggravations may continue for longer periods of time.

Antidotes

Most people as they begin their study of homeopathics obsess about **antidotes** to homeopathic remedies. I guess it's only natural to worry that all your good work would be for nothing if some evil substance came along and antidoted you just as you were feeling better. Although there are some substances that antidote homeopathic remedies, and temporarily put a stop to cure, there are not enough to panic over.

Coffee is a pretty sure antidote. It is not the caffeine, but something in the bean itself that makes it a sure antidote. Generally speaking, you will be antidoted by coffee in proportion to the impact that coffee normally has on your system. If you get a buzz from just one cup, chances are that one cup will antidote a dose of any homeopathic remedy. If your system is not affected by coffee, coffee will not have a great impact on your remedy dose.

Camphor is another pretty sure antidote. From tiger balm to mothballs, anything with camphor in it antidotes homeopathic remedies.

From your television to your computer, just about all electronic devices emit a radiation field. As homeopathic remedies are energy medicines, these electromagnetic fields can affect the potency of any remedy taken.

Other than that, it is a matter of sensitivity. Some people are so sensitive that they can be antidoted by any strong smell, particularly perfumes and mint. Some have problems with garlic. Others have problems with none of these.

As with most everything in homeopathy, it is an individual experience. When you start out on a cure, plan to avoid coffee and get rid of all camphor products. From there, check your own sensitivity to the many chemicals and toxins in your environment.

THE SIGNS OF CURE

Homeopathic cure always starts with today, with the totality of symptoms and with the being of the person who is being treated today. Homeopathic cure is based on the expression of symptoms that heretofore have been suppressed. Therefore, when a cold is treated homeopathically, the symptoms are not denied, as they are through the use of antihistamines and other traditional medicines. Rather, the symptoms move through very quickly, flush out of the patient's system, and are gone. In this way, in the homeopathic cure of chronic conditions, it is often necessary to revisit past symptoms, symptoms that have been suppressed by years of allopathic care. These symptoms, too, are revisited rapidly and with far less violence then they once held.

When under homeopathic treatment, the following signs show a movement to cure:

■ **An increase in energy.** Whether an aggravation takes place, and whether symptoms continue, the homeopath looks for the patient to say, "I just feel better. I have more energy. I can cope better with my condition."

■ **Increased clarity of the mind.** Again, homeopathic cure does not mean instant cure. But, as the well-selected remedy takes effect, the patient should report that he feels more like himself. Memory should clear. Concentration should improve.

■ **Improvement of the being.** While specific symptoms may take time to remove, the patient should report an increased wholeness, an improved sense of being.

■ **Clearing of symptoms.** As Hering states, the most recent symptoms are usually the first to be removed. Long-term symptoms are harder to remove and may require repeated constitutional care. The ailment moves from the mind down to the body and from the more important organs— brain, heart, lungs—to the less important organs—muscle, extremities, skin. When the ailment finally moves out onto the skin, usually with a rash of some sort, it is a sign that cure is nearby. Treating that rash now suppresses the work of cure that has been done to date. The rash allowed to run its course carries the disease away with it.

■ **The pentimento effect.** As a patient under constitutional care moves from remedy to remedy, the transitional state is one of pentimento. As with a painting that has been painted over another and after a period of time begins to bleed through the second work, so, too, when a patient is moving back through past suppressions, you see the clear picture of a constitutional remedy begin to be muddied by the expression of the symptoms of the chronic layer beneath the one now being cleared away. The wise practitioner knows when to move from one remedy to another and how to identify the clearing of each layer. This is perhaps the hardest part of constitutional care.

In short, the goal of homeopathic care is the total restoration of health as experienced by a unique and whole being. When health is achieved, homeopathic typing does not cease. It is not like a symptom, which is cleared away and disappeares. It is more like a sign of the zodiac. We are all born at a specific time and with our own unique astrological chart. In the same way, we are all born with a specific homeopathic type. And within the range of types, there is also a range of health and wholeness. Therefore, it is as possible to be a healthy, happy, and functioning Sulphur type as it is to be a sick, unhappy, and nonfunctioning Sulphur type. It is not the task of homeopathy to remove every unique symptom from the patient. It is the job of the homeopath to remove all *symptoms of illness* from the patient. The patient remains a unique, whole, and healthy individual, whose being is still described in the form of a homeopathic type.

BIBLIOGRAPHY

The books gathered here are all recommended reading on the topic of homeopathy. Each has informed and enlightened me in some way or other. While this list is certainly not exhaustive, I have tried my best to gather together the works on various aspects of homeopathy that I feel belong in the home of any serious student of homeopathy.

BOOKS ON HOMEOPATHIC PHILOSOPHY

Aubin, Michel, and Philippe Picard. *Homeopathy: A Different Way of Treating Common Ailments*. Bath, England: Ashgrove Press, 1989. An interesting work, which includes a fascinating section, "How I Became a Homeopathic Doctor." It avoids the oversimplification of remedies by listing their unique combination of symptoms as "syndromes."

Bach, Edward. *The Collected Writings of Edward Bach*. Hereford, England: Bach Educational Programme, 1987. Bach's writings span his work as an allopath, a homeopath, and the developer of the Bach flower remedies. More important, his writing style is readable and highly enjoyable, and his topic encompasses the basic principles of healing rather than just his own work as a physician. An excellent book.

Cook, Trevor M. *Homeopathic Medicine Today: A Modern Course of Study.* New Canaan, CT: Keats, 1989. A good basic guide to the philosophy of homeopathy and how it came to be. Cook is one of the leaders of the homeopathic revival worldwide and is particularly respected as a homeopathic educator.

Coulter, Harris. *Divided Legacy: A History of the Schism in Medical Thought.* 4 volumes. Berkeley: North Atlantic, 1975, 1977, 1981, 1994. While not strictly speaking a book of homeopathic philosophy, no student should be without this set. Coulter gives the political, cultural, and philosophical history of homeopathy as no one else has. His writing is fascinating, making this exhaustive history easy to read. Coulter is the most respected homeopathic historian now living and is a noted homeopathic educator.

Eizayaga, Francisco Xavier. *Treatise on Homeopathic Medicine.* Buenos Aires: Ediciones Marecel, 1991. Eizayaga is perhaps the most influential practitioner of homeopathy at work today. This thin volume gives his take on the history of homeopathic philosophy as well as his insights into case taking and practice.

Hahnemann, Samuel. *The Organon of Medicine.* Translated by William Boericke. New Delhi: B. Jain Publishers, 1991. There are several editions of *The Organon* available. The fifth edition was completed and published before Hahnemann's death, and it was several years until the sixth was published. It is important that students of homeopathy use either the sixth or the combined fifth and sixth editions. Different publishing houses publish the book. The Indian publisher B. Jain makes the book available at the lowest cost. This is the single most important book on homeopathic philosophy, without which the others could not exist.

————. *The Organon of Medicine.* Translated by Jost Kunzli, Alain Naude, and Peter Pendleton. Blaine, WA: Cooper Publishing, 1982. This edition of *The Organon* is a new translation of the work, not just a new edition. I suggest that this edition be used along with the older Boericke edition, in the way a modern-language Bible might be used alongside a King James.

Hardy, Mary, and Dotty Nonman. *The Alchemist's Handbook to Homeopathy.* Allegan, MI: Delta K Trust, 1994. A very odd book. It explains the philosophy and use of homeopathy based in alchemy. The second half of the book has an alphabetical listing of ailments, with a list of remedies for use with each. While I would not suggest this book to a beginner, it is of value to those who have already learned homeopathy as Hahnemann wrote it.

Kent, James Tyler. *Lectures on Homeopathic Philosophy.* Berkeley: North Atlantic, 1979. This book is second in importance only to Hahnemann's. Kent takes on the major points of homeopathic treatment, susceptibility, similarity, and the like and presents them in a format that is both readable and practical for professionals and laypersons alike.

Roberts, H. A. *The Principles and Art of Cure by Homeopathy.* New Delhi: B. Jain

Publishers. As do many Indian homeopaths, Roberts closely follows Kent's philosophy of homeopathic practice. He bases his book on Kent's and simplifies it for the layperson.

Vithoulkas, George. *The Science of Homeopathy*. New York: Grove, 1980. As the title suggests, this book is of particular interest to those who are well grounded in modern science and wish to understand homeopathy within that context.

Whitmont, Edward C. *The Alchemy of Healing: Psyche and Soma*. Berkeley: North Atlantic, 1993. This is deep philosophy that concerns itself with healing and uses homeopathy as a tool to that healing.

———. *Psyche and Substance: Essays on Homeopathy in the Light of Jungian Psychology*. Berkeley: North Atlantic, 1991. This book contains the principles of homeopathic philosophy and blends them with the principles of Jungian psychology and ancient alchemy. While this book is certainly not an easy read, it is valuable for its descriptions of constitutional remedies.

Wood, Matthew. *The Magical Staff: The Vitalist Tradition in Western Medicine*. Berkeley: North Atlantic, 1992. A very interesting book that is more of a history than an exact study of homeopathic philosophy. It is, however, an in-depth study of the vitalist tradition, which is a foundation of homeopathy. The book contains seven short histories of leading healers, each of whom contributed to our understanding of energy healing.

REPERTORIES

Beginning students of homeopathy often make the mistake of buying books only about acute remedies, and when household crises occur, run to their bookcase and open these books, hoping to match the symptoms of the crisis to the brief descriptions listed. But anyone who has any true interest in homeopathy must have a materia medica and a repertory on the shelf next to *The Organon*. Only by learning to use both the repertory and the materia medica can you ever really learn anything about using the remedies.

But remember, each repertory and each materia medica represents only the notes of an individual practitioner. There is no one definitive repertory or materia medica. Find the repertory that is structured in the manner that makes the most sense to you. The same with the materia medica. The more you think like the author of the book, the more easily you will be able to use that book. So look through several and then select the one that is easiest for you to use.

Kent, James Tyler. *Repertory of the Homeopathic Materia Medica*. New Delhi: B. Jain Publishers, 1986. This is the basic repertory and probably the one most often used worldwide. It is a good basic repertory and the least expensive of the group. It lists symptoms from the top of the head to the bottom of the feet, moving down the body.

Murphy, Robin. *Homeopathic Medical Repertory*. Pagosa Springs, CO: HANA, 1993. Murphy's repertory revolutionized the field. It is organized in an alphabetized dictionary format, making it much easier to use than early repertories. This book, however, is costly, and is not often recommended for beginners.

Schroyens, F. *Synthesis Repertorium*. London: Homeopathic Book Publishers, 1993. This work pulls together symptoms rubrics from several sources, making it the largest, if not the most complete, one-volume repertory. Although this is an excellent resource, it is most often used by homeopathic professionals and not by laypersons.

Van Zandvoort, Roger. *The Complete Repertory*. 3 volumes. Leidschendam, Netherlands: IRHIS, 1994. An extraordinarily detailed work generally considered to be the most complete repertory available.

MATERIA MEDICA

Again, there are a wide range of books available on homeopathic remedies. They are structured in many different ways and should be selected on the basis of this structure as well as on the number and type of remedies included. As all these books still represent the experience of one person concerning the remedies, it is wise for the serious student of homeopathy to own more than one. One author's insights into Lycopodium may be very different from another's.

Bailey, Philip. *Homeopathic Psychology: Personality Profiles of the Major Constitutional Remedies*. Berkeley: North Atlantic, 1995. An odd combination of materia medica and personal memoir. This work gives the author's insights into some three dozen remedy types, based on his work as a practitioner.

Boericke, William. *Pocket Manual of Materia Medica with Repertory*. New Delhi: B. Jain Publishers, 1996. This is the basic homeopathic materia medica, the one that most of us first own before going on to other, more complete volumes. As an inexpensive introduction to the remedies, it is excellent, although in the long run it leaves a lot to be desired. The repertory portion of the book is poor.

Coulter, Catherine. *Portraits of Homeopathic Medicines*. 2 volumes. Berkeley: North Atlantic, 1986, 1988. These two volumes give unique insights into the twenty or so remedies included. As much a memoir of her practice as a materia medica, Coulter's work gives casework and examples from popular culture in addition to listing symptoms and motivations of the types.

Hahnemann, Samuel. *Materia Medica Pura*. 2 volumes. New Delhi: B. Jain Publishers, 1989. You might think that Samuel Hahnemann's own two-volume materia medica would be the best, but, in that it contains only those sixty-odd remedies in use in Hahnemann's own practice, today it is more of a curiosity than a helpful materia medica. Some of our most used polycrests are included here, like

Suphur and Lyopodium, but some obscure and forgotten remedies have found their way in as well, like Magneis Polis Arcticus and Australis, remedies created from the north and south poles of a magnet.

Hering, Constantine. *Guiding Symptoms of Our Materia Medica.* 10 volumes. New Delhi: B. Jain Publishers. This is Hering's masterwork and one of the grand operas of homeopathy. It is, however, a rather burdensome work and well beyond the need of all but the most serious student or practitioner of homeopathy.

Jouanny, Jacques. *The Essentials of Homeopathic Materia Medica.* Boiron S A France: Boiron, 1984. Jouanny gives his insights into the homeopathic materia medica from the standpoint of a French physician. This is of particular interest to Americans who have been trained only in Kent's method of homeopathic treatment.

Kent, James Tyler. *Lectures on Homeopathic Materia Medica.* New Delhi: B. Jain Publishers, 1986. Sadly, Kent never wrote a materia medica. But this volume captures the lectures that Kent gave his students on specific remedies, and it is a great tool to understanding and using homeopathic remedies.

Mathur, K. N. *Systematic Materia Medica of Homeopathic Remedies with Totality of Characteristic Symptoms and Various Indications of Each Remedy.* New Delhi: B. Jain Publishers, 1988. The book is as long as its title and gives all the information promised. While other materia medicae are more in-depth, I probably turn to this volume, which combines the information so well and so simply, more than I do any other.

Morrison, Roger. *Desktop Guide to Keynotes and Confirmatory Symptoms.* Berkeley: Hahnemann, 1993. An excellent book. Morrison's text is clear and simple enough for laypersons and detailed enough for professionals. This is a book you will turn to again and again.

Murphy, Robin. *Lotus Materia Medica.* Pagosa Springs, CO: HANA, 1995. Murphy combines the listing of Hahnemann's remedies with Bach's and other floral remedies, as well as alchemical remedies. Although this makes for a very interesting study, with many anecdotes concerning the history and use of both substances and remedies, it can be confusing.

Nash, E. B. *Leaders in Homeopathic Therapies.* New Delhi: B. Jain Publishers. This is one of the real classics in the field of homeopathy. Although it does not list all the remedies, those listed (a hundred or so) are given a very clear and consise treatment. A great secondary volume for your library.

Tyler, Margaret. *Drug Pictures.* Saffron Walden, England: C. W. Daniel, 1952. This is sort of a combination materia medica and memoir. It is very much a classic volume and of great interest to any student of homeopathy.

Vermuelen, Frans. *Concordance Matieria Medica.* Haarlem, Netherlands: Merlijn Publishers, 1994. This is a modern work that seeks to update Boericke's materia medica and to draw upon several sources in making a complete guide to the remedies.

Vithoulkas, George. *Materia Medica Viva, Volume One.* Mill Valley, CA: Health and Habitat, 1992. This is the first of what promises to be a multivolume materia medica. Unlike his student, Ananda Zaren, Vithoulkas begins with the letter

A rather than the remedies he finds most needed or interesting. Thus the first volume contains several obscure remedies that are of little or no practical use to the student of homeopathy. When more volumes are completed, the collection will be of greater use.

Zaren, Ananda. *Core Elements of the Materia Medica of the Mind.* 2 volumes. Göttingen: Burgdorf, 1993, 1994. The first volumes of a planned multivolume work give psychological insight into the motivations of the various remedy types. Zaren has a unique approach to constitutional treatment.

SELF-CARE BOOKS

I am not a particular fan of the self-care book. They can, from time to time, be very helpful, but too often those students who begin their study of homeopathy with these books never move on to understanding the deeper issues of homeopathic healing.

Castro, Miranda. *The Complete Homeopathy Handbook.* New York: St. Martin's, 1990. The subtitle says it all: "Safe and Effective Ways to Treat Fevers, Coughs, Colds and Sore Throats, Childhood Ailments, Food Poisoning, Flu, and a Wide Range of Everyday Complaints." Castro is particularly good in explaining the emotional and mental symptoms that may accompany even the mildest physical complaint and that so often lead to the correct remedy.

———. *Homeopathy for Pregnancy, Birth and Your Baby's First Year.* New York: St. Martin's, 1993. Castro writes about homeopathy with a warmth and humor all too often missing from these books. This excellent guide lives up to its title, giving exhaustive information on the issues surrounding pregnancy and birth, as well as postnatal care and early childhood health care.

Curtis, Susan, and Romy Fraser. *Natural Healing for Women.* London: Pandora, 1991. This guide lists both homeopathic remedies and herbal treatments for women's common ailments. Nutritional suggestions are also given, as are aromatherapy treatments.

De Schepper, Luc. *Musculoskeletal Diseases and Homeopathy.* Santa Fe: Full of Life Publishing, 1994. This book is a bit limited in its scope, but it still is a helpful guide for the various diseases of the musculoskeletal system.

Lessell, Colin B. *The World Traveller's Manuel of Homeopathy.* Saffron Walden, England: C. W. Daniel, 1993. Of interest to those who travel a good deal. It gives remedies for the ailments that beset travelers in foreign lands. It is a good idea to pack this book, along with a kit of homeopathic remedies, in your suitcase.

Lockie, Andrew. *The Family Guide to Homeopathy: Symptoms and Natural Solutions.* New York: Simon and Schuster, 1993. This is an exhaustive work by a British practitioner. The book lists not only the remedies available to a specific crisis but the first-aid treatments that may also be required.

Lockie, Andrew, and Nicola Geddes. *The Women's Guide to Homeopathy*. New York: St. Martin's, 1994. The best and most complete guide of women's homeopathic health care. Care should be taken, however, as the book gives both acute and chronic conditions, as if the layperson were equipped to treat either or both on her own.

Moskowitz, Richard. *Homeopathic Medicine for Pregnancy and Childbirth*. Berkeley: North Atlantic, 1992. Women who are approaching childbirth would do well to buy and use this excellent guide as well as Castro's.

Nauman, Eileen. *Poisons that Heal*. Sedona, AZ: Light Technology Publishing, 1995. I love this book. It is a bit wackier than some of the others, but how can you not love a book with section titles like, "Killer Epidemics and How to Survive Them." This is the only book I know with remedies listed for ebola.

Panos, Maesimund B, and Jane Heimlich. *Homeopathic Medicine at Home: Natural Remedies for Everyday Ailments and Minor Injuries*. Los Angeles: Tarcher, 1976. This guide is somewhat confusing until you learn to work with the charts included. It can be very helpful for day-to-day ailments and injuries.

Ullman, Dana. *The Consumer's Guide to Homeopathy*. New York: Tarcher Putnam, 1995. Ullman is better known for his other general guide to homeopathic health care, *Everybody's Guide to Homeopathic Medicines* [New York: Tarcher Putnam, 1984]. This is Ullman's best work, giving a well-rounded understanding of how homeopathy works before diving in to dozens of uses for the remedies.

Zand, Janet, Rachel Walton, and Bob Roundtree. *Smart Medicince for a Healthier Child*. New York: Avery, 1994. Although limited to childhood ailments, this guide is rounded in its scope, dealing with any and all ailments of childhood. The book also travels outside the realm of homeopathy, offering nutritional tips and herbal remedies.

RESOURCES

The past decade has seen a dramatic rise both in the numbers of people interested in learning about homeopathy and in organizations and businesses standing ready to educate and to make available homeopathic products.

This list, divided into several sections, represents the most complete resource listing I could gather together. With the exception of those organizations listed in the first grouping, given in order of importance, I do not have firsthand knowledge of the organizations. Nor does my listing of a specific school or pharmacy constitute any direct recommendation.

HOMEOPATHIC ORGANIZATIONS

National Center for Homeopathy
801 North Fairfax, Suite 306
Alexandra, VA 22314
(703) 548-7790

The National Center offers memberships to professionals and laypersons alike. The organization publishes a monthly newsletter, *Homeopathy Today*, which is mailed free to members. In addition, the organization sponsors an annual conference, a summer school educational program for professionals and laypersons, and a study group project that has established a network of study groups nationwide.

The Connecticut Homeopathic Association
PO Box 1055
Greens Farms, CT 06846
(203) 327-6525

A not-for-profit corporation dedicated to making homeopathic education available to all interested parties. Sponsors monthly day-long classes in subjects related to homeopathy. Publishes a quarterly newsletter, *The HomeoPATH*, mailed free to all members. The organization also presents a monthly study group. Vinton McCabe, president of the association, has created five study guides on topics related to homeopathy that are available only through the organization. The association also has available tapes of McCabe's classes and lectures. Membership is open to laypersons and professionals.

The American Institute of Homeopathy
925 East 17th Avenue
Denver, CO 80218
(505) 989-1457

A professional organization with memberships available only to medical doctors, D.O.'s, podiatrists, and dentists who make use of homeopathics in their practice or who are supportive of homeopathy in general. The organization publishes a quarterly journal, *The Journal of the American Institute of Homeopathy*, and supports educational and research efforts in the field of homeopathy. The AIH is especially supportive to physicians who are newly establishing their homeopathic practice.

International Foundation for Homeopathy
2366 Eastlake Avenue East, #325
Seattle, WA 98102
(206) 324-8230

This organization dedicates itself to the training of homeopathic practitioners. It sponsors an annual conference for practitioners and serious students of homeopathy. The organization publishes a bimonthly journal, *Resonance*, which is sent free to the membership. This is a particularly fine magazine, with articles on the latest research in homeopathy as well as a listing of all upcoming events in the homeopathic community.

Homeopathic Academy of Naturopathic Physicians
14653 South Graves Road
Mulino, OR 97042

This organization is open only to naturopathic physicians who incorporate homeopathy into their practice. The academy publishes a professional journal. It also certifies naturopathic physicians in the practice of homeopathy.

Foundation for Homeopathic Education and Research
2124 Kittredge Street
Berkeley, CA 94704
(510) 649-8930

The organization's purpose is to educate the medical community as to new and ongoing scientific research in the field of homeopathy. It extends its educational process to the community at large, by providing speakers to hospitals, medical schools, and community groups. To my knowledge, there are no memberships, as such, available in this organization. This foundation is the not-for-profit wing of Dana Ullman's Homeopathic Educational Services, located at the same address. Homeopathic Educational Services is a leading supplier of tapes, books, and software on the subject of homeopathy.

HOMEOPATHIC PHARMACIES

All these sell homeopathic remedies, some by kit, some by single remedies, most by both. Many supply other homeopathic products as well, from books to tapes to software.

Arrowroot Standard Direct
83 East Lancaster Avenue
Paoli, PA 19301
(800) 234-8879

Biological Homeopathic Industries
11600 Cochiti Southeast
Albuquerque, NM 87123
(505) 293-3843

Boericke and Tafel
2381 Circadian Way
Santa Rosa, CA 95407
(707) 571-8202

Boiron-Bornemann, Inc.
6 Campus Boulevard, Building A
Newtown Square, PA 19073
1 (800) BOIRON-1
(610) 325-7464

Boiron-Bournemann, Inc.
98c West Cochran
Simi Valley, CA 93065
(805) 582-9091

Dolisos
3014 Rigel Road
Las Vegas, NV 89102
(702) 871-7153

Hahnemann Medical Clinic Pharmacy
828 San Pablo Avenue
Albany, CA 94706
(510) 527-3003

Homeopathic Educational Services
2124 Kittredge Street
Berkeley, CA 94704
(510) 649-0294

Longevity Pure Medicines
9595 Wilshire Boulevard, #502
Beverly Hills, CA 90212
(310) 273-7423

Santa Monica Homeopathic Pharmacy
629 Broadway
Santa Monica, CA 90401
(310) 395-1131

Luyties Pharmacal
4200 Laclede Avenue
St. Louis, MO 63108
(314) 533-9600

Similasan Corporation
1321-D South Central Avenue
Kent, WA 98032
(800) 426-1644

Medicine From Nature
10 Mountain Springs Parkway
Springville, UT 84663
(801) 489-1500

Standard Homeopathic Company
204-210 West 131st Street
Los Angeles, CA 90061
(310) 321-4284

New Vistas
5260 East 39th Street
Denver, CO 80207
(800) 283-4533

Washington Homeopathic Products
4914 Del Ray Avenue
Bethesda, MD 20814
(800) 336-1695

INTERNATIONAL RESOURCES

Aggarwal Book Centre
19 DDA, A-One Market
Mayapuri
New Delhi, India 110064
(0-91-11) 514-0430

One of the world's leading suppliers of homeopathic books. Virtually every book on homeopathy published worldwide is available through them.

Foundation for Homeopathic Research
8-5 Giriraj, Neelkanth Valley
Ghatkopar, Bombay 400 077
India

In addition to research, this organization sponsors month-long classes in homeopathic practice that have been especially created for American and European students. Open to both professionals and advanced students of homeopathy. The organization was created by a student of Rajan Sankaran.

Homeopathic Master Clinician Course
F-31
Bowen Island, B.C. V0N 1G0
Canada

This is an advanced training program, led by Louis Klein, a respected homeopathic educator who also teaches in San Francisco, Los Angeles, and Boston.

HomeoVia
8601 Warden Avenue
PO Box 56603
Markham, Ontario L3R 0M6
Canada
(800) 668-7543

Supplier of homeopathic software as well as books on homeopathy.

Oceanic Institute of Classical Homeopathy
404 Great Eastern Highway
West Midland 6056
Western Australia

Dedicated to classical homeopathic education. Primarily for professional homeopaths.

Royal London Homeopathic Hospital
Great Ormond Street
London WC1N 3HR
England

Offers courses for medical professionals on the uses of homeopathics.

Society of Homoeopaths
2 Artizan Road
Northampton NN1 4HU
England

A good umbrella organization for information concerning classes and study groups in England. It keeps tabs especially on weekend classes in homeopathy. It publishes *The Homoeopath: The Journal of the Society of Homoeopaths*, one of the most respected magazines of its kind in the world. Published quarterly, it dedicates equal amounts of space to articles on the philosophy and the practice of homeopathy.

INTERNATIONAL ENGLISH–LANGUAGE PUBLICATIONS

British Homoeopathic Journal
The Invicta Press
Ashford, Kent TN24 8HH
England
A quarterly journal known for its in-depth research and its reviews of other homeopathic journals.

European Journal for Classical Homeopathy
PO Box 56603, 8601 Warden A
Markham, Ontario L3R 0M6
Canada
Journal edited by George Vithoulkas. Known for its articles on clinical uses of homeopathics.

Health and Homoeopathy
Hahnemann House
2 Powis Place
Great Ormond Street
London WC1N 3HT
England
A glossy magazine that has been published with the layperson as the target reader. Made up mostly of anecdotal evidence as to the power of homeopathy.

Homeopathic Links
Bantigerstrasse 37
CH 3006 Bern
Switzerland
Quarterly journal of classical homeopathy geared to both practitioners and serious students of homeopathy.

Homeopathy International
243 The Broadway
Southall, Middlesex UB1 11NF
England
Published by the UK Homeopathic Medical Association, this quarterly journal is for both professionals and serious students of homeopathy.

INTERNATIONAL FOREIGN-LANGUAGE PUBLICATIONS

Allgemeine Homöopathische Zeitung
Karl F. Haug Verlag
Fritz-Frey-Str. 21
Postfach 10 28 40
D-6900 Heidelberg 1
Germany

Les Annales Homéopathiques Françaises
64800 Arrps-Nay
C.C.P. 2594-63, Bordeaux
France

Cahiers de Biothérapie
Société Medicale de Biothérapie
71 rue Beaubourg
75013 Paris
France

L'Homéopathie Européenne
1-3 rue de Depart
75014 Paris
France

L'Homéopathie Française
16 rue Mumont d'Urville
Paris 75116
France

La Homeopatia de México
Miro 26 y 28
Mexico 06400, D.F.

Révue Belge d'Homéopathie
av. Cardinal Micara 1
1160 Brussels
Belgium

Zeitschrift für Klassische Homöopathie
Karl F. Haug Verlag
Frita-Frey-St. 21
Postfach 10 28 40
D-6900 Heidelberg 1
Germany

INDEX

Twelve Healers (Bach), 75–76
twitches, 207, 211
type A personality, 206
typhoid fever, 144, 234

ulcers, 173, 219
unconscious, the, 200
Unger, Felix, 177, 183
unicist school, 301
uniqueness, of humans, and analysis of
    illness in, 14, 19–20, 29, 32, 34, 44,
    84, 90, 99, 294, 295
urine, 124
Urtica Urens (AR), 160–62
uterine fibroids, 267
uterus, 136, 267

vaccination, 22, 66, 74, 253, 255, 259;
    and homeopathic philosophy, 30, 31;
    ill effects of, 250, 251–52, 256, 257;
    principle of, 31–32, 60
vaccinosis, 251–52, 257, 265
valerian, 32
Valium, 32
Vannier, Leon, 272
vegetarian diet, 278
venereal disease, 255, 298
venom, 66, 122, 139–40
vertigo, 143, 146, 204–5, 227
victim role, 24–25, 95, 275; and
    Lycopodium, 193, 195; and
    Pulsatilla, 222
Victoria, Queen, 200
violent behavior, 252, 253, 254, 255–56,
    257, 266, 269
visible nature, of humans, 15, 34
vision therapy, 121
vital force, 14–15, 17, 44–45, 295–96;
    blockages of, as seat of illness, 20–22;
    failure of, 250; as link between spirit
    and body, 260; low, 249; as seat of
    healing, 15, 55; signs of, in body
    language, 85; and symptoms, 18

vitalism, 13–14
Vithoulkas, George, 21, 24, 293
vomiting, 155, 182, 219, 242

war, children of, 252
warts, 251, 257
wasting diseases, 183
water, fear of, 215
weakness, 199
weapons, desire for, 209
weather, 51, 233, 297
weight, excessive, 184
weight consciousness, 179
weight loss, 183, 270
well-being: improvement in, as sign of
    cure, 305; sense of, 115
Welles, Orson, 262
Western medicine. See allopathy
white bryony, 144
white cedar, 251
whooping cough, 161
widowhood, 200
wild hops, 144
wild rosemary, 156
Wilkes, Melanie, 228
windflower (anemone), 122, 220–21
wine, 197
winning, need for, 206–7, 208
wisdom of the body, 21
withdrawal, social, 245–46
wolfsbane, 137
work-oriented behavior, 140, 183–90,
    230, 237
worms, 189
worry, 187, 240
wounded ego, 261–63
wounds, 140, 147, 151, 157

X (decimal) scale, 58, 104, 301–2

yellow bile, 44, 47

zinc, 51